UPDATES IN THE DIAGNOSIS AND TREATMENT OF VASCULITIS

Edited by **Lazaros I. Sakkas**
and **Christina Katsiari**

Updates in the Diagnosis and Treatment of Vasculitis
http://dx.doi.org/10.5772/46068
Edited by Lazaros I. Sakkas and Christina Katsiari

Contributors

Reem Hamdy Mohammed, Lazaros Sakkas, Cheryl Barnabe, Aurore Fifi-Mah, Mohamed Abdgawad, Panagiota Boura, Konstantinos Tselios, Ioannis Gkougkourellas, Alexandros Sarantopoulos, Norbert Lukan, Mislav Radic, Josipa Radić, Dragos Catalin Jianu, Silviana Nina Jianu, Shaun Summers, Jacques Elias Choucair

Published by InTech
Janeza Trdine 9, 51000 Rijeka, Croatia

Publishing Process Manager Danijela Duric
Technical Editor InTech DTP team
Cover InTech Design team

Additional hard copies can be obtained from orders@intechopen.com

Updates in the Diagnosis and Treatment of Vasculitis, Edited by Lazaros I. Sakkas and Christina Katsiari
p. cm.
ISBN 978-953-51-1008-8

For EU product safety concerns:
IN TECH d.o.o., Prolaz Marije Krucifikse Kozulić 3, 51000 Rijeka, Croatia,
info@intechopen.com or visit our website at intechopen.com.

Meet the editors

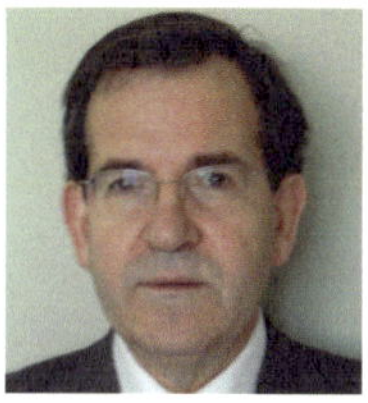

Dr Sakkas is Professor of Medicine and Rheumatology at the Faculty of Medicine, School of Health Sciences, University of Thessaly, and Director of Rheumatology Clinic, University General Hospital of Larissa, Larissa, Greece. He is also Adjunct Professor, Old Dominion University, Norfolk, VA, USA, and President of the Institute of Rheumatic Diseases, Greece. Dr Sakkas received his MD degree and his DM degree from the Medical School of National and Kapodistrian University, Athens, Greece, and his PhD degree from London University, UK. Since 1998 he has been at the Univesity of Thessaly and Director of the Rheumatology Clinic, and first as Assistant Professor, and then Associate Professor and Professor. Dr Sakkas has served as Editor of the Hellenic Rheumatology, the official journal of the Hellenic Society of Rheumatology (2007-present) and guest Editor of Current Rheumatology Reviews (2010). He has also served on the Editorial Boards of Clinical Immunology (2005-8), International Journal of Biomedical Sciences (2006-present), World Journal of Rheumatology (2011-present), and World Journal of Orthopedics (2011-present). His research interests include inflammation in rheumatic diseases and particularly rheumatoid arthritis, systemic sclerosis, and osteoarthritis where he has worked for nearly 10 years at Guy's Hospital, London, UK, and Temple University, Philadelphia, PA, USA. Dr Sakkas has published more than 140 articles, reviews, and chapters in international and Greek scientific journals and textbooks, with impact factor more than 237, and more than 1600 citations.

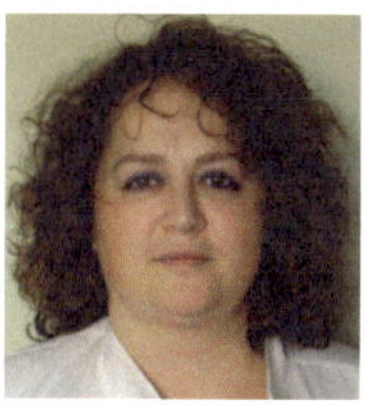

Dr Katsiari is a Lecturer of Medicine and Rheumatology at the Faculty of Medicine School of Health Sciences, University of Thessaly and Consultant of the Rheumatology Clinic, University General Hospital of Larissa, Larissa Greece. Dr Katsiari received her MD and PhD degree from the Medical School of National and Kapodistrian University, Athens, Greece. Following her degree she worked at the Walter Reed Army Institute of Research, Washington DC, USA, where her work under the mentorship of Professor George Tsokos launched the research on phosphatases in T cells in patients with lupus (RO1 grant). Dr Katsiari has served on the editorial board of Hellenic Rheumatology, as regular reviewer in several journals (Lupus, Clinical Immunology, Open Rheumatology, FEBS Journal, Neurology). Since 2010 she has been at the University of Larissa. Her research interests include pathophysiologic mechanisms and targeted treatment of autoimmune diseases and particularly systemic lupus erythematosus, systemic sclerosis and Adamandiades-Behcet's disease. Dr Katsiari has published more than 30 articles, reviews and chapters in international and Greek scientific journals and textbooks, with impact factor more than 100, and more than 800 citations.

Contents

Preface

Vasculitis, an inflammation of blood vessels, can be idiopathic or secondary to other conditions. Infections may also mimic idiopathic vasculitis and the differential diagnosis is of paramount importance for the practicing physician. Vasculitides are not uncommon diseases. In fact, some vasculitides, such as giant cell arteritis, cutaneous vasculitis, and ANCA-associated vasculitis, are relatively common in everyday practice. Vasculitis may rapidly lead to organ failure, and put patient's life in danger. Therefore, physicians of different specialties must diagnose systemic vasculitis early, because early treatment is crucial for the favorable outcome.

In recent years progress has been made in the pathophysiology and treatment of vasculitis. Understanding molecular mechanisms in the pathogenesis of vasculitis helps in the rational development of new treatments. Trials with biological agents have been published, and EULAR and ACR have issued guidelines for the treatment of various types of vasculitis. This book reflects new advances in pathogenetic mechanisms, diagnosis, and treatment of different types of vasculitis. The international panel of authors helps in achieving a balanced view on different aspects of vasculitis.

We hope that this book will be an enjoyable and useful reading.

Lazaros I. Sakkas, MD, DM, PhD
Professor and Chairman,
School of Medicine, University of Thessaly,
Larissa, Greece

Christina Katsiari, MD, DM,
Lecturer,
School of Medicine, University of Thessaly,
Larissa, Greece

Chapter 1

History, Classification and Pathophysiology of Small Vessel Vasculitis

Mohamed Abdgawad

Additional information is available at the end of the chapter

http://dx.doi.org/10.5772/55238

1. Introduction

Systemic vasculitides are a heterogenous group of disorders characterized by destructive inflammation and fibrinoid necrosis of the blood vessel wall, blood vessel occlusion and ischemia of surrounding tissue. Typical clinical manifestations vary depending on the size of the affected blood vessels, and include fever, weight loss, malaise, arthralgias and arthritis. Vasculitides can be idiopathic, primary, secondary to another disease such as Systemic Lupus Erythematosus (SLE) and Rheumatoid Artritis (RA), or associated with infections, such as infective endocarditis, pharmaceutical drug use, such as propylthiouracil and hydralazine, or other chemical exposures [1]. Vasculitis can be isolated to one organ or vessel and be relatively insignificant clinically or can present as a systemic life-treatening illness involving several organs and vessels [2].

ANCA- associated Systemic Vasculitis (AASV) is the most common primary systemic small-vessel vasculitis that occurs in adults. AASV is a small-vessel vasculitis affecting arterioles, venules, capillaries, and occasionally medium-sized arteries that commonly involves multiple organ systems. Although infrequent, the incidence of AASV is increasing. AASV is also called pauci-immune vasculitis, because no immunoglobulins or complement components are detected in the vasculitic lesions.

AASV is associated with significant morbidity and mortality, with almost all patients requiring aggressive immunosuppression. Without treatment, the mortality approaches 100% in 5 years [3]. Based upon the clinical presentation and the predominant organ involvement, AASV cases are classified as Wegener's granulomatosis (WG), microscopic polyangiitis (MPA), Churg-Strauss syndrome (CSS) and Renal Limited Vasculitis (RLV). ANCA are predominantly IgG antibodies that were first described in the 1980s by Davies et al. in patients with necrotizing glomerulonephritis [4]. These antibodies are directed against antigenic components of neutrophilic granules or lysosomes. Indirect immunofluorescence (IIF) of ethanol-fixed neutrophils reveals cytoplasmic (cANCA) or perinuclear (pANCA) staining. cANCA staining correlates with proteinase-3 (PR3) reactivity, while pANCA staining correlates with reactivity towards myeloperoxidase (MPO) or other antigens.

PR3-ANCAs are mainly detected in patients with WG, whereas MPO-ANCAs are predominantly detected in patients with MPA and CSS. These diseases exhibit similar pathological focal necrotizing lesions, though WG and CSS also have granulomatous lesions [5].

Henoch-Schönlein purpura (HSP) is the most common systemic small-vessel vasculitis in children [6]. HSP is a systemic vasculitis affecting small vessels and capillaries. HSP is characterized by palpable purpura, edema, abdominal pain, joint pain and renal symptoms [7]. The prognosis is good as long as the patients have no renal symptoms. Renal symptoms vary from intermittent hematuria and proteinuria to rapidly progressive glomerulonephritis.

In this chapter, we shall discuss the pathophysiology of the most common primary small vessel vasculitis in adults, AASV, as well as the most common small vessel vasculitis in children, HSP.

2. History

Purpura was the first manifestation of vasculitis in vessels smaller than arteries. In 1808, Willan clearly distinguished purpura caused by infections from non-infectious purpura [8]. Over the next century, Henoch and his teacher, Schönlein, described a broad spectrum of signs and symptoms that were associated with purpura, and with small vessel vasculitis, including arthritis, peripheral neuropathy, abdominal pain, pulmonary hemorrhage, epistaxis, iritis, and nephritis [9].

In 1866, Kussmaul and Maier described a patient with general weakness caused by vasculitic neuropathy accompanied by tachycardia, abdominal pain, and the appearance of cutaneous nodules over the trunk. The patient's muscle paralysis progressed quickly causing death. At autopsy, visible nodules were present along the medium-sized arteries of the patient [10]. Kussmaul and Maier named this disease "periarteritis nodosa" because they observed inflammation in the perivascular sheaths and outer layers of the arterial walls and nodular thickening of the vessels. However, the name was later changed to "polyarteritis nodosa" because of the widespread involvement of vessels and the fact that it affects the entire thickness of the vessel wall [1].

A disorder of necrotizing vasculitis, granulomatous lesions of the entire respiratory tract, and glomerulonephritis was first described in 1897 by Peter McBride [11]. In 1931, Heinz Klinger described the pathological anatomical picture of this disease in two patients who died of

http://dx.doi.org/10.5772/55238

systemic vasculitis [12]. In 1936, Friedrich Wegener, a German pathologist, described three patients with necrotizing granuloma and later interpreted the pathological and clinical findings to represent a distinctive disease entity in 1939 [13]. Goodman and Churg in 1954 wrote a detailed description of the disease known as "Wegener′s granulomatosis" (WG) presenting definite criteria: necrotizing granulomata of the respiratory tract, generalized vasculitis and necrotizing glomerulonephritis [14]. DeRemee and colleages in 1976 proposed the ELK classification (E= upper respiratory tract including paranasal sinuses; L= lung; K= kidney), allowing them to understand and manage cases that did not fit the strict criteria of Goodman and Churg [15]. In the early 1970s, Fauci and Wolff introduced treatment with cyclophosphamide and corticosteroids for WG, which resulted in a nearly complete and long-lasting remission of the disease [16]. In addition, DeRemee published in 1985 a report on the benefits of using cotrimoxazole (trimethoprim/ sulfamethoxazole) in WG with local disease [17]. In the same year, a major breakthrough was made by Van der Woude et al who reported autoantibodies sensitive and specific for the disease. These autoantibodies reacted with the cytoplasm of ethanol-fixed neutrophils, and monocytes and were called Anti-neutrophil Cytoplasmic Autoantibodies (ANCA) [18].

3. Classification

There are 20 recognized primary forms of vasculitis, which are classified according to the size of the affected blood vessels. The large vessel vasculitides, giant cell (temporal) arteritis and Takayasu arteritis, are caused by a granulomatous inflammation of the aorta and its major branches. In the case of giant cell arteritis, there is a particular predeliction for the extracranial branches of the carotid artery, often with involvement of the temporal artery and frequent association with polymyalgia rheumatica. The age of the patient is helpful in distinguishing between the two conditions, because giant cell arteritis is rare in patients under the age of 50 and Takayasu's disease is more common in younger patients [19].

Classical polyarteritis nodosa affects medium-sized vessels and therefore should not involve glomerulonephritis or vasculitis in arterioles, capillaries or venules. Kawasaki's disease is a medium-sized vessel vasculitis that frequently involves the coronary arteries, is associated with the mucocutaneous lymph node syndrome and is most common in children [2].

Small vessel vasculitides include the immune-complex associated vasculitis of Henoch-Shoenlein pupura and essential cryoglobulinemic vasculitis. Henoch-Schönlein pupura has predominantly IgA immune complex deposition and involves the skin, gut and glomeruli with arthritis and arthralgia, while essential cryoglobulinemic vasculitis is caused by the deposition of cryoglobulins predominantly in the small vessels of the skin and glomeruli and is frequently associated with Hepatitis C infection. Another small vessel vasculitis category is cutaneous leucocytoclastic vasculitis, which is confined only to the skin, has no systemic involvement and has a better prognosis than vasculitides with systemic involvement [2].

Examples of different types of vasculitis are depicted in Table 1.

Dominant vessel involved	Primary	Secondary
Large arteries	Giant cell arteritis	Aortitis associated with RA
	Takayasu's arteritis	Infection (eg. Syphilis)
Medium arteries	Classical PAN	Infection (eg. Hepatitis B)
	Kawasaki disease	
Small vessels and medium arteries	Wegener's granulomatosis*	Vasculitis 2 to RA, SLE, Sjögren's syndrome
	Churg-Strauss syndrome*	Drugs
	Microscopic polyangiitis*	Infection (e.g. HIV)
Small vessels (leukocytoclastic)	Henoch-Schönlein purpura	Drugs**
	Essential mixed cryoglobulinaemia	Infection (e.g. Hepatitis B, C)
	Cutaneous leukocytoclastic vasculitis	

(*) Diseases most commonly associated with ANCA, pausi-immune crescentic glomerulonepghritis and which are most responsive to immunosuppression with cyclophosphamide. (**) e.g. sulphonamides, penicillins, thiazide diuretics, and many others. PAN= Polyarteritis Nodosa. RA= Rheumatoid Arthritis. SLE= Systemic Lupus Erythematosus.

Table 1. Classification of systemic vasculitis.

ANCA-associated systemic vasculitis (AASV) are a group of diseases classified as small vessel vasculitides that are associated with anti-neutrophil cytoplasmic antibodies. AASV include microscopic polyangiitis, Wegener´s granulomatosis, Churg-Struass syndrome and renal limited vasculitis. Together they are responsible for 5-6% of cases presenting with renal failure. They are characterized histologically by necrotizing vasculitis preferentially affecting small blood vessels and often associated with pauci-immune necrotizing crescentic glomerulonephritis. Serologically, these diseases present autoantibodies directed against constituents of neutrophil granules [20].

In1990, three independent groups showed that azurophilic granule enzyme proteinase 3 was the target autoantigen recognized by ANCA (PR3-ANCA) [21,22,23]. Together with proteinase 3, another granule protein, myeloperoxidase (MPO) was also identified as a target autoantigen of ANCA (MPO-ANCA) [24]. The discovery of ANCA has been critical to understanding the pathogenesis of the disease, as well as providing a valuable diagnostic tool. The American College of Rheumatology published criteria for classifying vasculitides in 1990, leading to improved categorization of patients for clinical trials [25]. However, these criteria were not adequate for diagnosing patients with ANCA-associated vasculitides. An individual patient could simultaneously meet the criteria for WG, Churg Strauss Syndrome (CSS), Polyarteritis Nodosa (PAN), hypersensitivity vasculitis and Henoch-Schönlein pupura. In 1994 the Chapel Hill Consensus conference (CHCC) adopted standardized names and definitions of vasculitides, based on the size of the affected blood vessels [26].

Recently a group of physicians from multiple medical disciplines met at the European Medicines Agency (EMEA) in London in September 2004 and January 2006 and developed a stepwise algorithm for classifying AASV and PAN for epidemiological studies. Their aim was to develop a consensus approach for applying CHCC definitions and ACR criteria to AASV and PAN, in order to facilitate comparison between epidemiological data for different vasculitides [27].

Without treatment, patients with AASV have a very poor prognosis with a median survival time of 5 months [28]. Current treatment regimens based on cyclophosphamide and corticosteroids have dramatically improved the prognosis for these patients and increased the median survival time to 21.7 years [29]. Although this regimen achieves long-lasting remission and prolonged survival of patients with AASV, it has its drawbacks; the worst being life-threatening infections early in the course of the disease and risk of malignancy in late stages of the disease [30,31]. Furthermore, the disease has a high relapse rate in spite of heavy immunosuppression. Improved understanding of the mechanisms underlying AASV may help in the search for better treatment modalities for this serious and devastating illness.

4. Pathophysiology of ANCA-Associated Systemic Vasculitis (AASV)

The pathophysiology of AASV remains largely unknown. Clinical and laboratory evidence suggest a multifactorial origin. Although the association between ANCA and pauci-immune small vessel vasculitides has been established, the exact role of ANCA in the pathogenesis of AASV is yet not fully elucidated. It is not known whether ANCA play a direct role in disease manifestations, or whether the antibodies are secondary markers of the disease process. Available data suggest that neutrophils, B- and T- lymphocytes play a key role in the pathophysiology of AASV.

4.1. Pathogenic B-cell response and production of ANCA

B-cells are the direct precursors of antibody producing plasma cells. B-cells also produce autoantibodies and cytokines (Interleukin IL-6, Tumor Necrosis Factor alpha-TNFα, IL-10), act as antigen presenting cells, and differentiate into long lasting memory B-cells. Csernak et al. have shown that in WG patients, ANCA are produced following B-cell activation [32]. A polyclonal B-cell lymphoid infiltrate in the endonasal granulomatous lesion included PR3-ANCA-producing cells with copy number increase in three VH genes. The granulomatous lesions in WG consist of clusters of PR3 surrounded by an infiltrate consisting of maturing B-cells, antigen-presenting cells (APCs) and Th1-type CD4+CD28− T cells. This suggests that endonasal B-cell maturation is antigen-driven, and that B-cells generate ANCA via contact with PR3 or an antigenic microbial epitope [33].

B-cells recognize soluble antigens via specific B-cell receptors (BCR) and co-receptor CD19 that augments BCR downstream signaling. CD19 dysregulation has been reported in patients with AASV. Culton et al. showed that CD19 expression is 20% lower in naive B-cells from patients with AASV than from normal controls [34]. In contrast, the memory B-cells from some patients with AASV express more CD19 than normal controls. This subset of B-cells shows evidence of antigenic selection, suggesting that in AASV, mechanisms of self-tolerance may be lost leading to production of auto-reactive B-cells [34]. Experiments in transgenic mice indicate that defective B-cell regulation, specifically in pathways responsible for deletion (central and peripheral) of auto-reactive B-cells, may also play a role in generating autoantibodies in AASV [35]. Interestingly, expression of B-cell activating factor of the TNF family (BAFF) is increased in patients with WG [36]. It is postulated that BAFF may drive B-cell expansion, which then leads to ANCA production. B-cell depletion via rituximab in patients with AASV decreases ANCA levels and induces disease remission [37,38]. Conversely, clinical relapse correlates with increase levels of B cells [39]. These data support the conclusion that B cells play a central role in ANCA production and that ANCA play a significant role in the pathogenesis of AASV.

4.2. Pathogenic T-response, tissue damage, and granuloma formation

Under normal conditions, naïve T-cells are activated during an immune response to an antigen stimulus. Antigen-specific T-cells then differentiate into memory T-cells, while effector-T cells undergo apoptosis. Paucity of immunoglobulins in the vasculitic lesions, predominance of IgG1 and IgG4 subclasses of IgG, and the presence of granulomatous lesions indicate that T-cell-mediated immune responses play a role in the pathogenesis of AASV [40]. This is consistent with the fact that T cell-based treatment strategies produce clinically-relevant remission in AASV patients [41,42].

In patients with active WG, higher proportion of activated T-cells and higher concentration of soluble T cell activation markers (including soluble IL-2 receptor or CD30) are reported to correlate with disease activity [43]. High levels of activation markers also correlate with ANCA-positivity, which suggests persistent T cell activation, likely secondary to a persistent antigenic trigger, as an underlying pathogenic factor. This is consistent with reports of persistent expansion of CD4+ effector memory T-cells (Tem) combined with a decrease in naïve T-cells in patients with AASV [44,45]. A polarization of Th1 and Th2 response has also been reported in AASV. In particular, a Th2-type response is predominant in patients with active generalized WG or CSS, while a Th1 response is dominant in patients with localized WG or MPA, indicating that aberrant T cell response plays a role in the disease process [46,47]. CCR5 is also expressed on T-cells in early, localized WG, which might also favor recruitment of Th1-type cytokine secreting cells into inflammatory lesions in localized WG [48]. Conversion from Th1 to Th2 type response could underlie progression from localized to generalized WG. This shift could reflect B-cell expansion and T-cell-dependent PR3-ANCA production, secondary to interaction between neutrophils and auto-reactive T- and B-cells in inflammatory lesions, Figure 1.

The granulomas in AASV resemble a germinal centre, with a cluster of primed neutrophils surrounded by dendritic cells, T- and B-cells. CD4+ T cells are likely to play an important role in the granulomatous response in AASV. The decrease in CD4+CD28-- Tem subset of T-cells during active disease, in patients with WG, indicates an increased migration of these cells to sites of inflammation [44]. In an experimental model of autoimmune, anti-MPO-associated glomerulonephritis, it was noted that mice depleted of CD4+ T cells, at the time of administration of anti-mouse anti-GBM antibodies, developed significantly less crescent formation and cell response, compared to controls [49]. In patients with ANCA-associated glomerulonephritis, Tem cells are the predominant T-cell subtype in the glomerular infiltrate [50]. Together, these observations suggest that a cell mediated immune response contributes to the pathogenesis of renal lesions. Indeed, CD4+ Tem cells from WG patients lack NKG2A (inhibitory receptor) and demonstrate increased expression of NKG2D, which is a

http://dx.doi.org/10.5772/55238

member of the killer immunoglobulin-like receptor family [51]. A significant increase in the proportion of IL-17 producing CD4+ T cells (Th17 cells) in in vitro stimulated peripheral blood cells from WG patients has also been reported [52]. IL-17 induces secretion of neutrophil-attracting chemokines, and release of pro-inflammatory cytokines (IL-1β, TNF-α) capable of increasing expression of PR3 on the surface of neutrophils. Patients with ANCA-positive WG are reported to have more PR3-specific Th17 cells than ANCA-negative WG patients and healthy controls [52]. It is, therefore, likely that a Th1 response plays an important role in antibody production and granuloma formation in AASV.

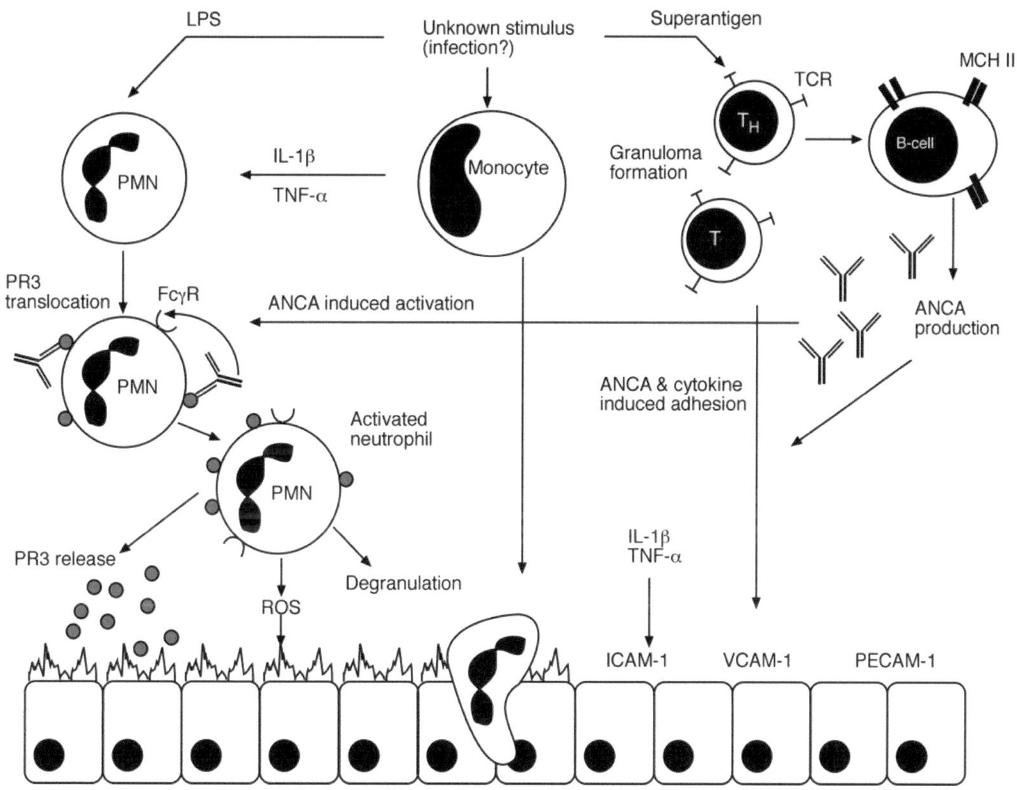

Figure 1. Pathophysiology of AASV. The stimulation of neutrophils by TNF-α or IL-1β (priming), e.g. during a preceding infection, leads to the translocation of the ANCA-antigens, PR3 and MPO, from the cytoplasmic granules (specific granules and secretory vesicels) to the cell surface, where they are accessible for ANCA, which leads to a further activation of the cell. ANCA-induced neutrophil activation initiates production of ROS, neutrophil degranulation with release of inflammatory cytokines and granule contents (e.g., PR3 and HLE) from azurophilic granules, leading to endothelial cell detachment and lysis. Furthermore, neutrophil activation leads to leukocyte adhesion (via ICAM-1, VCAM-1) and transmigration through endothelium (via PECAM-1), and release of ROS and proteases into tissues. Superantigen (e.g., Staphylococcal exotoxins) or PR3 presented to the T-cells directly or via dendritic cells, are capable of stimulating the proliferation of T-cells, leading to granuloma formation and finally to maturation of PR3-specific autoreactive B-cells, culminating in ANCA production. ROS= Reactive oxygen species. PR3= Proteinase 3, MPO= Myeloperoxidase, HLE= Human Leukocyte elastase, ICAM= Intercellular adhesion molecule-1, VCAM-1=Vascular cell adhesion molecule-1, PECAM-1= Platelet endothelial cell adhesion molecule-1, TCR= T-cell receptor, MHC-II= Major Histocompatibility complex-II, TNF-α=Tumor necrosis factor-alpha, IL-1β=Interleukin-1 Beta.

4.3. Monocyte activation and production of pro-inflammatory cytokines

Wickman et al compared monocytes and cytokine profiles in patients with acute anti-PR3 vasculitis and normal controls; monocytes from patients were reported to have a reduced capacity to produce oxygen radicals [53]. Ohlsson et al., from our group, reported a positive correlation between circulating levels of IL-8 and monocyte IL-8 mRNA in patients with AASV, suggesting prolonged immune activation [54]. Pathological analysis of renal tissue from patients with AASV revealed the presence of monocytes in the glomerular crescents and granulomas [55]. In-vitro studies demonstrated that ANCA are capable of stimulating monocytes, leading to release of cytokines including IL-8, MCP-1, TNF-, IL-1, IL-6 and thromboxane A2 [56,57]. On the other hand, membrane PR3 expression on monocytes does not correlate with disease activity. There are many possible explanations for the presence of activated monocytes in glomerular crescents. For example, it is possible that monocytes are activated by direct physical interaction with components of glomerular lesions once they reach site of lesion; alternatively, dysfunctional apoptosis may stimulate monocyte activation [58].

4.4. Endothelial cell activation and enhanced expression of adhesion molecules

Endothelial damage, neutrophil invasion and necrosis are histopathological features of AASV [59]. Activated endothelial cells express high levels of adhesion molecules. Increased circulating levels of endothelial proteins (thrombomodulin, vWF), and adhesion molecules (soluble intercellular adhesion molecule (sICAM)-1 and the soluble endothelial cell-leukocyte adhesion molecule (sELAM)-1) have been reported in vasculitis [60]. Woywodt et al. reported the presence of significant number of circulating endothelial cells and necrotic endothelial cell fragments in patients of active AASV [61]. A significant proportion of the circulating endothelial cells (EC) stain positive for tissue factor (TF), which links proinflammatory mechanisms with thrombosis [61]. Interestingly, TF expression can be induced in ECs by the release of PR3 and elastase from neutrophils; this may be mediated via PR3 receptors on the endothelial cell surface [62]. Endothelial cell necrosis, and release of TF, may play a role in development of vasculitic lesions. The mechanism of endothelial cell necrosis is not yet fully elucidated. Although anti-endothelial cell antibodies have been detected in AASV, their significance in this regard is not clear [63]. ANCA antigens, PR3 and MPO, can bind to endothelial cells via endothelial cell receptors [64,65]. ANCA can bind to endothelial cell bound antigens, leading to EC activation. It is possible that ANCA-induced neutrophil activation induces release of cytotoxic enzymes that damage endothelial cells. In AASV patients with renal involvement, the levels of circulating angiopoietin-2 (Ang-2) correlate with the increased number of circulating ECs. In-vitro studies suggeset that the endothelial-specific angiopoietin (Ang)-Tie ligand-receptor system regulates endothelial cell detachment. By analogy, Ang-2 might regulate endothelial cell detachment in AASV [66].

4.5. Environmental factors

Clinical and epidemiological evidence demonstrate that environmental factors, including silica, asbestos, drugs (anti-thyroid medications), and various infections (bacterial endocarditis, hepatitis C visrus), correlate with circulating ANCA and development of AASV [67,68].

Beaudreuil et al showed that exposure to silica is associated with a nearly seven-fold increased risk of being ANCA-positive [69]. ANCA, both PR3 and MPO, are detected in sera of patients with protracted infections; however, in most infections, ANCA are directed against a wide repertoire of antigens and tend to be dual [70]. Stegeman et al. described an association between nasal S. aureus and relapses of PR3-AAV [71]. Chronic infections may prime neutrophils, which can be further activated by PR3-ANCA, leading to vasculitis. It is also possible that some exogenous non-self proteins (i.e., bacterial, viral, fungal) mimic auto-antigens, which generates ANCA and an ANCA response. For example, PR3-ANCA has been detected in sera of patients with bacterial endocarditis [72]. Long standing exposure of the immune system to specific antigens, may set the stage for development of ANCA and subsequent AASV. Many theories have been made in line of this thought, including anti-complementary PR3 antibody theory [73] and Anti-LAMP (Lysosomal associated membrane protein) anatibody theory [74], which are out of the scope of this study.

4.6. Genetic predisposition

In general, autoimmune diseases display familial inheritance, suggesting that affected individuals carry genetic variation that contributes to disease susceptibility. Case reports show clusters of WG in siblings and close relatives, and specific HLA associations (DR1-DQw1) in AASV patients also suggest the existence of genetic susceptibility loci [75,76,77]. In patients with WG, neutrophils with positive expression of membrane-PR3 ($mPR3^+$) are more abundant than in healthy controls, leading to a skewed bimodal distribution of mPR3 towards a high $mPR3^+$ phenotype in WG [78]. This phenomenon may be genetically determined, because the proportion of $mPR3^+$neutrophils is a stable phenotype in the same individual over prolonged periods of time, it also runs in families and is similar between twins [79]. Furtherore, patients with WG carry a polymorphism that disrupts a putative transcription factor binding site in the PR3 promoter region [80]. This polymorphism may lead to increased expression of PR3 and explain the high $mPR3^+$ phenotype. Additional polymorphisms involving CTLA-4 (affecting T cell activation), alpha-1 antitrypsin level (protease inhibitor of PR3), and other genes/proteins have been reported in AASV patients [81,82,83,84].

5. Are ANCA pathogenic?

The subject of pathogenicity of ANCA is controversial. ANCA are absent in some patients with small vessel vasculitis, while MPO-ANCA are detected in patients with rheumatoid arthritis and other disorders [85]. Also, a paucity of immune complexes at sites of pathological lesions argues against a direct role for ANCA. However, animal models of small vessel vasculitis provide convincing evidence that ANCA are pathogenic in AASV. Xiao et al demonstrated that $Rag2^{-/-}$ mice, which are completely deficient in T- and B-lymphocytes with antigen receptors, developed a severe necrotizing glomerulonephritis and small vessel vasculitis when they were injected with anti-MPO splenocytes, while mice that received anti-BSA or normal splenocytes remained disease-free. Similarly, $Rag2^{-/-}$ and WT B6-mice injected with anti-MPO IgG developed focal glomerular necrosis and crescent formation, clearly indicating that the antibodies were pathogenic [86]. Neumann et al demonstrated excessive immune deposits in the early stages of life of SCG/Kinjoh mice (that spontaneously develop small vessel vasculitis and p-ANCA), and suggested that immune complex deposition leads to an inflammatory state, which when amplified by ANCA, likely lead to severe vasculitis [87]. In renal biopsies from AASV patients with renal involvement, Bajema et al showed that PR3, MPO, elastase and lactoferrin localized within or around fibrinoid necrotic lesions, and the lesions contained high levels of PR3 and elastase, which were also enriched inside the lesions [88]. Schlieben et al described a case of pulmonary renal syndrome in a newborn who received MPO-ANCA via passive transfer from the mother, supporting the idea that ANCA are pathogenic [89]. Animal models have not been developed to text the pathogenicity of PR3-ANCA, because human and murine PR3 share a low level of homology. However, an animal model of vasculitis and severe segmental and necrotizing glomerulonephritis, similar to WG, was recently developed in non-obese diabetic-severe combined immune deficiency (NOD-SCID) mice. In this model, splenocytes were isolated from NOD mice immunized with recombinant mouse PR3 and transferred into NOD-SCID mice, who developed disease pathology. These findings suggest that PR3-ANCA may play a direct role in PR3-ANCA-associated renal disease; however, in this model, a specific genetic background and autoimmune predisposition for kidney pathology are prerequisites for disease manifestation [90].

5.1. Role of neutrophil apoptosis in AASV

Increased neutrophil apoptosis has been observed in AASV. Pathological specimens from patients of WG show clear presence of apoptotic and necrotic neutrophils [91,92]. Leucocytes, with degraded nuclear material, undergoing disintegration and apoptotic cells have been observed in tissue specimens from ANCA-positive renal vasculitis [93]. Histologically, AASV is characterized by leukocytoclasis, with infiltration and accumulation of unscavenged apoptotic and necrotic neutrophils in tissues around blood vessels, and fibrinoid necrosis of the blood vessel walls [94]. E/M studies of the leukocytoclastic lesions, in patients with leukocytoclastic vasculitis, have suggested that there may be a defect in the clearance of apoptotic neutrophils. The minority of neutrophils in this study showed typical apoptotic changes of the condensed and marginated nuclei, while the majority showed intact nuclei with disintegrated cytoplasmic organelles and plasma membranes [95]. Apoptotic neutrophils may, in fact, be a source of immunologically exposed neutrophil antigens that promote the production of ANCAs. It has been speculated that the development of ANCA-positive vasculitis is a three step pathological process. The first step involves an exogenous stimulus that increases neutrophil and macrophage apoptosis. An example is exposure to an inhaled substance like silica, which is known to induce apoptosis in human peripheral blood lymphocytes and to also induce Fas-ligand expression in lung macrophages (in *vitro* and in *vivo*), promoting Fas-dependent macrophage apoptosis in a murine model of silicosis [96,97]. Similarly, other postulated etiological agents for AASV (propylthiouracil, *Streptococcus Pneumoniae*) have also been shown to induce/accelerate apoptosis [98,99]. There is also pathological evidence of leucocytes with degraded nuclear material undergoing disintegration in tissues and apoptotic cells have been observed in AASV. Therefore, it seems logical to suggest that defective clearance/increased exposure to apoptotic neutrophils may be the initiating factor for ANCA production and development of AASV (step two). Finally, environmental and genetic factors can also contribute to disease expression [100].

There are also experimental data that support this developmental model. There is evidence that in an inflammatory environment, autoantigens (nuclear/cytosolic) are presented by the opsonized cells, likely resulting in autoantibody formation. Kettritz et al used high doses of TNF-α to prime neutrophils, and demonstrated that caspase 3 dependent early neutrophil apoptosis was accompanied by increased surface expression of PR3 and MPO. In addition, these early apoptotic neutrophils showed a down-regulation of respiratory burst in response to ANCA [101].

Interestingly, Patry et al showed that injection of syngenic apoptotic neutrophils, but not freshly isolated neutrophils, into Brown Norway rats resulted in development of P-ANCA, with the majority being specific for elastase, again indicating that apoptotic neutrophils may boost an autoimmune response [102]. In another study, intraperitoneal infusion of live or apoptotic human neutrophils (but not formaline fixed or lysed neutrophils) into C57BL/6J mice resulted in development of ANCA specific for lactoferrin or myeloperoxidase. A second intravenous infusion of apoptotic neutrophils resulted in the development of PR3-specific ANCA. Again no vasculitic lesions were found in those mice developing ANCA [103].

As already known from general molecular biology knowledge, neutrophils migrating to inflamed sites undergo spontaneous apoptosis leading to their clearance without damage to the surrounding tissue. Macrophages in the blood recognize, among other surface membrane signals, the externalized Phosphatidyl Serine (PS) on the apoptotic neutrophils leading to their safe clearance. However, neutrophils that are not cleared in this manner progress to secondary necrosis, a process that triggers the release of pro-inflammatory cytokines. It appears that ANCAs dysregulate the process of neutrophil apoptosis. In an *in vitro* study conducted by Harper et al., ANCAs accelerated apoptosis of TNF--primed neutrophils by a mechanism dependent on NADPH oxidase and the generation of ROS. This was accompanied by uncoupling of the nuclear and cytoplasmic changes from the surface membrane changes. That is, while apoptosis progressed more rapidly, there was no corresponding change in the rate of externalization of PS following activation of neutrophils by ANCAs. This dysregulation created a 'reduced window of opportunity' for phagocyte clearance by macrophages, leading to a more pro-inflammatory environment [104]. It must be noted here that ANCAs were unable to accelerate apoptosis in unprimed neutrophils. Additionally, although there was increased expression of PR3 and MPO as apoptosis progressed, ANCAs were unable to activate these neutrophils. In fact, there was a time-dependent decrease in ROS generation as these neutrophils aged [104]. ANCA accelerates neutrophil apoptosis, in primed neutrophils, via generation of ROS that act as amplifying factors for apoptosis. ROS are critical since neutrophils isolated from patients with chronic granulomatous disease (having a defect in ROS production) do not show accelerated apoptosis after ANCA activation [104]. The same authors, in a later study, as well as another independent group showed that ANCA binding to apoptotic neutrophils enhanced phagocytosis by human monocyte-derived macrophages, but at the same time they increased the secretion of pro-inflammatory cytokines like IL-1, IL-8 and TNF-α [105,106]. IL-1 and IL-8 are capable of retarding apoptosis and are powerful chemo-attractants. The pro-inflammatory neutrophil clearance will result in further cell recruitment and perpetuation of inflammation. The autoimmune response may be promoted by aberrant phagocytosis of apoptotic neutrophils by dendritic cells. In a recent study it has been shown that anti-PR3 antibody can also penetrate into human neutrophils (*in vitro*) and lead to enhancement of the apoptotic process [107].

Understanding the pathogenesis of neutrophil apoptosis and clearance in AASV can help to rationalize existing therapies and indicate new approaches to therapy [108].

5.2. The role of netting Neutrophils (NETs)

A novel form of PMN death named "NETosis", characterized by the active release of chromatin, has been described recently [109]. Neutrophil extracellular traps (NETs) are extrusions of plasma membrane and nuclear material, containing granule components and histones. These structures bind gram-positive and negative bacteria, as well as fungi. In vitro, NETs have been shown to bind and kill extracellular microorganisms; *in vivo,* they have been documented in conditions, including appendicitis, sepsis, pre-eclampsia and experimental models of shigellosis [110]. The changes leading to NET formation follow a specific pattern, which is initiated by the loss of nuclear segregation into eu- and heterochromatin. Once the chromatin and granular components are mixed, NETs are released from the cell after cytoplasmic membrane rupture by a process distinct from necrosis or apoptosis, termed NETosis. NADPH oxidase plays a role in this process, via generation of ROS, which act as signaling molecules. Fuchs et al demonstrated that NET formation is a part of active cell death, and that NETs are released when the activated neutrophils dies [111].

Kessenbrock et al. demonstrated that ANCA-stimulated neutrophils release NETs, which contain PR3 and MPO in addition to chromatin and LL37 (an antimicrobial peptide with capabilities of activating dendritic cells) [112]. In-vivo presence of NETs was shown in tissues (kidney biopsies from patients with small vessel vasculitis), with maximal concentration in areas showing neutrophilic infiltration, which suggests that NET formation occurs predominantly during active disease [112]. In patients of AASV, increased levels of circulating nucleosomes has been reported [113]. It is likely that these may, in fact, be derived from and reflect NET formation in AASV. In short, NETs may incite production of ANCA, via presentation of antigen-chromatin complexes to the immune system, or ANCA may incite production of NETs, which then could aggravate the immune response, leading to perpetuation of the auto-immune response, Figure 2.

5.3. Recent updates

Experiments performed by our group, have shown that the plasma levels of mature PR3 as well as pro-PR3 are elevated in AASV [114,115,116]. It was also observed that $mPR3^{+}$ neutrophils are more abundant in AASV compared to healthy donors, which agrees with previous studies suggesting that a high percentage of $mPR3^{+}$cells may be a risk factor for vasculitis [78,115]. Circulating neutrophils and monocytes from patients with AASV display upregulated transcription of the PR3 gene [117]. It is likely that aberrant PR3/mPR3 expression may reflect, or be a marker of a specific functional defect in neutrophils. A possible origin of high plasma levels of PR3 is shedding of membrane PR3.

http://dx.doi.org/10.5772/55238

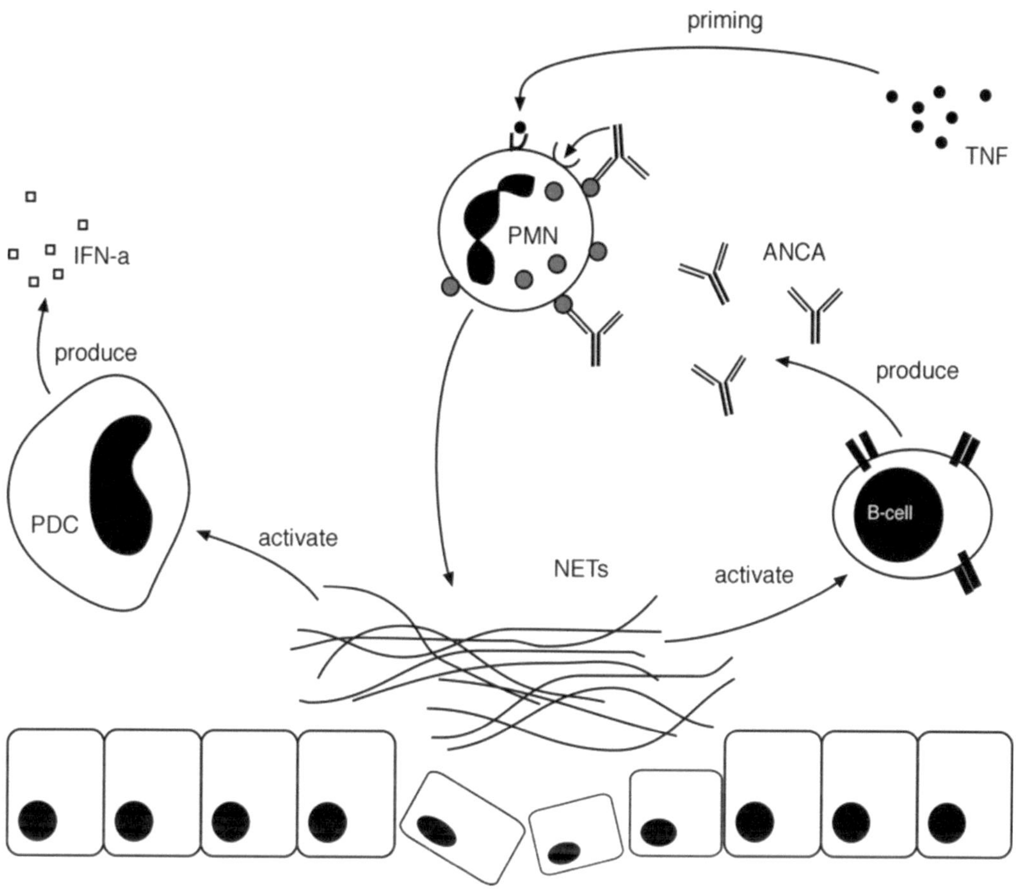

Figure 2. Pathophysiological model of neutrophil extracellular traps (NETs) in ANCAassociated vasculitis. ANCA can induce TNF-α-primed neutrophils to produce NETs. The deposition of NETs may activate plasmacytoid dendritic cells that produce large amounts of interferon-α driving the autoimmune response. In this context, NETs may activate autoreactive B cells to the production of ANCA, which results in a vicious circle of NET production that maintains the delivery of antigen–chromatin complexes to the immune system. Moreover, NETs may also stick to the endothelium and cause endothelial damage.

A significant recent finding is that mPR3 and CD177 are co-expressed on the same subset of circulating neutrophils in healthy subjects as well as in AASV patients [118,119]. Our group has demonstrated that the mPR3^{+}/CD177^{+}neutrophil subpopulation was larger in AASV patients as compared to healthy controls, which suggests a distinct pathophysiological neutrophil phenotype in AASV [116]. Interestingly, higher CD177–mRNA, but not PR3–mRNA was found to correlate with a higher proportion of mPR3+/CD177+cells, suggesting that overproduction of CD177 could lead to an increase in the proportion of mPR3+/CD177+neutrophils [116].

It is likely that these two subpopulations have distinct functions, which may have a direct bearing on pathophysiological processes. Membrane CD177 helps neutrophils adhere to the endothelium, while m-PR3 helps this positive subpopulation to migrate through the endothelium and interstitial tissues. It may be inferred that the mPR3+/CD177+ cells possess greater killing capabilities, including higher NET and ROS production, than the mPR3$^-$/CD177$^-$ subpopulation. In simplistic terms, the mPR3$^+$/CD177$^+$ neutrophils may be the designated "fighting" neutrophils, designed to migrate from blood into tissues and promote pro-inflammatory, microbicidal functions, while mPR3-negative neutrophils are destined to stay in the intra-vascular compartment, and function as anti-inflammatory cells, until they are needed for resolution of inflammation to produce anti-inflammatory mediators or to phagocytose tissue debris and other dead neutrophils at the site of inflammation.

Our group is the first to demonstrate a lower rate of spontaneous apoptosis and *longer in vitro* survival in neutrophils from AASV patients in remission as compared to neutrophils from healthy blood donors [120].

Contrary to our results, Harper et al. showed that neutrophils from AASV patients, especially those with active disease, have an accelerated rate of apoptosis [106].

6. Pathophysiology of Henoch-Schönlein Purpura (HSP)

The etiology of HSP as well as its pathogenesis are largely unknown.

6.1. Genetic factors

Familial clustering of HSP has been described and suggests a genetic background to the disease [121,122]. In several countries and ethnic groups different HLA types have been associated with susceptibility for HSP [123,124]. The different HLA type associations may explain differences in manifestations between different ethnic groups, but, so far, no conclusions could be drawn from these studies to explain the pathogenesis of HSP. Positivity for HLAB35 was found to increase the risk for the development of HSP [125].

A polymorphism in the angiotensinogen gene (M235T) may confer risk for the development of Henoch-Schönlein Nephritis [126,127].

Polymorphisms in the gene for angiotensin 1-converting enzyme (ACE) may be involved in the pathogenesis of HSP or HSN, although data are conflicting. The insertion (I)/deletion (D) genotype of a polymorphism in ACE may confer susceptibility to HSP [126,127]. The DD polymorphism was related to persistent proteinuria in patients with HSP in one study [128], whereas in another study no correlation was found between the prognosis of HSP and the ACE genotype [129].

Variations in the complement C4 protein gene may confer susceptibility to the development of HSP. C4 null isotypes have been described to be prevalent in a significantly higher proportion of patients with HSP and HSN than controls [130,131,132]. A partial or complete deficiency of C4 could be related to impaired clearance of immune complexes and thus play a role in the pathogenesis of HSP [133]. Complement deficiency is, however, uncommon and transient in patients with HSP [134].

Investigations addressing polymorphisms in genes encoding for proinflammatory cytokines (TNF-α, IL-1b, IL-8, TGF-β and VEGF) have so far not revealed any predisposing factors for HSP [135,136].

Familial mediterranean fever (FMF) is an autoinflammatory disease caused by a mutation in the MEFV gene, which in 7 % of cases is associated with HSP [137]. There is a high prevalence of children with MEFV mutations among HSP patients in countries with relative abundance of FMF [138,139]. The implication this association has on the general pathogenesis of HSP is, if at all, unclear.

6.2. Infectious and non-infectious agents

HSP is usually preceded by infections, in up to 95 % of cases localized in the upper respiratory tract, and appears in clusters in families [140,141,142]. The incidence of HSP is highest during early childhood and shows distinct seasonal variations with a peak during autumn and winter [6]. Both early childhood and the autumn-winter season are periods with frequent infections. Thus, clinical observations suggest an important role of infections in the etiology and pathogenesis of HSP.

Several studies have shown a circumstantial relation of infections with group A streptococci and the development of HSP [143,144,145]. Others found serological evidence for an association with infections with other bacteria such as Bartonella henselae or viruses such as parvovirus B19 and hepatitis C virus [146,147,148].

Non-infectious agents have been found to be associated with the development of HSP especially in adults. These include certain drugs such as angiotensin-converting enzyme inhibitors, angiotensin II-receptor antagonists, antibiotics, and non-steroidal anti-inflammatory drugs as well as insect bites, vaccinations or food allergies [149].

6.3. IgA1 in HSP

IgA deposits in HSP are composed of immune-complexes mainly consisting of IgA1 [150].

Serum samples from HSN patients were found to have elevated levels of underglycosylated polymeric IgA1 compared to controls [151]. However, in children with HSP without renal involvement the levels were not higher than those of controls [152]. Underglycosylated polymeric IgA1 has been found to exhibit an inflammatory and proliferative effect on mesangial cells (see IgA1 in IgAN). Taken together, underglycosylated polymeric IgA1 seems to be involved in the development of HSN, but its role in the pathogenesis of HSP per se remains unclear.

6.4. Mediators of inflammation

The acute phase of systemic vasculitis is generally characterized by vascular leukocytic infiltration and activation of innate immunity. Elevated levels of inflammatory cytokines are usually detectable in the serum and affected tissues in these diseases.

IL-6, TNF-α, tumor necrosis factor-like weak inducer of apoptosis (TWEAK), IL-8, TGF-β, and VEGF have been found to be up-regulated during the acute stage of HSP [153,154].

Tissue samples of affected skin areas from patients with HSP show epidermal staining with IL-6 [155]. Serum levels of IL-6 were significantly higher in patients with HSP during the acute phase of disease than in controls and also higher in patients with HSN than HSP without renal affection [153]. IL-6 displays a wide variety of pro-inflammatory properties and promotes the secretion of IgA [153,156].

IL-6 displays, besides its various pro-inflammatory effects, even anti-inflammatory effects by inhibiting TNF-α and IL-1 and activating IL-1ra as well as IL-10 [157].

TNF-α is produced by macrophages and T cells in affected skin areas during HSP. Serum levels of TNF-α were higher in patients with HSN than HSP without renal engagement [153].

It stimulates the presentation of adhesion molecules and receptors on leukocytes and endothelial cells thereby directing inflammatory events. Furthermore, endothelial cells stimulated with TNF-α were shown to bind IgA with higher affinity [155]. These findings suggest, that TNF-α could be involved in the accumulation of granulocytes and endothelial sequestration of IgA as seen in affected tissues in HSP [153].

TWEAK, a member of the TNF superfamily, which binds to specific receptors on endothelial cells, is involved in the regulation of cell growth, angiogenesis, apoptosis, and inflammation.

In vitro evidence suggests that TWEAK may induce cytokine production by human microvascular endothelial cells via up-regulation of the production of IL-8 and CCL-5 leading to a leucocyte migration into affected vessels [158,159] which are common aspects of the HSP lesion.

Sera and IgA from patients with HSP induce the secretion of IL-8 from endothelial cells invitro [160,161].

IL-8 is a potent chemoattractant for polymorphonuclear neutrophilic granulocytes (PMNs). Levels of leukotriene B4, also a potent chemo-attractant and activator of PMNs, are elevated both in serum and urine in patients with HSN compared to those with HSP.

Furthermore, the levels of leukotriene A4, which counter-balance the effects of leukotriene B4 and inhibit the synthesis of proinflammatory cytokines (e.g. IL-6, IL-8, TNF- α), are decreased in patients with HSN [162].

The role of VEGF in HSP is not clear-cut. Serum levels of VEGF were significantly higher during the acute phase of HSP than during remission. However tissue staining for VEGF showed more intense staining for VEGF in the epidermis and vascular bed during the resolution phase than during the acute phase of HSP [163]. High serum levels of VEGF could influence endothelial permeability, which may enhance capillary leakage and facilitate the extravasation and perivascular deposition of immune complexes. The increased tissue staining during the resolution phase, on the other hand, suggests a possible function of VEGF in the resolution of vascular damage.

T helper cells (Th) are a sub-population of lymphocytes, which have an important role in adaptive immune responses. Dependent on the surrounding cytokine environment naïve Th-cells differentiate into subtypes with different functions [164]. In patients with HSP an elevated number of Th2 and Th17 with increased synthesis of IL-5 and IL-13 have been found together with increased serum levels of IL-4, IL-6, and IL-17A [165]. The differentiation towards Th2 is stimulated by exposure to IL-4 and towards Th17 by TGF-β combined with IL-6. By secreting IL-4, Th2 exhibit a stimulatory effect on B cells and promote the generation of plasma cells. Further secretion of IL-5 or IL-13 from Th2 leads to an antibody switch in plasma cells towards the generation of IgA or IgE, respectively. Th17 secrete IL17, which in turn stimulates the expression of pro-inflammatory cytokines such as IL-1, IL-6, and cell adhesion factors and promotes leukocyte migration to the sites of inflammation. Th17 has been implicated in the pathogenesis of autoimmune diseases [164]. An imbalance of Th with Th2 and TH17 predominance, as seen in HSP, could explain elevated serum levels of IgA and IgE, the expression of pro-inflammatory cytokines and leukocyte infiltrations into affected tissues seen in HSP [166,167].

If the pieces of this puzzle are put together potential origins of cardinal symptoms of

HSP emerge. Neutrophilic infiltration of the perivascular region may be mediated by TNF-α, TWEAK, IL-8, chemo-attractant leukotrienes, VEGF and/or Th17 and the extravasation and deposition of IgA by IL-6, TNF-α, VEGF, and Th2. The development of HSN could be related to the prevalence of underglycosylated polymeric IgA1, the effect of IL-6, TNF-α, and a disturbed balance between chemo-attractant and counteracting leukotrienes.

The contact system, which induces liberation of bradykinin or other vasoactive kinins from high-molecular kininogen, has been found to be activated in HSP, which could contribute to the development of clinical features such as inflammation, vasodilatation, edema and pain [168].

Increased reactive oxygen species, lipid and protein oxidation, and nitric oxide level detectable during the acute phase of HSP are believed to reflect secondary events and vascular damage [169,170,171].

Author details

Mohamed Abdgawad*

Address all correspondence to: mohamed.abdgawad@med.lu.se

The Department of Medicine, Blekinge Hospital, Karlshamn, Sweden

References

[1] Firestein, G. S B. R. Harris Jr ED, McInnes IB, Ruddy S, Sergent JS ((2008). Vasculitis. The classification and epidemiology of systemic vasculitis. Kelley´s Tetbook of Rheumatology 8th edition Philadelphia, WB Saunders: Part 13, chapter 80.

[2] Watts, R S. D. (1995). Vasculitis. Baillière's clinical rheumatology , 9, 529-554.

[3] Booth, A. D, Almond, M. K, Burns, A, Ellis, P, Gaskin, G, et al. (2003). Outcome of ANCA-associated renal vasculitis: a 5-year retrospective study. Am J Kidney Dis , 41, 776-784.

[4] Davies, D. J, Moran, J. E, Niall, J. F, & Ryan, G. B. (1982). Segmental necrotising glomerulonephritis with antineutrophil antibody: possible arbovirus aetiology? Br Med J (Clin Res Ed) 285: 606.

[5] Savage, C. O, Harper, L, & Adu, D. (1997). Primary systemic vasculitis. Lancet , 349, 553-558.

[6] Gardner-medwin, J. M, Dolezalova, P, Cummins, C, & Southwood, T. R. (2002). Incidence of Henoch-Schonlein purpura, Kawasaki disease, and rare vasculitides in children of different ethnic origins. Lancet , 360, 1197-1202.

[7] Niaudet, P, Murcia, I, Beaufils, H, Broyer, M, & Habib, R. (1993). Primary IgA nephropathies in children: prognosis and treatment. Adv Nephrol Necker Hosp , 22, 121-140.

[8] Nunnelee, J. D. (2000). Henoch-Schonlein purpura: a review of the literature. Clin Excell Nurse Pract , 4, 72-75.

[9] Iglesias-gamarra, A, Penaranda, E, & Espinoza, L. R. (2011). Vasculitides throughout history and their clinical treatment today. Curr Rheumatol Rep , 13, 465-472.

[10] Kussmaul, A M. R. (1866). Ueber eine bisher nicht beschriebene eigenthumliche arterienerkrankung (periarteritis nodosa), die mit morbus brightii und rapid fortschreitender allgemeiner muskellähmung einhergeht. Deutsche Arch Klin Med , 1, 484-518.

[11] Mcbride, P. (1991). Photographs of a case of rapid destruction of the nose and face. 1897. J Laryngol Otol 105: 1120.

[12] Klinger, H. (1931). Grenzformen der Periarteriitis nodosa.. Frankfurter Zeitschrift für Pathologie, Wiesbaden , 42, 455-480.

[13] Wegener, F. (1939). Uber eine eigenartige rhinogene Granulomatose mit besonderer Beteiligung des Arteriensystems und der Nieren. Beitr Pathol Anat , 102, 36-68.

[14] Godman, G. C C. J. (1954). Wegener's granulomatosis: pathology and review of literature. AMA Arch Patholog , 58, 533-553.

[15] De Remee RA MDTHarrison EJ Jr, et al ((1976). Wegener's granulomatosis, anatomic correlates, a proposed classification. Mayo Clin Proc , 51, 777-781.

[16] Fauci, A. S W. S, & Johnson, J. S. (1971). Effect of cyclophosphamide upon the immune response in Wegener's granulomatosis. N Engl J Med 285.

[17] Deremee, R. A, Mcdonald, T. J, & Weiland, L. H. (1985). Wegener's granulomatosis: observations on treatment with antimicrobial agents. Mayo Clin Proc , 60, 27-32.

[18] Van Der Woude, F. J, Rasmussen, N, Lobatto, S, Wiik, A, Permin, H, et al. (1985). Autoantibodies against neutrophils and monocytes: tool for diagnosis and marker of disease activity in Wegener's granulomatosis. Lancet , 1, 425-429.

[19] Firestein, G. S B. R. Harris Jr ED, McInnes IB, Ruddy S, Sergent JS ((2008). Vasculitis. Giant cell arteritis, polymyalgia rheumatica, and Takayasu's arteritis. Kelley's Tetbook of Rheumatology 8th edition Philadelphia, WB Saunders: Part 13, chapter 81.

[20] Salama, A. D. (1999). Pathogenesis and treatment of ANCA-associated systemic vasculitis. J R Soc Med , 92, 456-461.

[21] Goldschmeding, R, & Van Der Schoot, C. E. ten Bokkel Huinink D, Hack CE, van den Ende ME, et al. ((1989). Wegener's granulomatosis autoantibodies identify a novel diisopropylfluorophosphate-binding protein in the lysosomes of normal human neutrophils. J Clin Invest , 84, 1577-1587.

[22] Niles, J. L, Mccluskey, R. T, Ahmad, M. F, & Arnaout, M. A. (1989). Wegener's granulomatosis autoantigen is a novel neutrophil serine proteinase. Blood , 74, 1888-1893.

[23] Ludemann, J, Csernok, E, Ulmer, M, Lemke, H, Utecht, B, et al. (1990). Anti-neutrophil cytoplasm antibodies in Wegener's granulomatosis: immunodiagnostic value, monoclonal antibodies and characterization of the target antigen. Neth J Med , 36, 157-162.

[24] Falk, R. J, & Jennette, J. C. (1988). Anti-neutrophil cytoplasmic autoantibodies with specificity for myeloperoxidase in patients with systemic vasculitis and idiopathic necrotizing and crescentic glomerulonephritis. N Engl J Med , 318, 1651-1657.

[25] Fries, J. F, Hunder, G. G, Bloch, D. A, Michel, B. A, Arend, W. P, et al. (1990). The American College of Rheumatology 1990 criteria for the classification of vasculitis. Summary. Arthritis Rheum , 33, 1135-1136.

[26] Jennette, J. C, Falk, R. J, Andrassy, K, Bacon, P. A, Churg, J, et al. (1994). Nomenclature of systemic vasculitides. Proposal of an international consensus conference. Arthritis Rheum , 37, 187-192.

[27] Watts, R, Lane, S, Hanslik, T, Hauser, T, Hellmich, B, et al. (2007). Development and validation of a consensus methodology for the classification of the ANCA-associated vasculitides and polyarteritis nodosa for epidemiological studies. Ann Rheum Dis , 66, 222-227.

[28] Fauci, A. S, Haynes, B. F, Katz, P, & Wolff, S. M. (1983). Wegener's granulomatosis: prospective clinical and therapeutic experience with 85 patients for 21 years. Ann Intern Med , 98, 76-85.

[29] Reinhold-keller, E, Beuge, N, Latza, U, De Groot, K, Rudert, H, et al. (2000). An interdisciplinary approach to the care of patients with Wegener's granulomatosis: long-term outcome in 155 patients. Arthritis Rheum , 43, 1021-1032.

[30] Westman, K. W, Bygren, P. G, Olsson, H, Ranstam, J, & Wieslander, J. (1998). Relapse rate, renal survival, and cancer morbidity in patients with Wegener's granulomatosis or microscopic polyangiitis with renal involvement. J Am Soc Nephrol , 9, 842-852.

[31] Gayraud, M, & Guillevin, L. le Toumelin P, Cohen P, Lhote F, et al. ((2001). Long-term followup of polyarteritis nodosa, microscopic polyangiitis, and Churg-Strauss syndrome: analysis of four prospective trials including 278 patients. Arthritis Rheum , 44, 666-675.

[32] Csernok, E, Moosig, F, & Gross, W. L. (2008). Pathways to ANCA production: from differentiation of dendritic cells by proteinase 3 to B lymphocyte maturation in Wegener's granuloma. Clin Rev Allergy Immunol , 34, 300-306.

[33] Voswinkel, J, Mueller, A, Kraemer, J. A, Lamprecht, P, Herlyn, K, et al. (2006). B lymphocyte maturation in Wegener's granulomatosis: a comparative analysis of VH genes from endonasal lesions. Ann Rheum Dis , 65, 859-864.

[34] Culton, D. A, Nicholas, M. W, Bunch, D. O, Zhen, Q. L, Kepler, T. B, et al. (2007). Similar CD19 dysregulation in two autoantibody-associated autoimmune diseases suggests a shared mechanism of B-cell tolerance loss. J Clin Immunol , 27, 53-68.

[35] Bunch, D. O, Silver, J. S, Majure, M. C, Sullivan, P, Alcorta, D. A, et al. (2008). Maintenance of tolerance by regulation of anti-myeloperoxidase B cells. J Am Soc Nephrol , 19, 1763-1773.

[36] Krumbholz, M, Specks, U, Wick, M, Kalled, S. L, Jenne, D, et al. (2005). BAFF is elevated in serum of patients with Wegener's granulomatosis. J Autoimmun , 25, 298-302.

[37] Keogh, K. A, Wylam, M. E, Stone, J. H, & Specks, U. (2005). Induction of remission by B lymphocyte depletion in eleven patients with refractory antineutrophil cytoplasmic antibody-associated vasculitis. Arthritis Rheum , 52, 262-268.

[38] Keogh, K. A, Ytterberg, S. R, Fervenza, F. C, Carlson, K. A, Schroeder, D. R, et al. (2006). Rituximab for refractory Wegener's granulomatosis: report of a prospective, open-label pilot trial. Am J Respir Crit Care Med , 173, 180-187.

[39] Ferraro, A. J, Day, C. J, Drayson, M. T, & Savage, C. O. (2005). Effective therapeutic use of rituximab in refractory Wegener's granulomatosis. Nephrol Dial Transplant , 20, 622-625.

[40] Brouwer, E, Tervaert, J. W, Horst, G, Huitema, M. G, Van Der Giessen, M, et al. (1991). Predominance of IgG1 and IgG4 subclasses of anti-neutrophil cytoplasmic autoantibodies (ANCA) in patients with Wegener's granulomatosis and clinically related disorders. Clin Exp Immunol , 83, 379-386.

[41] Lockwood, C. M, Thiru, S, Stewart, S, Hale, G, Isaacs, J, et al. (1996). Treatment of refractory Wegener's granulomatosis with humanized monoclonal antibodies. Qjm , 89, 903-912.

[42] Hagen, E. C, De Keizer, R. J, Andrassy, K, Van Boven, W. P, Bruijn, J. A, et al. (1995). Compassionate treatment of Wegener's granulomatosis with rabbit anti-thymocyte globulin. Clin Nephrol , 43, 351-359.

[43] Sanders, J. S, Huitma, M. G, Kallenberg, C. G, & Stegeman, C. A. (2006). Plasma levels of soluble interleukin 2 receptor, soluble CD30, interleukin 10 and B cell activator of the tumour necrosis factor family during follow-up in vasculitis associated with proteinase 3-antineutrophil cytoplasmic antibodies: associations with disease activity and relapse. Ann Rheum Dis , 65, 1484-1489.

[44] Abdulahad, W. H, Van Der Geld, Y. M, Stegeman, C. A, & Kallenberg, C. G. (2006). Persistent expansion of CD4+ effector memory T cells in Wegener's granulomatosis. Kidney Int , 70, 938-947.

[45] Marinaki, S, Kalsch, A. I, Grimminger, P, Breedijk, A, Birck, R, et al. (2006). Persistent T-cell activation and clinical correlations in patients with ANCA-associated systemic vasculitis. Nephrol Dial Transplant , 21, 1825-1832.

[46] Schonermarck, U, Csernok, E, Trabandt, A, Hansen, H, & Gross, W. L. (2000). Circulating cytokines and soluble CD23, CD26 and CD30 in ANCA-associated vasculitides. Clin Exp Rheumatol , 18, 457-463.

[47] Wang, G, Hansen, H, Tatsis, E, Csernok, E, Lemke, H, et al. (1997). High plasma levels of the soluble form of CD30 activation molecule reflect disease activity in patients with Wegener's granulomatosis. Am J Med , 102, 517-523.

[48] Lamprecht, P, Bruhl, H, Erdmann, A, Holl-ulrich, K, Csernok, E, et al. (2003). Differences in CCR5 expression on peripheral blood CD4+CD28- T-cells and in granulomatous lesions between localized and generalized Wegener's granulomatosis. Clin Immunol , 108, 1-7.

[49] Ruth, A. J, Kitching, A. R, Kwan, R. Y, Odobasic, D, Ooi, J. D, et al. (2006). Anti-neutrophil cytoplasmic antibodies and effector CD4+ cells play nonredundant roles in anti-myeloperoxidase crescentic glomerulonephritis. J Am Soc Nephrol , 17, 1940-1949.

[50] Sakatsume, M, Xie, Y, Ueno, M, Obayashi, H, Goto, S, et al. (2001). Human glomerulonephritis accompanied by active cellular infiltrates shows effector T cells in urine. J Am Soc Nephrol , 12, 2636-2644.

[51] Capraru, D, Muller, A, Csernok, E, Gross, W. L, Holl-ulrich, K, et al. (2008). Expansion of circulating NKG2D+ effector memory T-cells and expression of NKG2D-ligand MIC in granulomaous lesions in Wegener's granulomatosis. Clin Immunol , 127, 144-150.

[52] Abdulahad, W. H, Stegeman, C. A, Limburg, P. C, & Kallenberg, C. G. (2008). Skewed distribution of Th17 lymphocytes in patients with Wegener's granulomatosis in remission. Arthritis Rheum , 58, 2196-2205.

[53] Wikman, A, & Fagergren, A. Gunnar OJS, Lundahl J, Jacobson SH ((2003). Monocyte activation and relationship to anti-proteinase 3 in acute vasculitis. Nephrol Dial Transplant , 18, 1792-1799.

[54] Ohlsson, S, Wieslander, J, & Segelmark, M. (2004). Circulating cytokine profile in anti-neutrophilic cytoplasmatic autoantibody-associated vasculitis: prediction of outcome? Mediators Inflamm , 13, 275-283.

[55] Ferrario, F, & Rastaldi, M. P. (1999). Necrotizing-crescentic glomerulonephritis in ANCA-associated vasculitis: the role of monocytes. Nephrol Dial Transplant , 14, 1627-1631.

[56] Ralston, D. R, Marsh, C. B, Lowe, M. P, & Wewers, M. D. (1997). Antineutrophil cytoplasmic antibodies induce monocyte IL-8 release. Role of surface proteinase-3, alpha1-antitrypsin, and Fcgamma receptors. J Clin Invest , 100, 1416-1424.

[57] Hattar, K, Bickenbach, A, Csernok, E, Rosseau, S, Grandel, U, et al. (2002). Wegener's granulomatosis: antiproteinase 3 antibodies induce monocyte cytokine and prostanoid release-role of autocrine cell activation. J Leukoc Biol , 71, 996-1004.

[58] Lan, H. Y, Mitsuhashi, H, Ng, Y. Y, Nikolic-paterson, D. J, Yang, N, et al. (1997). Macrophage apoptosis in rat crescentic glomerulonephritis. Am J Pathol , 151, 531-538.

[59] Jennette, J. C O. J, Schwart, M. M, & Silva, F. G. (1998). Renal involvement in small-vessel vasculitis. Heptinstall's pathology of the kidney Philadelphia: Lippincott-Raven 5th Edition: 1059.

[60] Di Lorenzo GPacor ML, Mansueto P, Lo Bianco C, Di Natale E, et al. ((2004). Circulating levels of soluble adhesion molecules in patients with ANCA-associated vasculitis. J Nephrol , 17, 800-807.

[61] Woywodt, A, Streiber, F, De Groot, K, Regelsberger, H, Haller, H, et al. (2003). Circulating endothelial cells as markers for ANCA-associated small-vessel vasculitis. Lancet , 361, 206-210.

[62] Haubitz, M, Gerlach, M, Kruse, H. J, & Brunkhorst, R. (2001). Endothelial tissue factor stimulation by proteinase 3 and elastase. Clin Exp Immunol , 126, 584-588.

[63] Gobel, U, Eichhorn, J, Kettritz, R, Briedigkeit, L, Sima, D, et al. (1996). Disease activity and autoantibodies to endothelial cells in patients with Wegener's granulomatosis. Am J Kidney Dis , 28, 186-194.

[64] Ballieux, B. E, Zondervan, K. T, Kievit, P, Hagen, E. C, Van Es, L. A, et al. (1994). Binding of proteinase 3 and myeloperoxidase to endothelial cells: ANCA-mediated endothelial damage through ADCC? Clin Exp Immunol , 97, 52-60.

[65] Taekema-roelvink, M. E, Van Kooten, C, Heemskerk, E, Schroeijers, W, & Daha, M. R. (2000). Proteinase 3 interacts with a 111-kD membrane molecule of human umbilical vein endothelial cells. J Am Soc Nephrol , 11, 640-648.

[66] Kumpers, P, Hellpap, J, David, S, Horn, R, Leitolf, H, et al. (2009). Circulating angiopoietin-2 is a marker and potential mediator of endothelial cell detachment in ANCA-associated vasculitis with renal involvement. Nephrol Dial Transplant , 24, 1845-1850.

[67] Chen, M, & Kallenberg, C. G. (2010). The environment, geoepidemiology and ANCA-associated vasculitides. Autoimmun Rev 9: A, 293-298.

[68] Pelclova, D, Bartunkova, J, Fenclova, Z, Lebedova, J, Hladikova, M, et al. (2003). Asbestos exposure and antineutrophil cytoplasmic Antibody (ANCA) positivity. Arch Environ Health , 58, 662-668.

[69] Beaudreuil, S, Lasfargues, G, Laueriere, L, El Ghoul, Z, Fourquet, F, et al. (2005). Occupational exposure in ANCA-positive patients: a case-control study. Kidney Int , 67, 1961-1966.

[70] Bonaci-nikolic, B, Andrejevic, S, Pavlovic, M, Dimcic, Z, Ivanovic, B, et al. (2010). Prolonged infections associated with antineutrophil cytoplasmic antibodies specific to proteinase 3 and myeloperoxidase: diagnostic and therapeutic challenge. Clin Rheumatol , 29, 893-904.

[71] Stegeman, C. A, Tervaert, J. W, Sluiter, W. J, Manson, W. L, De Jong, P. E, et al. (1994). Association of chronic nasal carriage of Staphylococcus aureus and higher relapse rates in Wegener granulomatosis. Ann Intern Med , 120, 12-17.

[72] Choi, H. K, Lamprecht, P, Niles, J. L, Gross, W. L, & Merkel, P. A. (2000). Subacute bacterial endocarditis with positive cytoplasmic antineutrophil cytoplasmic antibodies and anti-proteinase 3 antibodies. Arthritis Rheum , 43, 226-231.

[73] Pendergraft, W. F. rd, Preston GA, Shah RR, Tropsha A, Carter CW, Jr., et al. ((2004). Autoimmunity is triggered by cPR-3(105-201), a protein complementary to human autoantigen proteinase-3. Nat Med , 10, 72-79.

[74] Kain, R, Matsui, K, Exner, M, Binder, S, Schaffner, G, et al. (1995). A novel class of autoantigens of anti-neutrophil cytoplasmic antibodies in necrotizing and crescentic glomerulonephritis: the lysosomal membrane glycoprotein h-lamp-2 in neutrophil

granulocytes and a related membrane protein in glomerular endothelial cells. J Exp Med , 181, 585-597.

[75] Stoney, P. J, Davies, W, Ho, S. F, Paterson, I. C, & Griffith, I. P. (1991). Wegener's granulomatosis in two siblings: a family study. J Laryngol Otol , 105, 123-124.

[76] Sewell, R. F, & Hamilton, D. V. (1992). Time-associated Wegener's granulomatosis in two members of a family. Nephrol Dial Transplant 7: 882.

[77] Hay, E. M, Beaman, M, Ralston, A. J, Ackrill, P, Bernstein, R. M, et al. (1991). Wegener's granulomatosis occurring in siblings. Br J Rheumatol , 30, 144-145.

[78] Witko-sarsat, V, Lesavre, P, Lopez, S, Bessou, G, Hieblot, C, et al. (1999). A large subset of neutrophils expressing membrane proteinase 3 is a risk factor for vasculitis and rheumatoid arthritis. J Am Soc Nephrol , 10, 1224-1233.

[79] Schreiber, A, Busjahn, A, Luft, F. C, & Kettritz, R. (2003). Membrane expression of proteinase 3 is genetically determined. J Am Soc Nephrol , 14, 68-75.

[80] Gencik, M, Meller, S, Borgmann, S, & Fricke, H. (2000). Proteinase 3 gene polymorphisms and Wegener's granulomatosis. Kidney Int , 58, 2473-2477.

[81] Steiner, K, Moosig, F, Csernok, E, Selleng, K, Gross, W. L, et al. (2001). Increased expression of CTLA-4 (CD152) by T and B lymphocytes in Wegener's granulomatosis. Clin Exp Immunol , 126, 143-150.

[82] Elzouki, A. N, Segelmark, M, Wieslander, J, & Eriksson, S. (1994). Strong link between the alpha 1-antitrypsin PiZ allele and Wegener's granulomatosis. J Intern Med , 236, 543-548.

[83] Fiebeler, A, Borgmann, S, Woywodt, A, Haller, H, & Haubitz, M. (2004). No association of G-463A myeloperoxidase gene polymorphism with MPO-ANCA-associated vasculitis. Nephrol Dial Transplant , 19, 969-971.

[84] Tse, W. Y, Abadeh, S, Jefferis, R, Savage, C. O, & Adu, D. (2000). Neutrophil FcgammaRIIIb allelic polymorphism in anti-neutrophil cytoplasmic antibody (ANCA)-positive systemic vasculitis. Clin Exp Immunol , 119, 574-577.

[85] Hoffman, G. S, & Specks, U. (1998). Antineutrophil cytoplasmic antibodies. Arthritis Rheum , 41, 1521-1537.

[86] Xiao, H, Heeringa, P, Hu, P, Liu, Z, Zhao, M, et al. (2002). Antineutrophil cytoplasmic autoantibodies specific for myeloperoxidase cause glomerulonephritis and vasculitis in mice. J Clin Invest , 110, 955-963.

[87] Neumann, I, Birck, R, Newman, M, Schnulle, P, Kriz, W, et al. (2003). SCG/Kinjoh mice: a model of ANCA-associated crescentic glomerulonephritis with immune deposits. Kidney Int , 64, 140-148.

[88] Bajema, I. M, Hagen, E. C, De Heer, E, Van Der Woude, F. J, & Bruijn, J. A. (2001). Colocalization of ANCA-antigens and fibrinoid necrosis in ANCA-associated vasculitis. Kidney Int , 60, 2025-2030.

[89] Schlieben, D. J, Korbet, S. M, Kimura, R. E, Schwartz, M. M, & Lewis, E. J. (2005). Pulmonary-renal syndrome in a newborn with placental transmission of ANCAs. Am J Kidney Dis , 45, 758-761.

[90] Primo, V. C, Marusic, S, Franklin, C. C, Goldmann, W. H, Achaval, C. G, et al. (2010). Anti-PR3 immune responses induce segmental and necrotizing glomerulonephritis. Clin Exp Immunol , 159, 327-337.

[91] Travis, W. D, Hoffman, G. S, Leavitt, R. Y, Pass, H. I, & Fauci, A. S. (1991). Surgical pathology of the lung in Wegener's granulomatosis. Review of 87 open lung biopsies from 67 patients. Am J Surg Pathol , 15, 315-333.

[92] Leigh, J, Wang, H, Bonin, A, Peters, M, & Ruan, X. (1997). Silica-induced apoptosis in alveolar and granulomatous cells in vivo. Environ Health Perspect 105 Suppl , 5, 1241-1245.

[93] Rastaldi, M. P, Ferrario, F, & Crippa, A. Dell'Antonio G, Casartelli D, et al. ((2000). Glomerular monocyte-macrophage features in ANCA-positive renal vasculitis and cryoglobulinemic nephritis. J Am Soc Nephrol , 11, 2036-2043.

[94] Barksdale, S. K, Hallahan, C. W, Kerr, G. S, Fauci, A. S, Stern, J. B, et al. (1995). Cutaneous pathology in Wegener's granulomatosis. A clinicopathologic study of 75 biopsies in 46 patients. Am J Surg Pathol , 19, 161-172.

[95] Yamamoto, T, Kaburagi, Y, Izaki, S, Tanaka, T, & Kitamura, K. (2000). Leukocytoclasis: ultrastructural in situ nick end labeling study in anaphylactoid purpura. J Dermatol Sci , 24, 158-165.

[96] Aikoh, T, Tomokuni, A, Matsukii, T, Hyodoh, F, Ueki, H, et al. (1998). Activation-induced cell death in human peripheral blood lymphocytes after stimulation with silicate in vitro. Int J Oncol , 12, 1355-1359.

[97] Borges, V. M, Falcao, H, Leite-junior, J. H, Alvim, L, Teixeira, G. P, et al. (2001). Fas ligand triggers pulmonary silicosis. J Exp Med , 194, 155-164.

[98] Zysk, G, Bejo, L, Schneider-wald, B. K, Nau, R, & Heinz, H. (2000). Induction of necrosis and apoptosis of neutrophil granulocytes by Streptococcus pneumoniae. Clin Exp Immunol , 122, 61-66.

[99] Kolaja, K. L, Hood, A. M, & Klaassen, C. D. (1999). The UDP-glucuronyltransferase inducers, phenobarbital and pregnenolone-16alpha-carbonitrile, enhance thyroid-follicular cell apoptosis: association with TGF-beta1 expression. Toxicol Lett , 106, 143-150.

[100] Esnault, V. L. (2002). Apoptosis: the central actor in the three hits that trigger anti-neutrophil cytoplasmic antibody-related systemic vasculitis. Nephrol Dial Transplant , 17, 1725-1728.

[101] Kettritz, R, Scheumann, J, Xu, Y, Luft, F. C, & Haller, H. (2002). TNF-alpha--accelerated apoptosis abrogates ANCA-mediated neutrophil respiratory burst by a caspase-dependent mechanism. Kidney Int , 61, 502-515.

[102] Patry, Y. C, Trewick, D. C, Gregoire, M, Audrain, M. A, Moreau, A. M, et al. (2001). Rats injected with syngenic rat apoptotic neutrophils develop antineutrophil cytoplasmic antibodies. J Am Soc Nephrol , 12, 1764-1768.

[103] Rauova, L, Gilburd, B, Zurgil, N, Blank, M, Guegas, L. L, et al. (2002). Induction of biologically active antineutrophil cytoplasmic antibodies by immunization with human apoptotic polymorphonuclear leukocytes. Clin Immunol , 103, 69-78.

[104] Harper, L, Ren, Y, Savill, J, Adu, D, & Savage, C. O. (2000). Antineutrophil cytoplasmic antibodies induce reactive oxygen-dependent dysregulation of primed neutrophil apoptosis and clearance by macrophages. Am J Pathol , 157, 211-220.

[105] Moosig, F, Csernok, E, Kumanovics, G, & Gross, W. L. (2000). Opsonization of apoptotic neutrophils by anti-neutrophil cytoplasmic antibodies (ANCA) leads to enhanced uptake by macrophages and increased release of tumour necrosis factor-alpha (TNF-alpha). Clin Exp Immunol , 122, 499-503.

[106] Harper, L, Cockwell, P, Adu, D, & Savage, C. O. (2001). Neutrophil priming and apoptosis in anti-neutrophil cytoplasmic autoantibody-associated vasculitis. Kidney Int , 59, 1729-1738.

[107] Deutsch, M, Guejes, L, Zurgil, N, Shovman, O, Gilburd, B, et al. (2004). Antineutrophil cytoplasmic autoantibodies penetrate into human polymorphonuclear leukocytes and modify their apoptosis. Clin Exp Rheumatol 22: S, 35-40.

[108] Harper, L. (2006). ANCA-associated vasculitis: is there a role for neutrophil apoptosis in autoimmunity? Expert Rev Clin Immunol , 2, 237-244.

[109] Brinkmann, V, Reichard, U, Goosmann, C, Fauler, B, Uhlemann, Y, et al. (2004). Neutrophil extracellular traps kill bacteria. Science , 303, 1532-1535.

[110] Brinkmann, V, & Zychlinsky, A. (2007). Beneficial suicide: why neutrophils die to make NETs. Nat Rev Microbiol , 5, 577-582.

[111] Fuchs, T. A, Abed, U, Goosmann, C, Hurwitz, R, Schulze, I, et al. (2007). Novel cell death program leads to neutrophil extracellular traps. J Cell Biol , 176, 231-241.

[112] Kessenbrock, K, Krumbholz, M, Schonermarck, U, Back, W, Gross, W. L, et al. (2009). Netting neutrophils in autoimmune small-vessel vasculitis. Nat Med , 15, 623-625.

[113] Holdenrieder, S, Eichhorn, P, Beuers, U, Samtleben, W, Schoenermarck, U, et al. (2006). Nucleosomal DNA fragments in autoimmune diseases. Ann N Y Acad Sci , 1075, 318-327.

[114] Ohlsson, S, Wieslander, J, & Segelmark, M. (2003). Increased circulating levels of proteinase 3 in patients with anti-neutrophilic cytoplasmic autoantibodies-associated systemic vasculitis in remission. Clin Exp Immunol , 131, 528-535.

[115] Abdgawad, M, Hellmark, T, Gunnarsson, L, Westman, K. W, & Segelmark, M. (2006). Increased neutrophil membrane expression and plasma level of proteinase 3 in systemic vasculitis are not a consequence of the- 564 A/G promotor polymorphism. Clin Exp Immunol , 145, 63-70.

[116] Abdgawad, M, Gunnarsson, L, Bengtsson, A. A, Geborek, P, Nilsson, L, et al. (2010). Elevated neutrophil membrane expression of proteinase 3 is dependent upon CD177 expression. Clin Exp Immunol , 161, 89-97.

[117] Ohlsson, S, Hellmark, T, Pieters, K, Sturfelt, G, Wieslander, J, et al. (2005). Increased monocyte transcription of the proteinase 3 gene in small vessel vasculitis. Clin Exp Immunol , 141, 174-182.

[118] Bauer, S, Abdgawad, M, Gunnarsson, L, Segelmark, M, Tapper, H, et al. (2007). Proteinase 3 and CD177 are expressed on the plasma membrane of the same subset of neutrophils. J Leukoc Biol , 81, 458-464.

[119] Von Vietinghoff, S, Tunnemann, G, Eulenberg, C, & Wellner, M. Cristina Cardoso M, et al. ((2007). NB1 mediates surface expression of the ANCA antigen proteinase 3 on human neutrophils. Blood , 109, 4487-4493.

[120] Abdgawad, M, Pettersson, A, Gunnarsson, L, Bengtsson, A. A, Geborek, P, et al. (2012). Decreased neutrophil apoptosis in quiescent ANCA-associated systemic vasculitis. PLoS One 7: e32439.

[121] Levy, M. (2001). Familial cases of Berger's disease and anaphylactoid purpura. Kidney Int , 60, 1611-1612.

[122] Motoyama, O, & Iitaka, K. (2005). Familial cases of Henoch-Schonlein purpura in eight families. Pediatr Int , 47, 612-615.

[123] Saulsbury, F. T. (2010). Henoch-Schonlein purpura. Curr Opin Rheumatol , 22, 598-602.

[124] Ren, S. M, Yang, G. L, Liu, C. Z, Zhang, C. X, Shou, Q. H, et al. (2012). Association between HLA-A and-B polymorphisms and susceptibility to Henoch-Schonlein purpura in Han and Mongolian children from Inner Mongolia. Genet Mol Res , 11, 221-228.

[125] Amoli, M. M, Thomson, W, Hajeer, A. H, Calvino, M. C, Garcia-porrua, C, et al. (2002). HLA-B35 association with nephritis in Henoch-Schonlein purpura. J Rheumatol , 29, 948-949.

[126] Ozkaya, O, Soylemezoglu, O, Gonen, S, Misirlioglu, M, Tuncer, S, et al. (2006). Renin-angiotensin system gene polymorphisms: association with susceptibility to Henoch-Schonlein purpura and renal involvement. Clin Rheumatol , 25, 861-865.

[127] Desong, L, Fang, L, Songhui, Z, Liu, W, Shi, M, et al. (2010). Renin-angiotensin system gene polymorphisms in children with Henoch-Schonlein purpura in West China. J Renin Angiotensin Aldosterone Syst , 11, 248-255.

[128] Yoshioka, T, Xu, Y. X, Yoshida, H, Shiraga, H, Muraki, T, et al. (1998). Deletion polymorphism of the angiotensin converting enzyme gene predicts persistent proteinuria in Henoch-Schonlein purpura nephritis. Arch Dis Child , 79, 394-399.

[129] Amoroso, A, Danek, G, Vatta, S, Crovella, S, Berrino, M, et al. (1998). Polymorphisms in angiotensin-converting enzyme gene and severity of renal disease in Henoch-Schoenlein patients. Italian Group of Renal Immunopathology. Nephrol Dial Transplant , 13, 3184-3188.

[130] Ault, B. H, Stapleton, F. B, Rivas, M. L, Waldo, F. B, Roy, S, et al. (1990). Association of Henoch-Schonlein purpura glomerulonephritis with C4B deficiency. J Pediatr , 117, 753-755.

[131] Mclean, R. H, Wyatt, R. J, & Julian, B. A. (1984). Complement phenotypes in glomerulonephritis: increased frequency of homozygous null C4 phenotypes in IgA nephropathy and Henoch-Schonlein purpura. Kidney Int , 26, 855-860.

[132] Stefansson Thors V, Kolka R, Sigurdardottir SL, Edvardsson VO, Arason G, et al. ((2005). Increased frequency of C4B*Q0 alleles in patients with Henoch-Schonlein purpura. Scand J Immunol , 61, 274-278.

[133] Atkinson, J. P. (1989). Complement deficiency: predisposing factor to autoimmune syndromes. Clin Exp Rheumatol 7 Suppl 3: S, 95-101.

[134] Motoyama, O, & Iitaka, K. (2005). Henoch-Schonlein purpura with hypocomplementemia in children. Pediatr Int , 47, 39-42.

[135] Brogan, P. A. (2007). What's new in the aetiopathogenesis of vasculitis? Pediatr Nephrol , 22, 1083-1094.

[136] Yang, Y. H, Chuang, Y. H, Wang, L. C, Huang, H. Y, Gershwin, M. E, et al. (2008). The immunobiology of Henoch-Schonlein purpura. Autoimmun Rev , 7, 179-184.

[137] Ozdogan, H, Arisoy, N, Kasapcapur, O, Sever, L, Caliskan, S, et al. (1997). Vasculitis in familial Mediterranean fever. J Rheumatol , 24, 323-327.

[138] Gershoni-baruch, R, Broza, Y, & Brik, R. (2003). Prevalence and significance of mutations in the familial Mediterranean fever gene in Henoch-Schonlein purpura. J Pediatr , 143, 658-661.

[139] Ozcakar, Z. B, Yalcinkaya, F, Cakar, N, Acar, B, Kasapcopur, O, et al. (2008). MEFV mutations modify the clinical presentation of Henoch-Schonlein purpura. J Rheumatol , 35, 2427-2429.

[140] Farley, T. A, Gillespie, S, Rasoulpour, M, Tolentino, N, Hadler, J. L, et al. (1989). Epidemiology of a cluster of Henoch-Schonlein purpura. Am J Dis Child , 143, 798-803.

[141] Allen, D. M, Diamond, L. K, & Howell, D. A. (1960). Anaphylactoid purpura in children (Schonlein-Henoch syndrome): review with a follow-up of the renal complications. AMA J Dis Child , 99, 833-854.

[142] Levy-khademi, F, Korman, S. H, & Amitai, Y. (2000). Henoch-Schonlein purpura: simultaneous occurrence in two siblings. Pediatr Dermatol , 17, 139-140.

[143] Al-sheyyab, M, Shanti, H, Ajlouni, S, Batieha, A, & Daoud, A. S. (1996). Henoch-Schonlein purpura: clinical experience and contemplations on a streptococcal association. J Trop Pediatr , 42, 200-203.

[144] Al-sheyyab, M, Batieha, A, Shanti, H, & Daoud, A. (1999). Henoch-Schonlein purpura and streptococcal infection: a prospective case-control study. Ann Trop Paediatr , 19, 253-255.

[145] Masuda, M, Nakanishi, K, Yoshizawa, N, Iijima, K, & Yoshikawa, N. (2003). Group A streptococcal antigen in the glomeruli of children with Henoch-Schonlein nephritis. Am J Kidney Dis , 41, 366-370.

[146] Frankum, B, & Katelaris, C. H. (1995). Hepatitis C infection and Henoch-Schonlein purpura. Aust N Z J Med 25: 176.

[147] Ayoub, E. M, Mcbride, J, Schmiederer, M, & Anderson, B. (2002). Role of Bartonella henselae in the etiology of Henoch-Schonlein purpura. Pediatr Infect Dis J , 21, 28-31.

[148] Cioc, A. M, Sedmak, D. D, Nuovo, G. J, Dawood, M. R, Smart, G, et al. (2002). Parvovirus B19 associated adult Henoch Schonlein purpura. J Cutan Pathol , 29, 602-607.

[149] Gonzalez, L. M, Janniger, C. K, & Schwartz, R. A. (2009). Pediatric Henoch-Schonlein purpura. Int J Dermatol , 48, 1157-1165.

[150] Conley, M. E, Cooper, M. D, & Michael, A. F. (1980). Selective deposition of immunoglobulin A1 in immunoglobulin A nephropathy, anaphylactoid purpura nephritis, and systemic lupus erythematosus. J Clin Invest , 66, 1432-1436.

[151] Lau, K. K, Wyatt, R. J, Moldoveanu, Z, Tomana, M, Julian, B. A, et al. (2007). Serum levels of galactose-deficient IgA in children with IgA nephropathy and Henoch-Schonlein purpura. Pediatr Nephrol , 22, 2067-2072.

[152] Allen, A. C, Willis, F. R, Beattie, T. J, & Feehally, J. (1998). Abnormal IgA glycosylation in Henoch-Schonlein purpura restricted to patients with clinical nephritis. Nephrol Dial Transplant , 13, 930-934.

[153] Besbas, N, Saatci, U, Ruacan, S, Ozen, S, Sungur, A, et al. (1997). The role of cytokines in Henoch Schonlein purpura. Scand J Rheumatol , 26, 456-460.

[154] Tahan, F, Dursun, I, Poyrazoglu, H, Gurgoze, M, & Dusunsel, R. (2007). The role of chemokines in Henoch Schonlein Purpura. Rheumatol Int , 27, 955-960.

[155] Yang, Y. H, Wang, S. J, Chuang, Y. H, Lin, Y. T, & Chiang, B. L. (2002). The level of IgA antibodies to human umbilical vein endothelial cells can be enhanced by TNF-alpha treatment in children with Henoch-Schonlein purpura. Clin Exp Immunol , 130, 352-357.

[156] Kunimoto, D. Y, Nordan, R. P, & Strober, W. (1989). IL-6 is a potent cofactor of IL-1 in IgM synthesis and of IL-5 in IgA synthesis. J Immunol , 143, 2230-2235.

[157] Petersen, A. M, & Pedersen, B. K. (2005). The anti-inflammatory effect of exercise. J Appl Physiol , 98, 1154-1162.

[158] Chen, T, Guo, Z. P, Li, M. M, Li, J. Y, Jiao, X. Y, et al. (2011). Tumour necrosis factor-like weak inducer of apoptosis (TWEAK), an important mediator of endothelial inflammation, is associated with the pathogenesis of Henoch-Schonlein purpura. Clin Exp Immunol , 166, 64-71.

[159] Sanchez-nino, M. D, Benito-martin, A, Goncalves, S, Sanz, A. B, Ucero, A. C, et al. TNF superfamily: a growing saga of kidney injury modulators. Mediators Inflamm (2010).

[160] Yang, Y. H, Lai, H. J, Huang, C. M, Wang, L. C, Lin, Y. T, et al. (2004). Sera from children with active Henoch-Schonlein purpura can enhance the production of interleukin 8 by human umbilical venous endothelial cells. Ann Rheum Dis , 63, 1511-1513.

[161] Yang, Y. H, Huang, Y. H, Lin, Y. L, Wang, L. C, Chuang, Y. H, et al. (2006). Circulating IgA from acute stage of childhood Henoch-Schonlein purpura can enhance endothelial interleukin (IL)-8 production through MEK/ERK signalling pathway. Clin Exp Immunol , 144, 247-253.

[162] Wu, S. H, Liao, P. Y, Yin, P. L, Zhang, Y. M, & Dong, L. (2009). Inverse temporal changes of lipoxin A4 and leukotrienes in children with Henoch-Schonlein purpura. Prostaglandins Leukot Essent Fatty Acids , 80, 177-183.

[163] Topaloglu, R, Sungur, A, Baskin, E, Besbas, N, Saatci, U, et al. (2001). Vascular endothelial growth factor in Henoch-Schonlein purpura. J Rheumatol , 28, 2269-2273.

[164] Afzali, B, Lombardi, G, Lechler, R. I, & Lord, G. M. (2007). The role of T helper 17 (Th17) and regulatory T cells (Treg) in human organ transplantation and autoimmune disease. Clin Exp Immunol , 148, 32-46.

[165] Li, Y. Y, Li, C. R, Wang, G. B, & Yang, J. Zu Y Investigation of the change in CD4(+) T cell subset in children with Henoch-Schonlein purpura. Rheumatol Int.

[166] Mccarthy, H. J, & Tizard, E. J. (2010). Clinical practice: Diagnosis and management of Henoch-Schonlein purpura. Eur J Pediatr , 169, 643-650.

[167] Davin, J. C, Pierard, G, Dechenne, C, Grossman, D, Nagy, J, et al. (1994). Possible pathogenic role of IgE in Henoch-Schonlein purpura. Pediatr Nephrol , 8, 169-171.

[168] Kahn, R, Herwald, H, Muller-esterl, W, Schmitt, R, Sjogren, A. C, et al. (2002). Contact-system activation in children with vasculitis. Lancet , 360, 535-541.

[169] Demircin, G, Oner, A, Unver, Y, Bulbul, M, & Erdogan, O. (1998). Erythrocyte superoxide dismutase activity and plasma malondialdehyde levels in children with Henoch Schonlein purpura. Acta Paediatr , 87, 848-852.

[170] Ece, A, Kelekci, S, Hekimoglu, A, Kocamaz, H, Balik, H, et al. (2007). Neutrophil activation, protein oxidation and ceruloplasmin levels in children with Henoch-Schonlein purpura. Pediatr Nephrol , 22, 1151-1157.

[171] Soylemezoglu, O, Ozkaya, O, Erbas, D, Akkok, N, Buyan, N, et al. (2002). Nitric oxide in Henoch-Schonlein purpura. Scand J Rheumatol , 31, 271-274.

Chapter 2

The Pathogenesis of Antineutrophil Cytoplasmic Antibody Renal Vasculitis

Sharon Lee Ford, Stephen Roger Holdsworth and
Shaun Andrew Summers

Additional information is available at the end of the chapter

http://dx.doi.org/10.5772/54637

1. Introduction

The vasculitides comprise a heterogeneous group of diseases characterized by inflammation and destruction of blood vessels. Vessels of any size can be involved which explains the diverse spectrum of clinical diseases attributed to vasculitis. While the immunological basis of disease for vasculitis was recognized over thirty years ago,[1] a standardized classification system was only adopted nearly twenty years later. The initial classification system proposed by the American College of Rheumatology attempted to classify vasculitis according to standardized criteria.[2] The subsequent system described by the Chapel Hill Conference on the Nomenclature of Systemic Vasculitis[3] introduced a system which coupled contemporary commonly used disease names and the size of vessel(s) involved.

1.1. Small vessel vasculitis

Necrotizing arteritis is common to many forms of vasculitis, but involvement of vessels smaller than arteries is unique to small vessel vasculitis.[4] A clinical report of 'Vasculitis' originated from the mid-nineteenth century[5] and clinical descriptions of these diseases were published in the 1930s,[6] however it was not until the 1950s that Wegener's Granulomatosis, Churg Strauss Syndrome and Microscopic polyangiitis were identified as unique clinical entities.[7] In the 1980s it was appreciated that the small vessel vasculitides represented a clinically distinct form of disease.[8] These small vessel vasculitides will be the primary focus of this chapter.

Classification	Disease Name
Large Vessel Vasculitis	Giant Cell (Temporal) Arteritis
	Takayasu's Arterits
Medium Sized Vessel Vasculitis	Polyarteritis Nodosa
	Kawasaki's disease
Small Vessel Vasculitis	Wegener's Granulomatosis*
	Churg Strauss Syndrome*
	Microscopic Polyangiitis*
	Henoch Schonlein Purpura
	Essential Cryoglobulinaemic Vasculitis
	Cutaneous Leukocytoclastic Angiitis

*These diseases have subsequently been renamed.

Table 1. The Chapel Hill Conference on the Nomenclature of Systemic Vasculitis

2. Antineutrophil cytoplasmic antibody associated vasculitis

2.1. Background and chapter overview

Glomerulonephritis is a common cause of renal failure both worldwide and in Australia. Rapidly progressive or crescentic glomerulonephritis represents the most severe form of the disease and antineutrophil cytoplasmic antibody (ANCA) associated vasculitis (AAV) accounts for >50% and more likely up to 80% of all cases of rapidly progressive glomerulonephritis. The AAVs are considered a heterogenous group of systemic autoimmune conditions characterised by necrotising inflammation of small to medium sized arteries, capillaries and venules. The disease is diagnosed by detecting ANCA in the serum which characteristically is directed against myeloperoxidase (MPO) or proteinase 3 (PR3). The two most severe clinical manifestations of disease are rapidly progressive glomerulonephritis and pulmonary haemorrhage due to pulmonary capillaritis. These syndromes are associated with significant morbidity and untreated have a mortality that approaches 100%. Renal vasculitis occurs in more than 50% of patients at presentation but in 70-85% of patients with AAV during the course of their disease [9]. While current treatments for active ANCA vasculitis are often life-saving they are toxic and more than 1 in 3 patients will suffer a significant treatment related adverse event.[10] A better understanding of the *critical molecular events* which underlie the disease process will help identify more specific targeted therapies.

In the early 1980s two Australian groups based in Melbourne, from St Vincent's Hospital[11] and the Austin Hospital[12] described the association of antibodies directed against the neutrophil cytoplasm in patients with rapidly progressive glomerulonephritis. These reports represented key advances in our understanding of the pathogenesis of autoimmune small vessel vasculitis. Subsequent work by a Dutch group helped establish the correlation between ANCAs and the three clinical syndromes; Wegener's granulomatosis, microscopic polyangiits and Churg-Strauss syndrome.[13] More recently these syndromes have been renamed to generate nomenclature free from the use of eponyms.[14-16] The new nomenclature proposed and adopted into the literature and clinical practice in 2011 is as follows; Microscopic Polyangiitis (MPA), Granulomatosis with polyangiitis, (GPA), formally known as Wegener's, Allergic Granulomatosis and Angiitis (AGA) formally known as Churg Strauss Disease and Renal Limited Vasculitis (RLV).[14] This new terminology will be adopted for the remainder of this chapter.

In this chapter, we will concentrate on renal injury resulting from AAV which has formed the basis for clinical and experimental studies. For both MPA and GPA target autoantigens have been identified which are constituents of neutrophils. For MPA, myeloperoxidase (MPO) is usually the target autoantigen, while antibodies to proteinase 3 (PR3) are usually detectable in patients with clinical features of GPA. In both clinical and experimental AAV (GPA or MPA) two separate key steps are required for the development of glomerulonephritis and renal injury. The first critical step involves the development of systemic autoimmunity to the target antigen, MPO or PR3. The second step involves antigen specific nephritogenic immune responses driving glomerular injury and renal disease.

2.2. The development of systemic autoimmunity in MPA and GPA

The development of autoimmunity is a complex process, multifactorial in origin, which involves the loss of tolerance and enhanced cellular and humoral activity.[17] In AAV, disease is defined and characterized by antibodies detected against MPO or PR3. While antibodies form the diagnostic hallmark of disease, cellular immunity is critical and is required for the development of humoral immunity and the subsequent generation of B cells and production of ANCAs. A role for cellular immunity has been defined in both clinical and experimental ANCA vasculitis. In addition to adaptive immune cells, innate immune cells contribute to the generation of autoimmunity with evidence for involvement of different cell types in this disease process.

2.3. The initiation and progression of rapidly progressive glomerulonephritis and renal injury in AAV

Enhanced cellular autoimmunity and innate cells stimulate B cells resulting in the production of antigen specific ANCAs. These auto-antibodies bind to and activate circulating neutrophils. These activated neutrophils are recruited to glomerular capillaries,[18] where they degranulate and initiate renal injury. Degranulating neutrophils release their noxious constituents and also deposit MPO [19] and probably PR3 in the glomerulus. Later, CD4+ T cells recognise the autoantigen (MPO/PR3) in the glomerulus and attract additional immune effector cells; this results in severe renal injury. In both clinical and experimental settings cellular nephritogenic immunity, humoral immunity and innate immune cells are critical for the development of rapidly progressive glomerulonephritis.[20-24] Our current treatment regimes were designed to target these cells, or combinations of them.

In this chapter we will focus on the pathogenesis of the ANCA associated vasculitides, focussing on AAV attributable to MPA and GPA. We will pay attention to the development of autoimmunity and concentrate on end organ injury in the kidney, a critical target of the small vessel vasculitides. Interestingly, while GPA and MPA share many diagnostic and clinical features and patients with these diseases have been grouped together in many clinical trials, more recent evidence including a landmark genetic study, suggests that GPA and MPA represent two different diseases. While we will discuss GPA and MPA separately, there is stronger experimental evidence linking MPO with disease. This includes several small animal studies which have confirmed pathogenic roles for cellular and humoral autoimmunity, directed against MPO, which closely resemble human disease. Our discussion will focus on the disease pathogenesis of AAV and attempt to define future directions for study which ultimately may lead to therapeutic interventions. Information has been made available from human studies assessing mechanisms of disease as well as experimental studies, utilizing rodent models of vasculitis. Further insights into disease pathogenesis can be gained from clinical trials, including those with negative results.

3. Genetic and epigenetic basis of disease in ANCA vasculitis

Consistent with improved mechanistic studies the last decade has witnessed significant advances in our understanding of the role of both the genetic and epigenetic factors driving AAV. While a detailed description and discussion of these factors is beyond the scope of this chapter it would be remiss not to discuss several recent key studies. It is important to note that all results discussed in this section are from clinical studies. It should also be noted that while the varying genetic background of commonly used laboratory rodents may contribute to a particular pattern and severity of disease in experimental AAV, the relevance and correlation of this to human disease is less clear.

A genetic basis for AAV has long been suspected, however this was recently confirmed by a publication which demonstrated a relative risk of 1:56 for first degree relatives of patients with GPA.[25] This rate is similar to that seen in other autoimmune diseases with an established genetic component which contributes to injury. This study followed on from previous studies which had suggested a genetic link into AAV. Many of the candidate genes identified as being over represented in vasculitis patients are associated with genes which encode proteins involved in the immune system. These include several genes encoded in the human leukocyte antigen (HLA) as well as genes encoding protein tyrosine phosphatase non-receptor type 22 (*PTPN22*), cytotoxic T-lymphocyte antigen 4 (*CTLA4*), Interleukin (*IL*)-2, *PRTN3* which encodes PR3, α1 anti-trypsin (*AAT*), complement related genes, *CD18*, *IL-10*, *CD226* as well as the Fc gamma receptors; *FCGR2A*, *FCGR3B* (for both copy number high and copy number low). For a detailed review of the individual genes linked with clinical disease, the authors recommend the review by Willcocks and colleagues, whose work with Ken Smith has been instrumental in advancing knowledge in this field.[26] It is important to acknowledge that while genetic variation of these genes has been associated with an increased incidence of AAV, many of these genes display aberrant expression in several autoimmune diseases. This is not surprising considering several of these genes encode proteins critical for maintenance of the immune system, including the function of innate immune cells, T lymphocytes, B lymphocytes and regulatory cells. There are several limitations to these studies. Some studies which linked aberrant gene expression with AAV included patients with only one form of the disease (i.e. GPA, MPA, RLV or AGA), while other studies were less specific and included all patients who had detectable ANCA levels. Furthermore several of these associations were not confirmed when assessing disease in different population groups and hence results from these early studies suggested that there was, at best, a modest link between genetic background and disease.[26-27]

In a genome wide association study with over 10 000 patients (including controls), not only was a genetic component confirmed but the antigenic specificity for AAV, i.e. for MPO or PR3 was found to have distinct genetic associations. For patients with ANCA directed against PR3, there was a strong genetic association with *HLA-DP and* genes encoding *α1-AT-SERPINA1* and *PTN3*. Conversely patients with antibodies directed against MPO showed a strong association with *HLA-DQ*.[28] The observation that there were different genetic associations for MPO-ANCA and PR3-ANCA strengthens the proposal that these diseases represented two different clinical entities. Furthermore the stronger genetic component to PR3 related disease identified in earlier studies was substantiated.

An epigenetic basis for disease has also been proposed. Neutrophil levels of the chromatin modification protein complex, H3K27me3, required for gene silencing were decreased in patients with AAV, at both the MPO and PR3 loci. This phenomenon was dependent on the transcription factor encoding gene, RUNX3. Interestingly RUNX3 message was found to be decreased in patients with AAV compared to healthy controls. These studies provided the first evidence that epigenetic modifications present in AAV patients could impair gene silencing and result in aberrant expression of the target auto-antigens, MPO and PR3.[29] These recently published genetic and epigenetic studies have added considerably to our understanding of AAV.

4. Environmental factors driving disease in ANCA vasculitis

In addition to genetic factors, environmental factors contribute to the loss of tolerance, the development of autoimmunity (to MPO or PR3) and subsequent organ injury. Environmental triggers that have been implicated in disease pathogenesis include environmental toxins, pharmacological therapies and infections, for which there is the strongest evidence.

Epidemiological studies have demonstrated increased incidence of ANCA vasculitis, and more specifically MPA, is increased in patients exposed to a variety of environmental toxins,[30] in particular silica.[31] This is thought to result from environmental toxins serving as adjuvants to the immune system.[32] The development of ANCAs, in particular those reactive to MPO, is not uncommon after treatment with propylithiouracil,[33] although systemic disease following treatment is uncommon. Overt MPA with focal necrotising glomerulonephritis has been described in patients treated with penicillamine[34] and hydralazine.[35] The rarity of these phenomena has prevented us from learning more about disease pathogenesis.

Links between infection and ANCA vasculitis have been suggested for some time, with seasonal variation in disease presentation suggesting a correlation with microbial infection.[36] Moreover results from several studies suggested that infection(s) may predate disease initiation and/or relapse in GPA, MPA and pulmonary vasculitis.[37-40] It must be noted that these results are contentious and other studies have not confirmed them.[30] However, nasal colonization with *Staphylococcus Aureus* is significantly increased in patients with GPA and increases the relative risk of relapse over 7 fold.[37] In a key study, published more than 15 years ago, it was shown that prophylactic antibiotic therapy (co-trimoxazole) successfully decreased disease relapses in ANCA vasculitis. This effect was presumed to result from decreased nasal carriage of *Staphylococcus Aureus*.[41] Interestingly, despite this finding long-term maintenance therapy with co-trimoxazole is not the standard of care in many centres, which may reflect concerns about the long-term safety of the drug. Consistent with an infective trigger to the development of AAV; features of vasculitis have been described in patients with bacterial endocarditis.[42-43] Despite the strong evidence linking infection with the development of autoimmunity (MPO/ PR3) and the ensuing organ injury few mechanistic links have been provided, until recently.

Several mechanisms have been proposed to link infection with the development of AAV, including the use of complementary proteins, molecular mimicry and the ligation of Toll like receptors (TLRs) which heighten innate and adaptive immune responses as well as activating resident kidney cells. A series of clinical and experimental studies have supported each of these concepts, however it is likely that these mechanisms act, at least partially, in combination.

Molecular mimicry refers to the development of antibodies to host proteins after (repeated) exposure to foreign antigens, this occurs due to structural similarities between host and foreign proteins. Molecular mimicry has been proposed as a reason for the loss of tolerance to self and the subsequent development of autoimmunity.[44] In a series of elegant experiments it was demonstrated that antibodies to the lysosomal associated membrane protein-2 (LAMP-2) were highly prevalent in patients with ANCA vasculitis. Furthermore LAMP-2 was pathogenic and administration of polyclonal LAMP-2 to rodents resulted in a characteristic pattern of AAV, with focal necrotising glomerulonephritis, similar to that observed in human renal vasculitis. We will discuss LAMP-2 in more detail later in this chapter. There is homology between the immunodominant LAMP-2 epitope and the peptide of FimH, which is a component of the fimbriae of Gram negative bacteria. It is hypothesized that certain patients infected with Gram negative bacteria would generate antibodies to LAMP-2 and develop vasculitis, through the process of molecular mimicry.[45] This highly plausible theory provides one explanation for the clinical association between infection and the development of ANCAs or LAMP-2 antibodies.

An earlier study reported that a form of molecular mimicry could link *Staphylococcus Aureus* infection with the development of AAV. This process was more complex and involved the use of complementary proteins. The authors observed that patients who were PR3-ANCA positive also had antibodies to a complementary PR3. Complementary PR3 is the protein sequence resulting from transcription of the antisense DNA strand of the PR3 gene. Subsequently it was found that mice immunized with complementary PR3 also developed PR3-ANCA, suggesting a form of molecular mimicry. Pendergraft et al proposed that loss of tolerance, with the development of autoantibodies, could develop as a consequence of immune responses directed against a complementary protein to the autoantigen.[46]

Both of these studies utilized human samples and elegant rodent models to propose infections as initiators of autoimmunity and renal vasculitis. Further work in this field is required to facilitate a better understanding of how molecular mimicry functions in humans and what organisms could be involved.

Infections activate and ligate Toll-like receptors (TLRs). These receptors are innate pattern and danger recognition receptors, ubiquitously expressed on immune cells, and resident tissue cells. which heighten innate and adaptive immune responses in response to infection or danger signals. Ligation of TLRs after infection can stimulate host immune responses, promoting auto-inflammatory and auto-immune responses. Furthermore TLR ligation can stimulate endothelial cells and other resident kidney cells to generate a cytokine milieu conducive to the recruitment of inflammatory leukocytes.

5. The role of adaptive immunity in the development of ANCA autoimmunity and glomerulonephritis

5.1. The role of humoral immunity in AAV pathogenesis

Since their description in the 1980s antibodies directed against MPO and PR3 have formed the diagnostic hallmark of AAV. While not entirely specific there is a strong association between MPO-ANCA and MPA, while PR3 is commonly associated with GPA. Clinical and experimental studies have supported the notion that ANCA are pathogenic. Furthermore therapies targeting (humoral immunity and) ANCAs, including plasma exchange[47] and the anti-CD20 monoclonal antibody Rituximab,[48-49] have been successful in clinical practice. Most of the experimental evidence has supported a role for MPO in disease, but more recently an animal model of PR3-associated vasculitis has also been developed. This represents a significant advance and it is anticipated that this model will facilitate an improved understanding of the pathogenesis of PR3-AAV. In this section, we will also discuss other roles for B cells including their function as antigen presenting cells (APCs) and as potential regulators of disease.

Are ANCAs pathogenic? There has been increasing evidence supporting a pathogenic role for ANCAs. Results from *in vitro* studies demonstrate that ANCAs activate primed neutrophils which degranulate and deposit autoantigens in glomeruli. Similarly results from *in vivo* studies, including an expanding number of animal models, have confirmed a pathogenic role for ANCAs. *In vitro* studies have consistently demonstrated that neutrophils from patients with AAV express increased amounts of the target antigens (MPO/PR3) on their cell surface.[50] These auto-antigens are targets for ANCA binding. Furthermore, several cytokines including tumor necrosis factor (TNF), IL-18 and granulocyte macrophage colony stimulating factor can prime neutrophils in AAV, increasing auto-antigen expression which facilitates ANCA binding.[51-53] Binding of ANCA to the neutrophil is associated with increased adherence to the endothelium, superoxide generation and cytokine production.[51, 54] The effect of neutrophils and their interaction with the endothelium will be discussed in greater detail later in this chapter.

Animal studies have demonstrated a pathogenic role for ANCAs. The model described by Xiao et al was one of the first murine models of AAV, which produced severe renal injury. The observed renal injury bore considerable resemblance to that seen in human rapidly progressive glomerulonephritis. In this model MPO deficient mice were immunized with MPO. Subsequently the spleens of these MPO deficient mice were transferred into recombinant activation gene knockout (RAG2-/-) mice, which lack adaptive immunity. After transfer of splenocytes (from MPO immunized MPO-/- mice) RAG2-/- mice developed humoral autoimmunity with the production of MPO-ANCAs. Kidneys from these mice displayed the hallmarks of severe crescentic glomerulonephritis. The authors also performed a passive transfer experiment, administering MPO-ANCAs to RAG2-/- mice. The passive transfer of MPO-ANCA to RAG2-/- mice resulted in a milder form of glomerular injury compared to that seen after splenocyte transfer.[55] These experiments highlighted the pathogenic role for MPO-ANCAs, however, it should be noted that the severe injury occurring after the transfer of splenocytes could reflect cellular immunity contributing to renal injury. None the less, the passive transfer of ANCAs to mice has consistency resulted in a degree of renal injury, which is neutrophil,[56] lipopolysaccharide[57], TLR4[58] and complement [59] dependent.

Additional evidence for a pathogenic role for MPO in driving AAV and renal injury was demonstrated in Wistar-Kyoto rats. Rats developed focal necrotizing glomerulonephritis and pulmonary vasculitis after immunization with purified human MPO. Furthermore a pathogenic role for the chemokine CXCL1 (the rodent homolog of human IL-8) in neutrophil-endothelial interactions was demonstrated, by analysis of neutrophil migration in the capillary beds.[60] Recently Little has described a model of vasculitis, dependent on PR3-ANCA, which develops in mice with a humanised immune system. This model was generated by treating irradiated NOD-scid-IL-2Rγ-/- mice with human haematopoietic cells. In NOD-scid-IL-2Rγ-/- mice there are multiple deficiencies in the function of both innate and adaptive immune cells. These chimeric mice were then treated with human immunoglobulin from patients with PR3-ANCA vasculitis or control serum. In control treated mice no glomerular injury was observed, however mice treated with PR3-ANCA demonstrated (at least mild) glomerulonephritis, while more severe injury was observed in 17% of PR3-ANCA treated mice.[61] While further work is required to confirm that this murine model is robust, it is anticipated that it will provide a good basis to explore the pathogenic nature of PR3-ANCA in clinical practice.

Another potential antigenic target is LAMP-2. Antibodies to LAMP-2 were reliably detected in more than 90% of patients with active ANCA associated necrotising crescentic glomerulonephritis. LAMP-2 antibodies were detected even when MPO-ANCA and PR3-ANCA could not be detected, suggesting this test may have improved diagnostic sensitivity and could possibly be useful for serological diagnosis in patients with renal limited vasculitis, who traditionally are found to be ANCA negative. Antibodies to LAMP-2 were also pathogenic and administration of human LAMP-2 antibodies to Wistar Kyoto rats resulted in pauci-immune focal necrotizing glomerulonephritis.[45] Subsequently, the authors working with several collaborative groups, have verified the prevalence of antibodies to LAMP-2 in cohorts of ANCA patients from a range of European countries. Three different techniques; enzyme linked immunosorbent assay; western blotting and an indirect immunofluorescence assay were all readily able to detect antibodies. Interestingly antibodies were undetectable shortly after treatment, although they were detectable during clinical relapse, highlighting the potential usefulness of these antibodies in clinical practice.[62] However studies from the United States could not confirm these findings, where the sensitivity of detecting LAMP-2 antibodies was much lower than that seen within the European studies.[63] The divergence of results is interesting and suggests that further work is required to facilitate assays which could result in the development of better diagnostic tools.

Most studies examining the pathogenic role of B cells in AAV have focussed on their role as effector cells, however B cells have a more diverse range of functions than autoantibody production alone. In other scenarios B cells are considered antigen presenting cells, while they possibly influence T cell responses.[64]

The B cell activating factor (BAFF) has also been shown to be elevated in patients with AAV,[65] which is exciting considering the therapeutic promise shown with BAFF inhibitors in systemic lupus erythematosus (SLE).[66] B cells may also contribute to disease in other ways and a detailed analysis of renal biopsies from patients with AAV demonstrated significant B cell infiltration, including organized B cell clusters.[67] In addition to proinflammatory responses B cell also display regulatory function and produce IL-10, a regulatory cytokine. Interestingly in patients with SLE regulatory B cells (Bregs) are impaired and are unable to suppress effector T cells.[68] While this has not been explored to date in vasculitis, it remains possible that heightened humoral and cellular immunity occurs as a consequence of impaired Bregs.

In concluding, B cells form the diagnostic hallmarks of ANCA vasculitis and are pathogenic. The success observed in clinical practice with therapies which chiefly target B cells has not been fully elucidated and may extend beyond autoantibody inhibition. Interestingly, Rituximab was shown to treat the clinical symptoms of GPA, even when ANCAs were not detectable. [69] An in-depth understanding of the role of humoral immunity is awaited and may help direct future therapies.

5.2. The role of cellular immunity in AAV pathogenesis

While ANCAs are diagnostic and pathogenic in AAV, cellular immunity is an essential requirement for the initiation and continued production of auto-reactive B cell responses and for driving effector cell responses in the kidney. Evidence for a key role for cellular autoimmunity in AAV comes from several lines of evidence, including observational studies in humans, reports of refractory disease responding to treatments targeting T cells and extensive murine studies showing a pathogenic role for T cells in the development of autoimmunity. Vasculitis involving the glomerular capillary bed has little or no antibody deposition, but rather demonstrates delayed type hypersensitivity responses, including fibrin deposition. This is most likely to be a consequence of auto-reactive CD4+ effector cells recognizing MPO, which is present in glomeruli in both human and experimental ANCA vasculitis [70-72]. In addition to enhancing inflammation, regulatory T cells (Tregs) are likely to have an important role in modulating immune responses and glomerular injury.

T cells are active participants in the loss of tolerance and the development of autoimmunity in AAV. Firstly we know that ANCAs are class switched high affinity antibodies which are (therefore) dependent on T cells for their generation.[73] Secondly, in proliferation studies, it has been demonstrated that auto-reactive T cells from patents with AAV respond to MPO and PR3,[74] while markers of T cell activity are increased in parallel with disease activity.[75-76] Furthermore, in renal biopsy samples from patients with AAV, the number of infiltrating T cells correlates with the severity of injury. Additional evidence supporting a pathogenic role for T cells was provided when 15 patients with refractory vasculitis, resistant to other therapies, were successfully treated with anti-thymocyte globulin, which targets T cells.[77]

Early studies supported a role for T helper (Th) 1 (and possibly Th2) cells in the pathogenesis of AAV. Peripheral blood lymphocytes from patients with MPO-ANCA were shown to produce IFNγ when stimulated.[78] The more recently defined Th17 cells represent a distinct lineage of CD4+ T cells, which are characterized by the production of IL-17A.[79] Two key human studies supported a role for Th17 cells in ANCA vasculitis. Firstly it was demonstrated that when peripheral blood from GPA patients was stimulated with PR3, there was an increased percentage of IL-17A producing CD4+ T cells (Th17). After stimulation no difference in IFNγ production was seen, suggesting that Th1 cells were not involved. The authors proposed that this skewed Th17 response supported a role for Th17 cells in disease.[80] A subsequent study demonstrated that sera from patients with active AAV consistently displayed a Th17 phenotype. Cytokines associated with Th17 cells, including IL-17A and IL-23, were increased in patients with acute AAV, while levels of IFNγ were unchanged. Interestingly immunosuppressive therapy did not consistently decrease IL-23 or IL-17 production.[23] In a study of human ANCA biopsies it has been shown that IL-17A producing CD4+ T cells constitute part of the inflammatory infiltrate and correspond with disease severity.[81] In addition, murine models have provided strong evidence for a pathogenic role for CD4+ T cells in glomerulonephritis.

An MPO-dependent murine model which demonstrates considerable homology to human ANCA vasculitis, where mice develop autoimmunity to MPO and focal necrotising glomerulonephritis was described. Immunization of C57BL/6 wild type mice with MPO results in cellular and humoral autoimmunity to MPO. A small dose of sheep anti-mouse glomerular basement membrane serum is subsequently administered. Treatment of chicken ovalbumin (OVA) immunized mice with this dose of sheep anti-mouse glomerular basement membrane serum does not result in significant renal injury. However in mice immunized with MPO and then sheep anti-mouse glomerular basement membrane serum significant renal injury is seen. Depletion of CD4+ effector cells significantly attenuated glomerular injury in this model, while experiments performed in B cell-deficient mice did not show renal protection.[72] These results provide strong evidence for a pathogenic role for CD4+ effector cells contributing to rapidly progressive glomerulonephritis in MPO-ANCA vasculitis. Subsequent work from this group has supported a role for both Th1 and Th17 cells in disease. Firstly, using IL-17A-/- mice it was shown that the development of cellular autoimmunity and necrotizing glomerulonephritis was IL-17A dependent. Secondly in the absence of IL-17A there was a decrease in glomerular neutrophil and macrophage recruitment and renal injury was attenuated. These results highlight the potential therapeutic benefits of IL-17A blockade in AAV.[24] This group has also elucidated that both IL-17A and IFNγ can drive nephritogenic autoimmunity and renal injury in AAV. Interestingly ligation of different TLRs dictated the pattern of cytokine production, TLR2 ligation promoted the development of Th17 autoimmunity, while TLR9 ligation drove Th1 autoimmunity. Mice which developed Th17 induced renal injury were successfully treated with anti-IL-17A monoclonal antibody (mAb). Conversely in mice that developed predominant Th1 driven injury, administration of anti-IFNγ mAb attenuated renal injury.[82] Work from Richard Kitching's group has further refined our understanding of the role of CD4+ T cells in the pathogenesis of AAV. Using 20 amino acid sequence peptides they identified the immunodominant MPO CD4+ T cell epitope. Subsequently they produced T cell clones which were specific for this immunodominant MPO epitope, which were then injected into mice. Using three different techniques it was demonstrated that when the MPO peptide (or whole MPO) was deposited in glomeruli focal necrotising glomerulonephritis was driven by antigen specific CD4+ T cells.[83] These key studies have helped define how effector T cells drive glomerular injury.

6. The role of Th17 cells in autoimmunity and glomerulonephritis

The original description of Th1, IFNγ producing and Th2, IL-4 producing, T helper cells by Mosmann and Coffman [84] has been expanded to include a new subset of Th cells, the IL-17A producing Th17 cells.[79, 85-86] While the prototypic cytokine produced by Th17 cells is IL-17A, these cells produce numerous other cytokines, including the ubiquitous IL-6, TNF and IL-1β.[85] Two transcription factors are critical for the development of Th17 cells; STAT3 and Rorγt.[87-88] For the induction and maintenance Th17 cells, several cytokines are required, these include; IL-23,[89] IL-6, TGF-β,[90-93] while IL-21 is required for amplification of Th17 cells.[94-96]

Prior to the discovery of Th17 cells, autoimmunity was believed to be predominantly a Th1-mediated phenomenon. There were inconsistencies, however, in this paradigm, for example IFNγ$^{-/-}$ mice developed exaggerated organ inflammation and injury in experimental autoimmune models.[97-98] Subsequently it was demonstrated that organ injury (in the most common autoimmune model, experimental autoimmune encephalomyelitis [EAE]) was unchanged in IL-12p35$^{-/-}$ mice (functionally Th1 deficient), while injury was significantly attenuated in IL-12p40$^{-/-}$ (functionally Th1 and Th17 deficient) and IL-12p19$^{-/-}$ (functionally Th17 deficient) mice.[99] Similarly IL-17A$^{-/-}$ mice were protected from EAE, [100] while increased IL-17 expression was seen in patients with multiple sclerosis, [101] a common autoimmune disease seen in clinical practice, which is the human equivalent of EAE. Further studies have implicated Th17 cells in several autoimmune diseases including rheumatoid arthritis,[102] consistent with this finding IL-17A$^{-/-}$ mice are protected from murine experimental arthritis.[103-104] IL-17A has been implicated in inflammatory bowel disease, both experimental[105] and clinical[106] as well as human inflammatory skin conditions.[107-108]

7. Th17 cells in the kidney

Early studies performed in gene deficient mice supported a role for Th17 related cytokines in the development of experimental autoimmune glomerulonephritis[109] and sheep anti-mouse glomerular basement membrane disease.[110] A pathogenic role for RORγt, the key IL-17A transcription factor, was also demonstrated in a murine model of crescentic glomerulonephritis.[111] A direct role for Th17 cells acting as effectors was subsequently published. The antigen, ovalbumin (OVA), was planted in the kidneys of RAG1-/- mice, after the conjugation of OVA to a non-nephritogenic antibody specific for the glomerular basement membrane. This was followed by the administration of Th-17 polarized ovalbumin specific CD4+ T cells, which resulted in neutrophil mediated proliferative glomerulonephritis.[112] Detailed reviews of the role of Th17 cells in kidney disease have recently been published.[113-114]

Th17 cells are a distinct line of CD4+ T helper cells with unique transcription factors and effector cytokines. These cells are active participants in the development of autoimmunity but are also involved as effector cells in autoimmune conditions including rapidly progressive glomerulonephritis.

In addition to CD4+ effector T cells other T cells are likely to contribute to AAV. Several years ago it was demonstrated that CD4+ effector memory cells (Tem) were increased in the blood of GPA patients in remission, compared to those with active disease.[115] While Tem were decreased in the blood, they were increased in the urine of patients with active disease - suggesting that these cells may influence renal injury during active disease.[116] Further *in vitro* studies suggested that in GPA patients these cells could mediate endothelial injury and thus play a role in driving glomerular injury.[117] Fewer studies have assessed potential pathogenic roles of CD8+ T cells in AAV, however it would seem likely that these cells are involved. A study assessing gene expression and outcome in AAV and SLE patients suggested that CD8+ T cell signatures and increased CD8+ T cell memory populations were associated with poorer outcomes.[118] It was hoped that results from these studies would facilitate more individualised treatments. It would seem important that we further explore the role of CD8+ T cells in AAV.

Regulatory T cells (Tregs) represent a subset of CD4+ CD25+ T cells which perform a key role in regulating inflammation and tissue injury. These cells are identified through the expression of FoxP3, which is considered a master regulator of Tregs. In several autoimmune diseases, including Goodpasture's disease, Tregs are required for the maintenance of tolerance and loss of Treg function can result in the development of autoimmunity and organ injury.[119] In GPA clinical studies have shown that although circulating FoxP3-expressing Tregs vary in number their suppressive capacity is reduced.[120] In MPA patients (and experimentally) FoxP3-expressing Tregs display diminished capacity to suppress antigen specific MPO responses an effect mediated through tryptophan.[121] Our current understanding of the role of Tregs in AAV is limited and further studies are required to improve our knowledge of their role in disease pathogenesis in order to facilitate treatments aimed at optimizing their therapeutic potential. It is well known that Th17 cells and Tregs require many of the same cytokines for growth and development and it has been postulated that they have an inverse relationship. Whilst this explanation may be simplistic it is attractive to hypothesise that both the initiation of disease and flares seen in AAV could be attributed to an imbalance in the Th17: Treg ratio; with Th17 overactivity promoting disease. This imbalance could be targeted in future treatment protocols.

8. Innate immune responses in ANCA associated vasculitis

8.1. Neutrophils, key effector cells, in ANCA associated vasculitis

Neutrophils play a critical role in the pathogenesis of ANCA vasculitis. Not only are neutrophils the primary effector cells in the kidney but neutrophils also contain the target autoantigens, MPO, PR3 (and LAMP-2) and hence are directly involved in the auto-immune process. We will discuss three different aspects of neutrophil involvement in disease, (a) The role of the Neutrophil in the development of Autoimmunity, (b) Neutrophil Activation by ANCAs and (c) Neutrophil Endothelial Interactions, which initiate glomerular injury.

8.1.1. The role of the neutrophil in the development of autoimmunity

It is well established that ANCAs bind to the autoantigens, MPO or PR3, located on the cell surface of the neutrophil. How and why these autoantigens translocate to the cell surface is poorly understood. We know that neutrophils die through apoptosis or necrosis and data suggests that neutrophil death through apoptosis can promote the loss of tolerance to MPO or PR3. After cell death neutrophils release granule constituents, including MPO and PR3, which translocate to the cell surface[122-123] where they serve as antigenic targets. This phenomenon was thought to occur exclusively after neutrophil death through apoptosis, which is possibly related to a slower mechanism of cell death, although the operational mechanisms of this system require further clarification.

An additional pathway linking neutrophil cell death and autoimmunity has recently been proposed, involving a distinct method of neutrophil death involving neutrophil extracellular traps (NETs). Neutrophils extrude NETs which consist of chromatin structures and include anti-microbial peptides such as; MPO, PR3 elastin, cathepsin, and lactoferrin.[124] Dying neutrophils extrude NETs to kill invading pathogens in a process recently named NETosis. It is understood that neutrophils, through NETosis, contribute to the development of autoimmunity, a concept well established in SLE. In SLE, in response to chronic autoantibody stimulation neutrophils and their NETs activate plasmacytoid dendritic cells which secrete IFNα.[125-127] NETosis has been linked with glomerular injury in AAV, through the enhancement of endothelial-leukocyte interaction,[71] however only recently have NETs been implicated in the development of ANCA autoimmunity. NETotic neutrophils interacted with myeloid dendritic cells (mDC). This interaction was not observed when neutrophils died by necrosis or apoptosis. This process was dependent on both TNF and IFNγ and in their absence NETosis did not occur. The interaction between the NETotic neutrophil and the mDC resulted in the transfer of MPO and PR3 to the mDC, which potentially could induce and promote adaptive immune responses. This process was confirmed to be pathogenic *in* vivo. Mice were immunized with mDCs co-cultured with NETotic neutrophils (6 times intraperitoneally) and three months later they developed ANCAs and showed evidence of renal injury. The mice also displayed features consistent with systemic auto-immune disease. A similar process was thought to be present in human AAV. Assessing skin lesions from patients with MPO-ANCA vasculitis revealed an interaction between mDCs and neutrophils, with uploading of the auto-antigens.[128] While this process is not yet completely understood, NETosis potentially explains how autoantigens are recognized by antigen presenting cells, activating cellular and humoral autoimmunity in AAV.

While neutrophil apoptosis and NETosis provide some insight into the role of the neutrophil in the development of AAV, there remain several 'gaps' in our knowledge. Why AAV patients develop autoimmunity to MPO/PR3, with an associated clinical syndrome and yet they do not develop autoantibodies to other neutrophil constituents which are released after cell death is unclear. The driving factors behind apoptosis and NETosis have not been well established. Further studies in this area are required before definitive conclusions can be reached. In addition to promoting autoimmunity the ANCA-neutrophil interaction is a key to two other mechanisms of injury, ANCA binding to neutrophils leading to neutrophil activation and an oxidative burst, and the recruitment of ANCA bound neutrophils to the glomerulus where they initiate renal injury.

8.1.2. Neutrophil activation by ANCAs

The first paper suggesting a role for ANCA in activating neutrophils was published over 20 years ago. In this landmark paper it was shown that both MPO-ANCA and PR3-ANCA could bind to primed neutrophils. After neutrophil priming by tumour necrosis factor (TNF) MPO and PR3 were translocated to the cell surface, providing an autoantibody antigenic target. Neutrophil binding by ANCAs produced an oxidative burst and resulted in degranulation. [115] Other authors have confirmed this process and shown that it is also Fcgamma RII-dependent.[129] Cytokine priming of neutrophils is important for ANCA binding as it increases surface expression of the autoantigens and mobilizes the NADPH oxidase complex, further increasing ANCA binding.[27, 53] In addition to TNF, IL-18 and granulocyte macrophage colony stimulating factor can prime neutrophils and enhance ANCA binding.[52]

The pathogenic role of TNF in AAV has attracted significant interest both experimentally and clinically. In a passive transfer model of MPO-ANCA vasculitis pre-treatment with lipopolysaccharide (LPS) increased systemic inflammation and glomerular injury. The *in vitro* oxidative burst induced by MPO-ANCA required TNF and anti-TNF mAb treatment attenuated renal injury *in vivo.[57]* Similar results were found by other authors who demonstrated that mAb directed against TNF successfully attenuated established glomerulonephritis in a rat model of AAV. Despite intact humoral responses there was a decrease in functional and histological injury in rats receiving the treatment.[130] The anti-TNF mAb, Infliximab, has been used with some success in patients with AAV. While Infliximab therapy was useful in treating patients with refractory disease,[131-132] disappointingly the addition of TNF blockade (Infliximab[133] or Adalimumab[134]) to standard treatment regimes did not result in an improvement in clinical outcomes and Etanercept, (a fusion protein TNF inhibitor) could not decrease relapse rates in GPA.[115] Despite the lack of efficacy of TNF blockade in these trials, it would seem that TNF has a central role in the pathogenesis and in selected patients the use of TNF blockade may be associated with clinical improvement. In addition to TNF other cytokines and chemokines are likely to be important in AAV. Interestingly it was first appreciated over 15 years ago that neutrophils stimulated by ANCA produce IL-1β.[135] Few studies have further investigated this observation. Recently the Inflammasome, which is a pattern recognition receptor which is characterized by the production of IL-1β, has been shown to promote auto-inflammatory and auto-immune disease. It is possible that the Inflammasome is involved in vasculitis. This is clinically relevant because diseases resulting from overstimulation of the Inflammasome have been successfully treated with monoclonal antibody therapy.[136] This warrants further investigation.

The intracellular signalling pathways activated by ANCA neutrophil binding are multiple, although several pathways are shared. Whereas the Fc portion of ANCA IgG activates tyrosine kinase pathways,[137] the F(ab')2 portion activates a G protein pathway.[138] Despite initiating two separate pathways, these pathways converge on the $p21^{ras}$ GTPase, which is essential for many neutrophil functions.[139] The identification of these pathways, combined with the development of antibodies directed against specific components of these pathways, predominantly used in preclinical models, has increased expectations of their potential therapeutic use in autoimmune diseases including renal vasculitis.[140-141]

8.1.3. Neutrophil- endothelial interactions

The interaction between neutrophils and endothelial cells is important in the initiation of glomerular lesions, including fibrinoid necrosis, which is frequently observed in patients with renal vasculitis. Under normal physiological conditions neutrophils do not interact with the endothelium, however when the endothelium is activated resulting in increased expression of adhesion molecules and chemokines (and neutrophils are activated) neutrophil recruitment, binding and transmigration is increased. Our understanding of this complex dynamic has been improved through the use of in vitro systems, which include flow chambers mimicking blood flow in human capillaries. For these studies neutrophils from healthy controls and patients with AAV have been compared. Further information has been gleaned from experimental models using live imaging of the kidney, including intravital microscopy.

It is likely that TNF production and complement activation in AAV patients results in a persistent low grade activation of neutrophils.[142] Results from in vitro studies have shown that neutrophils exposed to ANCA bind to human umbilical vein endothelial cells (HUVECs), [143-144] with up-regulation of CD11b, an adhesion molecule.[145-146] In a flow system set up to mirror blood flow in human capillaries, ANCA treated neutrophils demonstrated increased adhesion and transmigration which was β2 integrin and CXCR2 (neutrophil cell surface receptors) dependent.[146] This is likely to resemble what happens in human AAV, where expression of both β1 and β2 integrins are increased in circulating neutrophils,[147] and the adhesion molecules ICAM and VCAM are expressed on glomerular endothelial cells.[148] Additional results from human studies have implicated IL-8 in leukocyte recruitment which was also shown to correlate with glomerular injury.[51] Neutrophil degranulation with the accompanying release of reactive oxygen species, proteases[149-150] and an oxidative burst[151-152] directly leads to endothelial injury. Evidence for enhanced endothelial injury includes increased levels of endothelial cell microparticles in active disease, which subsequently reduce when the disease remits.[153-154] This is in direct contrast to the restorative endothelial progenitor cells which are decreased when disease is active.[155-156] It has been suggested that the pro-angiogenic protein, angiopoietin-2, may act locally to promote inflammation and endothelial cell injury.[154] It is likely that several mechanisms combine to result in endothelial injury. We know that neutrophil degranulation also results in deposition of the neutrophil constituents, MPO and PR3 in the glomerular bed,[157] and these deposited autoantigens provide targets for antigen specific T and B cells, which recruit additional effector cells, promoting a vicious cycle of injury.

Many of the original studies assessing neutrophil recruitment to the capillaries used intravital imaging of mesenteric and cremasteric vessels. These vessels are more accessible and provide some parallels with leukocyte recruitment seen in renal and lung vasculitis. More recently Michael Hickey's group have pioneered new methods for assessing neutrophil physiology in the inflamed glomerulus, which has considerably improved our understanding of leukocyte behaviour in glomerulonephritis.[158-159].

In vitro studies performed in a flow chamber have shown that human neutrophils treated with ANCA display altered patterns of rolling, adhesion and transmigration.[146, 160] Using intravital microscopy to visualise mesenteric postcapillary venules Little et al found that administration of MPO-ANCA induced neutrophil adhesion and transmigration. Similarly studies using intravital microscopy to visualize murine cremasteric postcapillary venules demonstrated increased neutrophil adhesion and transmigration after the passive transfer of MPO-ANCA. Neutrophil recruitment was both Fcgamma receptor and β2 integrin dependent.[161] While these studies provided valuable insight into neutrophil recruitment and transmigration in inflamed tissues in AAV, it remained unclear if the observations seen in the postcapillary venules could be replicated in the glomerulus. The use of live imaging of the murine kidney has facilitated the study of leukocyte behaviour in models of glomerular injury. Differences in neutrophil behaviour in the inflamed glomerulus have been noted. In the heterologous phase of renal injury induced after administration of sheep anti-mouse GBM serum, neutrophil recruitment occurred via rapid arrest and occurred in the absence of rolling.[158] Relevant to AAV, in mice treated with LPS and MPO-ANCA glomerular neutrophil recruitment occurred in a lymphocyte function-associated antigen (LFA-1)(a leukocyte integrin) dependent manner. However if an increased dose of MPO-ANCA was used (without LPS priming), neutrophil recruitment was α4-integrin dependent, but β2-integrin independent.[18] These studies highlight how MPO-ANCA can induce glomerular neutrophil recruitment through many different pathways and furthermore demonstrate that the glomerulus is a unique organ in which neutrophil migration differs from other postcapillary venules. While it is likely that injury in humans with renal vasculitis is a consequence of several mechanisms (discussed above) acting in tandem, direct visualization of the kidney appears to be the best technique to assess glomerulonephritis. In addition to the mechanisms detailed above there are likely to be several other factors which contribute to pathogenic neutrophil-endothelial interaction and the ensuing rapidly progressive glomerulonephritis, several of these are discussed later in this chapter.

8.1.3.1. The role of NETs in neutrophil-endothelial interactions and glomerulonephritis in AAV

The role of neutrophil extracellular traps (NETs) in the development of autoimmunity to MPO and PR3 has been discussed earlier. A further role for NETs in driving effector responses in renal vasculitis was described in an innovative paper published in 2009. In this manuscript, Kessenbrock et al, found that primed neutrophils cultured with ANCAs resulted in the development of NETs and these chromatin fibres contained the auto-antigens MPO and PR3. When neutrophils were recruited to inflamed glomeruli, degranulation of the neutrophil and NETs resulted in the deposition of these autoantigens in the glomerulus. Furthermore they demonstrated that in human kidney biopsies, from patients with AAV, NET formation was associated with areas of high neutrophil influx and acute injury.[71] It is likely that deposition of MPO and PR3 could directly result in glomerular injury, however these autoantigens could also serve as targets for auto-reactive CD4+ T cells and B cells further increasing the influx of inflammatory cells and exacerbating glomerular injury.

8.1.3.2. A pathogenic role for neutrophil microparticles in AAV

Microparticles in neutrophils contain an abundance of adhesion molecules and proteases which include the ANCA auto-antigens PR3 and MPO.[162] Recent data has shown ANCAs can induce the release of neutrophil microparticles from primed neutrophils. These microparticles bind to endothelial cells through an up-regulation of adhesion molecules and result in increased endothelial reactive oxygen species and released pro-inflammatory cytokines including, IL-6 and IL-8. The clinical relevance of this was supported by data which demonstrated that neutrophil microparticles were more readily detected in patients (children) with active AAV, while levels were suppressed in healthy controls and patients with inactive disease.[163] Several other mechanisms of neutrophil microparticle release have been described, including those triggered by the complement system, which is also active in renal vasculitis. These studies further highlight the complex nature of neutrophil induced glomerular injury in renal vasculitis. It is likely that that the synchrony of many innate immune cells and adaptive immunity result in the severe injury observed in rapidly progressive glomerulonephritis and acute kidney injury.

8.2. The role of Toll Like Receptors (TLRs) in ANCA associated vasculitis

The innate pattern recognition receptors, TLRs, recognise molecular patterns commonly found in bacterial and viral organisms.[164] In response to invading microbes, TLR ligation results in a 'hard-wired' activation of the innate immune system and heightened adaptive immune responses. While TLRs are required for protection from invading microbes, inappropriate stimulation can result in the development of autoimmunity and organ injury,[165] including renal disease.[166] In several experimental models of kidney disease, including acute kidney injury,[167] lupus nephritis[168] and crescentic glomerulonephritis,[169] we and others have demonstrated pathogenic roles for TLRs. However their role in AAV is likely to be dual. Firstly ligation of TLRs heightens innate and adaptive immune response, which in turn leads to the loss of tolerance and the development of autoimmunity. Secondly, TLRs activate both effector cells and resident kidney cells, increasing glomerular inflammation and renal injury. This is important as infections are known to promote injury in AAV, with TLRs providing a link between infection and the development of AAV and disease relapses. While many TLRs have been implicated in autoimmunity studies in AAV have largely concentrated on the surface receptors, TLR2 and TLR4, as well as the intracellular TLR9.

There is clinical evidence implicating TLRs in the loss of tolerance in AAV. Stimulation of peripheral blood mononuclear cells (PBMCs) from GPA patients with a TLR9 ligand resulted in increased ANCA production.[170] Moreover in patients with AAV in remission TLR9 expression is increased on B lymphocytes and when these B lymphocytes were cultured with a TLR9 ligand they produced ANCA.[171] These studies support a role for infection (through ligation of TLR9) promoting humoral autoimmunity. Expression of TLR2, TLR4 and TLR9 on B lymphocytes, T lymphocytes, natural killer (NK) cells, monocytes and granulocytes from AAV patients (and controls) was assessed. Amongst AAV patient's monocytes and NK cells had increased TLR expression.[172] We have provided supporting evidence for a pathogenic role for TLRs using experimental models of AAV. Immunization of WT mice with a TLR ligand and MPO resulted in the loss of tolerance with the development of cellular and humoral autoimmune responses and later necrotising glomerulonephritis. Interestingly immunization with a TLR9 ligand and MPO resulted in T-bet dependent IFNγ production and macrophage mediated renal injury. Conversely autoimmunity induced by a TLR2 ligand and MPO resulted in ROR-γ dependent Th17 autoimmunity and neutrophil mediated renal injury.[82]

However, TLRs are also likely to be involved in effector responses. While TLRs are expressed at low and often undetectable levels in normal kidney biopsies, increased expression has been seen in glomerulonephritis. In lupus nephritis glomerular and tubular TLR9 expression was shown to be increased in both children and adults.[173-174] In studies assessing patterns of TLR2, TLR4 and TLR9 in glomerulonephritis, strong TLR2 and TLR4 staining was seen in the inflammatory infiltrates of patients with AAV.[175] We have stained renal biopsies from patients with AAV and found that TLR9 staining is positive in the glomeruli (unpublished data), as illustrated.

Further studies have supported an interaction between AAV and TLRs, when epithelial cells, from kidney and lung, primed with PR3-ANCA serum produced exaggerated cytokine levels after TLR stimulation.[176] While early studies suggested that lipopolysaccharide (LPS) enhanced effector responses in AAV,[57] our understanding of this process has increased. We demonstrated that highly purified LPS, a pure TLR4 ligand, increased neutrophil recruitment and glomerular injury after the passive transfer of MPO-ANCA, in a TLR4 dependent manner.

We used bone marrow chimeras to define the relative contributions of bone marrow cell TLR4 and intrinsic renal cell TLR4 to the disease process. We found that both bone marrow and resident kidney cell TLR4 were required for maximal neutrophil recruitment and renal injury. [58] These studies highlighted the importance of TLR4 (and potentially other TLRs) in driving effector responses in ANCA vasculitis.

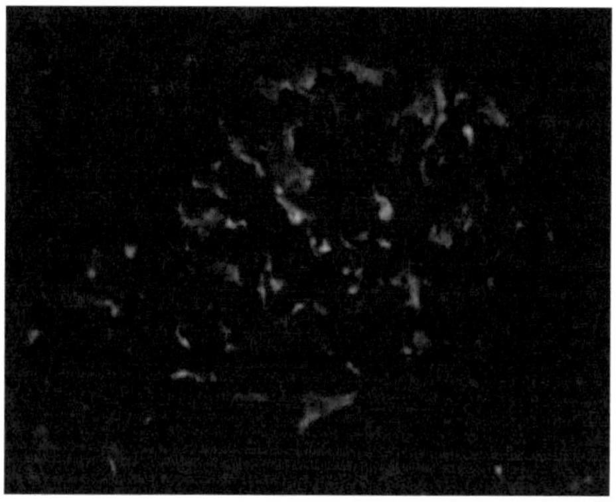

Figure 1. TLR9 staining in a kidney biopsy from a patient with PR3-ANCA vasculitis. While TLR9 staining was not detectable in normal kidney samples stained with a mAb directed against TLR9 and visualized under immunofluorescent light, TLR9 staining was readily detectable in patients with crescentic glomerulonephritis and PR3-ANCA vasculitis.

8.3. The role of complement in ANCA associated vasculitis

The complement system is recognized as one of the phylogenetically oldest components of human immune defence. This highly regulated system of proteins (together with their regulatory inhibitors) compromise an important part of host defence. In response to either innate or adaptive stimuli activation of the complement system results in a cascade of amplification and cleavage steps with the generation of anaphylatoxins (C5a and C3a) and a terminal attack complex capable of lying cells.[177] Three complement pathways are well described, namely, the classical pathway, the alternate pathway which is initiated by recognition of foreign surfaces and the mannose binding lectin pathway.[178] More recently a pathway which is initiated by coagulation and fibrinolytic proteins has been described.[179] In addition to its role in host defence, activation of the complement cascade can result in tissue injury and has been implicated in many forms of glomerulonephritis and kidney injury. Traditionally complement was not considered critical to the pathogenesis of AAV as renal injury was considered 'pauci immune' in nature and hence free from complement (and immune complex) deposition. Interestingly complement is frequently observed in renal and skin biopsies from patients with AAV,[180-182] while in vitro studies have demonstrated a role for complement in ANCA-neutrophil interactions.

From historical data we know that when neutrophils are activated by ANCA, the complement cascade is triggered and C3a is produced.[183] We also know that priming neutrophils with C5a enhances ANCA-neutrophil interactions,[184] an effect mediated by p38 mitogen-activated protein kinase, extracellular signal-regulated kinase and phosphoinositol 3-kinase.[185] Results from clinical studies have shown that serum and urine levels of C5a are elevated in patients with active disease strongly supporting the notion that the complement cascade is activated in active AAV.[186] Strong support for a pathogenic role for complement has also been provided from experimental studies. In an extensive set of experiments, the North Carolina group robustly demonstrated that complement depletion (achieved through the use of cobra venom serum) abrogated disease, an effect mediated through C5 and Factor B.[183] Factor B is critical for alternative pathway activation. Similarly inhibition of C5 using a mAb successfully attenuated experimental anti-MPO induced glomerulonephritis.[59] These studies detailing a pathogenic role for the alternative pathway in ANCA induced glomerulonephritis have helped improve our understanding of the disease. More recently a mAb directed against C5, Eculuzimab (also known as Soliris and manufactured by Alexion Pharmaceuticals) has been licensed for the treatment of several complement mediated diseases, including paroxysmal nocturnal hemoglobinuria. There is growing interest that C5 inhibition could be used for the treatment of glomerulonephritis and organ injury induced by AAV and this has formed the basis of a clinical trial currently underway in the United States.

8.4. Dendritic cells as antigen presenting cells and effector cells in AAV

Evidence from experimental models has supported a role for dendritic cells (DCs) in initiating and promoting immune responses in autoimmune diseases.[187] These specialised antigen presenting cells (APCs) recognise antigens through pattern-recognition receptors and co-ordinate the initiation and maintenance of the immune response.[188] Little is currently known about antigen presentation and the subsequent development of autoimmunity in AAV. It is likely that DCs are involved in two processes, firstly in the development of autoimmunity through interaction with dying neutrophils and also, acting locally, promoting kidney injury where their presence in renal biopsy samples positively correlates with injury.

A pathogenic role for DCs in human AAV was recognised several years ago. When immature DCs were isolated from GPA patients and cultured with PR3, markers of DC activation, CD80 and CD86 were increased. These antigen primed DCs were able to produce IFNγ, consistent with a Th1 phenotype.[189] In an experimental model of MPO induced ANCA vasculitis, we have shown that pulsing DCs with MPO is an effective means of inducing cellular and humoral autoimmunity directed against MPO. Furthermore, using our murine model of focal necrotising glomerulonephritis, these mice developed severe functional and histological renal injury (unpublished data). It is likely that up-regulation of DCs is (at least partially) TLR mediated and in AAV this could result from infection. After immunizing WT mice with a TLR2 or TLR9 ligand and MPO we found an increase in DC maturation (assessed as an increase in CD86 expression), compared to mice immunized with MPO alone.[82] In additional unpublished work, pilot studies have shown that stimulation of DCs with a TLR9 ligand and MPO results in increased CD40, CD80 and CD86 expression, compared to DCs stimulated with MPO alone, this is demonstrated below. These clinical and experimental studies implicate DCs in the loss of tolerance to MPO.

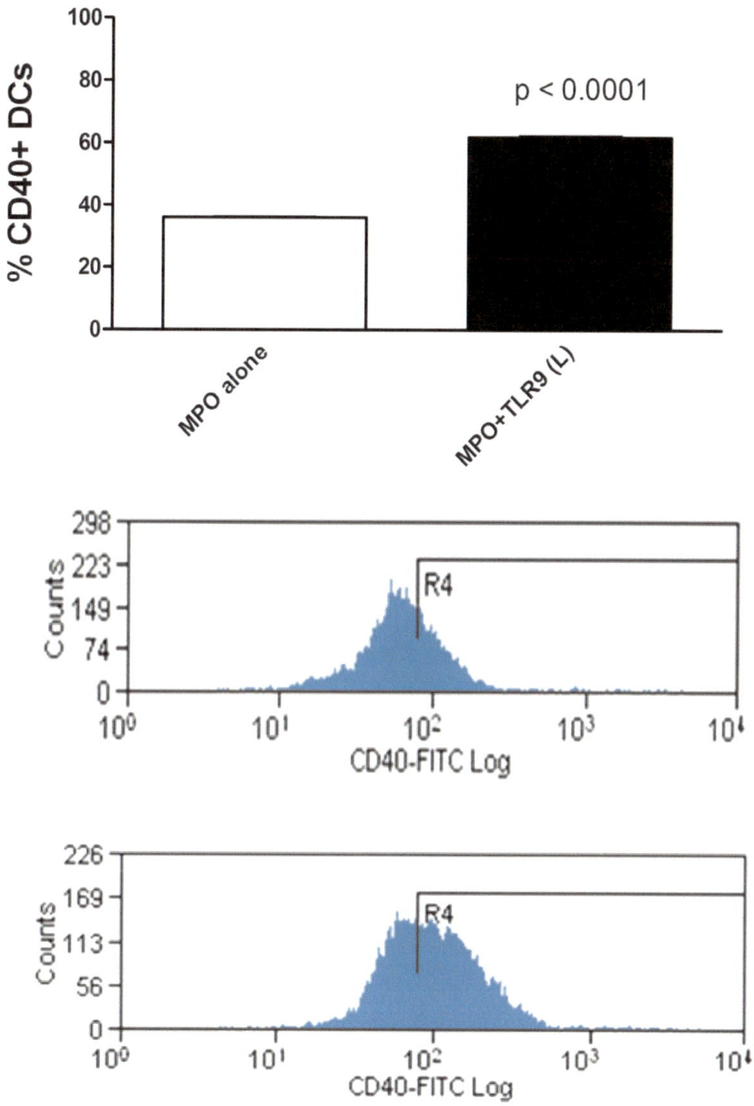

Figure 2. Dendritic cell (DC) activation after culturing DCs with MPO and a TLR9 ligand. After culturing DCs with MPO and control or a TLR 9 ligand, there was an increase on CD40+ DCs shown schematically in the top figure. In the middle figure we see representative CD40 expression from DCs treated with control and MPO, while the bottom figure shows the increase in CD40 expression after treatment with MPO and a TLR9 ligand.

A limitation of both the clinical and experimental studies is that these studies have largely focussed on myeloid DCs and not plasmacytoid DCs. In other diseases, including systemic lupus erythematosus, plasmacytoid DCs have been shown to be potent inducers of Type 1 IFNs and drive the development of autoimmunity.[190] In addition to their role in the development of autoimmune responses DCs represent a component of the characteristic inflammatory infiltrate see on renal biopsy samples from patients with AAV. Increased numbers of immature (CD209+) and mature (CD208+) DCs were found in renal biopsies from patients with AAV.[191] While these studies do not prove that DCs are pathogenic in renal vasculitis, their association with the inflammatory infiltrate suggests that they may be involved in the promotion of renal inflammation and injury.

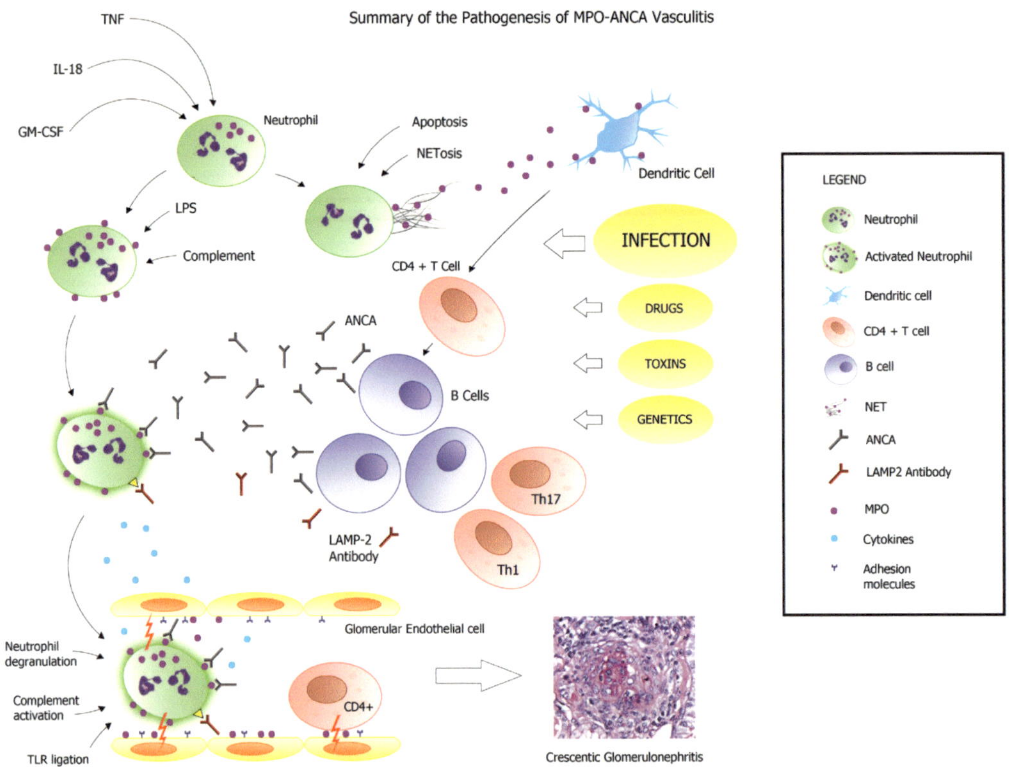

Figure 3. Summary of the Pathogenesis of MPO-ANCA Vasculitis. A summary of the events which contribute to the loss of tolerance to MPO, with the development of autoimmunity resulting in rapidly progressive crescentic glomerulonephritis

9. The role of resident kidney cells in ANCA associated renal vasculitis

Results from many of the studies discussed above have demonstrated that he kidney is not an 'innocent bystander' in the disease process. Rather the kidney provides an anatomic and physiological milieu which is well suited to recruit inflammatory cells. In our studies we have found that TLR ligation increased ANCA induced glomerular neutrophil recruitment and injury, which required contributions from both bone marrow and resident kidney cells.[58]

http://dx.doi.org/10.5772/54637

Our studies strongly supported a role for glomerular endothelial cells in this disease process and the role of the endothelium in promoting inflammation and injury is well known. It is likely that other glomerular cell types contribute to injury and immunofluorescent staining of kidney biopsies from patients with AAV has demonstrated that podocytes and tubulo-interstitial cells are major producers of IL-18, which is involved in neutrophil recruitment.[52] Similarly after staining human biopsies from AAV patients with crescentic glomerulonephritis the pathogenic isoform of the stress response protein kinase p38MAPK was detected in the podocyte, further implicating the role of this specialised cell in driving glomerular injury.[192] In addition to the glomerular injury observed in ANCA associated renal vasculitis tubular lesions, most notably peritubular inflammatory capillaritis, are common and are associated with a poor prognosis.[193] The interstitium is a prime target for inflammatory cells as many of the tubular epithelial cells express MHCII, TLRs and complement receptors, with which they can interact.[194] Furthermore peritubular capillaries display physiological characteristics similar to postcapillary venules which further increases the recruitment of inflammatory cells commonly observed in crescentic glomerulonephritis.[195-196] In conclusion it is apparent that the kidney harbours a particular environment which facilitates the recruitment of inflammatory cells and subsequent renal injury making it the key target for injury in AAV.

10. Conclusions

As new concepts of autoimmunity and cellular functions are elucidated in both innate and humoral immunity our scope of understanding of this complex disease entity continues to expand. Whilst an appreciation of the involvement of the adaptive immune dysfunction that contributes to AAV is well established new and varied innate immune system mechanisms of pathogenesis are emerging. Recent work investigating neutrophil functions and life cycle including the newly identified and described NETosis, along with imaging modalities allowing accurate characterisation of neutrophil trafficking and interactions with endothelial cells of the vessel wall provide us with a better understanding of the important role these cells have to play in this multifactorial disease process. The huge range of new biologic agents and advancing therapeutic technologies bring with them the possibilities of more effective, targeted, less toxic therapies for our patients.

Author details

Sharon Lee Ford[1,2], Stephen Roger Holdsworth[1,2] and Shaun Andrew Summers[1,2]

1 Centre for Inflammatory Diseases, Department of Medicine, Monash University, Australia

2 Department of Nephrology, Monash Medical Centre, Australia

References

[1] Fauci, A. S, Haynes, B, & Katz, P. The spectrum of vasculitis: clinical, pathologic, immunologic and therapeutic considerations. Ann Intern Med. (1978). Nov;89(5 Pt 1): 660-76.

[2] Hunder, G. G, Arend, W. P, Bloch, D. A, Calabrese, L. H, Fauci, A. S, Fries, J. F, Leavitt, R. Y, Lie, J. T, & Lightfoot, R. W. Jr., Masi AT, et al. The American College of Rheumatology 1990 criteria for the classification of vasculitis. Introduction. Arthritis Rheum. (1990). Aug;, 33(8), 1065-7.

[3] Jennette, J. C, Falk, R. J, Andrassy, K, Bacon, P. A, Churg, J, Gross, W. L, Hagen, E. C, Hoffman, G. S, Hunder, G. G, Kallenberg, C. G, et al. Nomenclature of systemic vasculitides. Proposal of an international consensus conference. Arthritis Rheum. (1994). Feb;, 37(2), 187-92.

[4] Jennette, J. C, & Falk, R. J. Small-vessel vasculitis. N Engl J Med. (1997). Nov 20;, 337(21), 1512-23.

[5] Kussmaul, A, & Maier, R. Ueber eine bisher nicht beschreibene eigenthümliche Arterienerkrankung (Periarteriitis nodosa), die mit Morbus Brightii und rapid fortschreitender allgemeiner Muskellähmung einhergeht. Dtsch Arch Klin Med. (1866). , 1, 484-518.

[6] Klinger, H. Grenzformen der Periarteriitis nodosa Frankf Z Pathol. (1931). , 42, 455-80.

[7] Godman, G. C, & Churg, J. Wegener's granulomatosis: pathology and review of the literature. AMA Arch Pathol. (1954). Dec;, 58(6), 533-53.

[8] Alarcón-segovia, D. Classification of the necrotizing vasculitides in man.. Clin Rheum Dis. (1980). , 6, 223-31.

[9] Booth, A. D, Almond, M. K, Burns, A, Ellis, P, Gaskin, G, Neild, G. H, Plaisance, M, Pusey, C. D, & Jayne, D. R. Pan-Thames Renal Research G. Outcome of ANCA-associated renal vasculitis: a 5-year retrospective study. Am J Kidney Dis. [Multicenter Study Review]. (2003). Apr;, 41(4), 776-84.

[10] Hoffman, G. S, Kerr, G. S, Leavitt, R. Y, Hallahan, C. W, Lebovics, R. S, Travis, W. D, Rottem, M, & Fauci, A. S. Wegener granulomatosis: an analysis of 158 patients. Ann Intern Med. (1992). Mar 15;, 116(6), 488-98.

[11] Davies, D. J, Moran, J. E, Niall, J. F, & Ryan, G. B. Segmental necrotising glomerulonephritis with antineutrophil antibody: possible arbovirus aetiology? Br Med J (Clin Res Ed). (1982). Aug Sep 4;285(6342):606., 28.

[12] Hall, J. B, Wadham, B. M, Wood, C. J, Ashton, V, & Adam, W. R. Vasculitis and glomerulonephritis: a subgroup with an antineutrophil cytoplasmic antibody. Aust N Z J Med. (1984). Jun;, 14(3), 277-8.

[13] Van Der Woude, F. J, Rasmussen, N, Lobatto, S, Wiik, A, Permin, H, Van Es, L. A, Van Der Giessen, M, Van Der Hem, G. K, & The, T. H. Autoantibodies against neutrophils and monocytes: tool for diagnosis and marker of disease activity in Wegener's granulomatosis. Lancet. (1985). Feb 23;, 1(8426), 425-9.

[14] Falk, R. J, Gross, W. L, Guillevin, L, Hoffman, G, Jayne, D. R, Jennette, J. C, Kallenberg, C. G, Luqmani, R, Mahr, A. D, Matteson, E. L, Merkel, P. A, Specks, U, & Watts, R. Granulomatosis with polyangiitis (Wegener's): an alternative name for Wegener's granulomatosis. J Am Soc Nephrol. [Editorial Historical Article]. (2011). Apr;, 22(4), 587-8.

[15] Falk, R. J, Gross, W. L, Guillevin, L, Hoffman, G. S, Jayne, D. R, Jennette, J. C, Kallenberg, C. G, Luqmani, R, Mahr, A. D, Matteson, E. L, Merkel, P. A, Specks, U, & Watts, R. A. Granulomatosis with polyangiitis (Wegener's): an alternative name for Wegener's granulomatosis. Arthritis Rheum. (2011). Apr;, 63(4), 863-4.

[16] Falk, R. J, Gross, W. L, Guillevin, L, Hoffman, G, Jayne, D. R, Jennette, J. C, Kallenberg, C. G, Luqmani, R, Mahr, A. D, Matteson, E. L, Merkel, P. A, Specks, U, & Watts, R. Granulomatosis with polyangiitis (Wegener's): an alternative name for Wegener's granulomatosis. Ann Rheum Dis. (2011). Apr;70(4):704.

[17] Goodnow, C. C. Multistep pathogenesis of autoimmune disease. Cell. (2007). Jul 13;, 130(1), 25-35.

[18] Kuligowski, M. P, Kwan, R. Y, Lo, C, Wong, C, James, W. G, Bourges, D, Ooi, J. D, Abeynaike, L. D, Hall, P, Kitching, A. R, & Hickey, M. J. Antimyeloperoxidase antibodies rapidly induce alpha-4-integrin-dependent glomerular neutrophil adhesion. Blood. (2009). Jun 18;, 113(25), 6485-94.

[19] Morgan, M. D, Harper, L, Williams, J, & Savage, C. Anti-neutrophil cytoplasm-associated glomerulonephritis. J Am Soc Nephrol. (2006). May;, 17(5), 1224-34.

[20] Neale, T. J, Tipping, P. G, Carson, S. D, & Holdsworth, S. R. Participation of cell-mediated immunity in deposition of fibrin in glomerulonephritis. Lancet. (1988). Aug 20;, 2(8608), 421-4.

[21] Cunningham, M. A, Huang, X. R, Dowling, J. P, Tipping, P. G, & Holdsworth, S. R. Prominence of cell-mediated immunity effectors in "pauci-immune" glomerulonephritis. J Am Soc Nephrol. (1999). Mar;, 10(3), 499-506.

[22] Holdsworth, S. R, Kitching, A. R, & Tipping, P. G. Th1 and Th2 T helper cell subsets affect patterns of injury and outcomes in glomerulonephritis. Kidney Int. (1999). Apr;, 55(4), 1198-216.

[23] Nogueira, E, Hamour, S, Sawant, D, Henderson, S, Mansfield, N, Chavele, K. M, Pusey, C. D, Salama, A. D, Serum, I. L, & Levels, I. L. and autoantigen-specific Th17 cells are elevated in patients with ANCA-associated vasculitis. Nephrol Dial Transplant. (2010). Jul;, 25(7), 2209-17.

[24] Gan, P. Y, Steinmetz, O. M, Tan, D. S, Sullivan, O, Ooi, K. M, Iwakura, J. D, Kitching, Y, Holdsworth, A. R, & Th, S. R. cells promote autoimmune anti-myeloperoxidase glomerulonephritis. J Am Soc Nephrol. (2010). Jun;, 21(6), 925-31.

[25] Knight, A, Sandin, S, & Askling, J. Risks and relative risks of Wegener's granulomatosis among close relatives of patients with the disease. Arthritis Rheum. (2008). Jan;, 58(1), 302-7.

[26] Willcocks, L. C, Lyons, P. A, Rees, A. J, & Smith, K. G. The contribution of genetic variation and infection to the pathogenesis of ANCA-associated systemic vasculitis. Arthritis Res Ther. (2010).

[27] Savage, C. O. Pathogenesis of anti-neutrophil cytoplasmic autoantibody (ANCA)-associated vasculitis. Clin Exp Immunol. (2011). May;164 Suppl , 1, 23-6.

[28] Lyons, P. A, Rayner, T. F, Trivedi, S, Holle, J. U, Watts, R. A, Jayne, D. R, Baslund, B, Brenchley, P, Bruchfeld, A, & Chaudhry, A. N. Cohen Tervaert JW, Deloukas P, Feighery C, Gross WL, Guillevin L, Gunnarsson I, Harper L, Hruskova Z, Little MA, Martorana D, Neumann T, Ohlsson S, Padmanabhan S, Pusey CD, Salama AD, Sanders JS, Savage CO, Segelmark M, Stegeman CA, Tesar V, Vaglio A, Wieczorek S, Wilde B, Zwerina J, Rees AJ, Clayton DG, Smith KG. Genetically distinct subsets within ANCA-associated vasculitis. N Engl J Med. (2012). Jul 19;, 367(3), 214-23.

[29] Ciavatta, D. J, Yang, J, Preston, G. A, Badhwar, A. K, Xiao, H, Hewins, P, Nester, C. M, & Pendergraft, W. F. rd, Magnuson TR, Jennette JC, Falk RJ. Epigenetic basis for aberrant upregulation of autoantigen genes in humans with ANCA vasculitis. J Clin Invest. (2010). Sep;, 120(9), 3209-19.

[30] Mahr, A. D, Neogi, T, & Merkel, P. A. Epidemiology of Wegener's granulomatosis: Lessons from descriptive studies and analyses of genetic and environmental risk determinants. Clin Exp Rheumatol. (2006). Mar-Apr;24(2 Suppl 41):S, 82-91.

[31] Hogan, S. L, Cooper, G. S, Savitz, D. A, Nylander-french, L. A, Parks, C. G, Chin, H, Jennette, C. E, Lionaki, S, Jennette, J. C, & Falk, R. J. Association of silica exposure with anti-neutrophil cytoplasmic autoantibody small-vessel vasculitis: a population-based, case-control study. Clin J Am Soc Nephrol. (2007). Mar;, 2(2), 290-9.

[32] Aikoh, T, Tomokuni, A, Matsukii, T, Hyodoh, F, Ueki, H, Otsuki, T, & Ueki, A. Activation-induced cell death in human peripheral blood lymphocytes after stimulation with silicate in vitro. Int J Oncol. (1998). Jun;, 12(6), 1355-9.

[33] de Lind van Wijngaarden RAvan Rijn L, Hagen EC, Watts RA, Gregorini G, Tervaert JW, Mahr AD, Niles JL, de Heer E, Bruijn JA, Bajema IM. Hypotheses on the etiology of antineutrophil cytoplasmic autoantibody associated vasculitis: the cause is hidden, but the result is known. Clin J Am Soc Nephrol. (2008). Jan;, 3(1), 237-52.

[34] Mathieson, P. W, Peat, D. S, Short, A, & Watts, R. A. Coexistent membranous nephropathy and ANCA-positive crescentic glomerulonephritis in association with penicillamine. Nephrol Dial Transplant. (1996). May;, 11(5), 863-6.

[35] Short, A. K, & Lockwood, C. M. Antigen specificity in hydralazine associated ANCA positive systemic vasculitis. QJM. (1995). Nov;, 88(11), 775-83.

[36] Tidman, M, Olander, R, Svalander, C, & Danielsson, D. Patients hospitalized because of small vessel vasculitides with renal involvement in the period 1975-95: organ involvement, anti-neutrophil cytoplasmic antibodies patterns, seasonal attack rates and fluctuation of annual frequencies. J Intern Med. (1998). Aug;, 244(2), 133-41.

[37] Stegeman, C. A, Tervaert, J. W, Sluiter, W. J, Manson, W. L, De Jong, P. E, & Kallenberg, C. G. Association of chronic nasal carriage of Staphylococcus aureus and higher relapse rates in Wegener granulomatosis. Ann Intern Med. (1994). Jan 1;, 120(1), 12-7.

[38] Pinching, A. J, Rees, A. J, Pussell, B. A, Lockwood, C. M, Mitchison, R. S, & Peters, D. K. Relapses in Wegener's granulomatosis: the role of infection. Br Med J. (1980). Sep 27;, 281(6244), 836-8.

[39] Capizzi, S. A, & Specks, U. Does infection play a role in the pathogenesis of pulmonary vasculitis? Semin Respir Infect. (2003). Mar;, 18(1), 17-22.

[40] Arimura, Y, Minoshima, S, Kamiya, Y, Tanaka, U, Nakabayashi, K, Kitamoto, K, Nagasawa, T, Sasaki, T, & Suzuki, K. Serum myeloperoxidase and serum cytokines in anti-myeloperoxidase antibody-associated glomerulonephritis. Clin Nephrol. (1993). Nov;, 40(5), 256-64.

[41] Stegeman, C. A, Tervaert, J. W, De Jong, P. E, & Kallenberg, C. G. Trimethoprim-sulfamethoxazole (co-trimoxazole) for the prevention of relapses of Wegener's granulomatosis. Dutch Co-Trimoxazole Wegener Study Group. N Engl J Med. (1996). Jul 4;, 335(1), 16-20.

[42] Chirinos, J. A, Corrales-medina, V. F, Garcia, S, Lichtstein, D. M, Bisno, A. L, & Chakko, S. Endocarditis associated with antineutrophil cytoplasmic antibodies: a case report and review of the literature. Clin Rheumatol. (2007). Apr;, 26(4), 590-5.

[43] Hellmich, B, Ehren, M, Lindstaedt, M, Meyer, M, Pfohl, M, & Schatz, H. Anti-MPO-ANCA-positive microscopic polyangiitis following subacute bacterial endocarditis. Clin Rheumatol. (2001). , 20(6), 441-3.

[44] Oldstone, M. B. Molecular mimicry, microbial infection, and autoimmune disease: evolution of the concept. Curr Top Microbiol Immunol. (2005). , 296, 1-17.

[45] Kain, R, Exner, M, Brandes, R, Ziebermayr, R, Cunningham, D, Alderson, C. A, Davidovits, A, Raab, I, Jahn, R, Ashour, O, Spitzauer, S, Sunder-plassmann, G, Fukuda, M, Klemm, P, Rees, A. J, & Kerjaschki, D. Molecular mimicry in pauci-immune focal necrotizing glomerulonephritis. Nat Med. (2008). Oct;, 14(10), 1088-96.

[46] Pendergraft, W. F. rd, Preston GA, Shah RR, Tropsha A, Carter CW, Jr., Jennette JC, Falk RJ. Autoimmunity is triggered by cPR-3(105-201), a protein complementary to human autoantigen proteinase-3. Nat Med. (2004). Jan;, 10(1), 72-9.

[47] Jayne, D. R, Gaskin, G, Rasmussen, N, Abramowicz, D, Ferrario, F, Guillevin, L, Mirapeix, E, Savage, C. O, Sinico, R. A, Stegeman, C. A, Westman, K. W, & Van Der

Woude, F. J. de Lind van Wijngaarden RA, Pusey CD. Randomized trial of plasma exchange or high-dosage methylprednisolone as adjunctive therapy for severe renal vasculitis. J Am Soc Nephrol. (2007). Jul;, 18(7), 2180-8.

[48] Jones, R. B, Tervaert, J. W, Hauser, T, Luqmani, R, Morgan, M. D, Peh, C. A, Savage, C. O, Segelmark, M, Tesar, V, Van Paassen, P, Walsh, D, Walsh, M, Westman, K, & Jayne, D. R. Rituximab versus cyclophosphamide in ANCA-associated renal vasculitis. N Engl J Med. (2010). Jul 15;, 363(3), 211-20.

[49] Stone, J. H, Merkel, P. A, Spiera, R, Seo, P, Langford, C. A, Hoffman, G. S, & Kallenberg, C. G. St Clair EW, Turkiewicz A, Tchao NK, Webber L, Ding L, Sejismundo LP, Mieras K, Weitzenkamp D, Ikle D, Seyfert-Margolis V, Mueller M, Brunetta P, Allen NB, Fervenza FC, Geetha D, Keogh KA, Kissin EY, Monach PA, Peikert T, Stegeman C, Ytterberg SR, Specks U. Rituximab versus cyclophosphamide for ANCA-associated vasculitis. N Engl J Med. (2010). Jul 15;, 363(3), 221-32.

[50] Harper, L, Cockwell, P, Adu, D, & Savage, C. O. Neutrophil priming and apoptosis in anti-neutrophil cytoplasmic autoantibody-associated vasculitis. Kidney Int. (2001). May;, 59(5), 1729-38.

[51] Cockwell, P, Brooks, C. J, Adu, D, & Savage, C. O. Interleukin-8: A pathogenetic role in antineutrophil cytoplasmic autoantibody-associated glomerulonephritis. Kidney Int. (1999). Mar;, 55(3), 852-63.

[52] Hewins, P, Morgan, M. D, Holden, N, Neil, D, Williams, J. M, Savage, C. O, & Harper, L. IL-18 is upregulated in the kidney and primes neutrophil responsiveness in ANCA-associated vasculitis. Kidney Int. (2006). Feb;, 69(3), 605-15.

[53] Kettritz, R, Falk, R. J, Jennette, J. C, & Gaido, M. L. Neutrophil superoxide release is required for spontaneous and FMLP-mediated but not for TNF alpha-mediated apoptosis. J Am Soc Nephrol. (1997). Jul;, 8(7), 1091-100.

[54] Harper, L, Ren, Y, Savill, J, Adu, D, & Savage, C. O. Antineutrophil cytoplasmic antibodies induce reactive oxygen-dependent dysregulation of primed neutrophil apoptosis and clearance by macrophages. Am J Pathol. (2000). Jul;, 157(1), 211-20.

[55] Xiao, H, Heeringa, P, Hu, P, Liu, Z, Zhao, M, Aratani, Y, Maeda, N, Falk, R. J, & Jennette, J. C. Antineutrophil cytoplasmic autoantibodies specific for myeloperoxidase cause glomerulonephritis and vasculitis in mice. J Clin Invest. (2002). Oct;, 110(7), 955-63.

[56] Xiao, H, Heeringa, P, Liu, Z, Huugen, D, Hu, P, Maeda, N, Falk, R. J, & Jennette, J. C. The role of neutrophils in the induction of glomerulonephritis by anti-myeloperoxidase antibodies. Am J Pathol. (2005). Jul;, 167(1), 39-45.

[57] Huugen, D, Xiao, H, Van Esch, A, Falk, R. J, Peutz-kootstra, C. J, Buurman, W. A, Tervaert, J. W, Jennette, J. C, & Heeringa, P. Aggravation of anti-myeloperoxidase antibody-induced glomerulonephritis by bacterial lipopolysaccharide: role of tumor necrosis factor-alpha. Am J Pathol. (2005). Jul;, 167(1), 47-58.

[58] Summers, S. A, Van Der Veen, B. S, Sullivan, O, Gan, K. M, Ooi, P. Y, Heeringa, J. D, Satchell, P, Mathieson, S. C, Saleem, P. W, Visvanathan, M. A, Holdsworth, K, & Kitching, S. R. AR. Intrinsic renal cell and leukocyte-derived TLR4 aggravate experimental anti-MPO glomerulonephritis. Kidney Int. (2010). Dec;, 78(12), 1263-74.

[59] Huugen, D, Van Esch, A, Xiao, H, Peutz-kootstra, C. J, Buurman, W. A, Tervaert, J. W, Jennette, J. C, & Heeringa, P. Inhibition of complement factor C5 protects against anti-myeloperoxidase antibody-mediated glomerulonephritis in mice. Kidney Int. (2007). Apr;, 71(7), 646-54.

[60] Little, M. A, Smyth, C. L, Yadav, R, Ambrose, L, Cook, H. T, Nourshargh, S, & Pusey, C. D. Antineutrophil cytoplasm antibodies directed against myeloperoxidase augment leukocyte-microvascular interactions in vivo. Blood. (2005). Sep 15;, 106(6), 2050-8.

[61] Little, M. A, Al-ani, B, Ren, S, Al-nuaimi, H, & Leite, M. Jr., Alpers CE, Savage CO, Duffield JS. Anti-proteinase 3 anti-neutrophil cytoplasm autoantibodies recapitulate systemic vasculitis in mice with a humanized immune system. PLoS One. (2012). e28626.

[62] Kain, R, Tadema, H, Mckinney, E. F, Benharkou, A, Brandes, R, Peschel, A, Hubert, V, Feenstra, T, Sengolge, G, Stegeman, C, Heeringa, P, Lyons, P. A, Smith, K. G, Kallenberg, C, & Rees, A. J. High prevalence of autoantibodies to hLAMP-2 in anti-neutrophil cytoplasmic antibody-associated vasculitis. J Am Soc Nephrol. (2012). Mar;, 23(3), 556-66.

[63] Roth, A. J, Brown, M. C, Smith, R. N, Badhwar, A. K, Parente, O, Chung, H, Bunch, D. O, Mcgregor, J. G, Hogan, S. L, Hu, Y, Yang, J. J, Berg, E. A, Niles, J, Jennette, J. C, Preston, G. A, & Falk, R. J. Anti-LAMP-2 antibodies are not prevalent in patients with antineutrophil cytoplasmic autoantibody glomerulonephritis. J Am Soc Nephrol. (2012). Mar;, 23(3), 545-55.

[64] Lepse, N, Abdulahad, W. H, Kallenberg, C. G, & Heeringa, P. Immune regulatory mechanisms in ANCA-associated vasculitides. Autoimmun Rev. (2011). Dec;, 11(2), 77-83.

[65] Schneeweis, C, Rafalowicz, M, Feist, E, Buttgereit, F, Rudolph, P. E, Burmester, G. R, & Egerer, K. Increased levels of BLyS and sVCAM-1 in anti-neutrophil cytoplasmatic antibody (ANCA)-associated vasculitides (AAV). Clin Exp Rheumatol. (2010). Jan-Feb; 28(1 Suppl 57):62-6.

[66] Stohl, W, & Hilbert, D. M. The discovery and development of belimumab: the anti BLyS-lupus connection. Nat Biotechnol. (2012). Jan;, 30(1), 69-77.

[67] Steinmetz, O. M, Velden, J, Kneissler, U, Marx, M, Klein, A, Helmchen, U, Stahl, R. A, & Panzer, U. Analysis and classification of B-cell infiltrates in lupus and ANCA-associated nephritis. Kidney Int. (2008). Aug;, 74(4), 448-57.

[68] Blair, P. A, Norena, L. Y, Flores-borja, F, Rawlings, D. J, Isenberg, D. A, Ehrenstein, M. R, Mauri, C, Hi, C. D19(+)C. D, & Hi, C. D. B cells exhibit regulatory capacity in healthy

individuals but are functionally impaired in systemic Lupus Erythematosus patients. Immunity. (2010). Jan 29;, 32(1), 129-40.

[69] Khan, A, Lawson, C. A, Quinn, M. A, Isdale, A. H, & Green, M. J. Successful Treatment of ANCA-Negative Wegener's Granulomatosis with Rituximab. Int J Rheumatol. (2010).

[70] Brouwer, E, Huitema, M. G, Klok, P. A, De Weerd, H, Tervaert, J. W, Weening, J. J, & Kallenberg, C. G. Antimyeloperoxidase-associated proliferative glomerulonephritis: an animal model. J Exp Med. (1993). Apr 1;, 177(4), 905-14.

[71] Kessenbrock, K, Krumbholz, M, Schonermarck, U, Back, W, Gross, W. L, Werb, Z, Grone, H. J, Brinkmann, V, & Jenne, D. E. Netting neutrophils in autoimmune small-vessel vasculitis. Nat Med. (2009). Jun;, 15(6), 623-5.

[72] Ruth, A. J, Kitching, A. R, Kwan, R. Y, Odobasic, D, Ooi, J. D, Timoshanko, J. R, Hickey, M. J, & Holdsworth, S. R. Anti-neutrophil cytoplasmic antibodies and effector CD4+ cells play nonredundant roles in anti-myeloperoxidase crescentic glomerulonephritis. J Am Soc Nephrol. (2006). Jul;, 17(7), 1940-9.

[73] Brouwer, E, Tervaert, J. W, Horst, G, Huitema, M. G, Van Der Giessen, M, Limburg, P. C, & Kallenberg, C. G. Predominance of IgG1 and IgG4 subclasses of anti-neutrophil cytoplasmic autoantibodies (ANCA) in patients with Wegener's granulomatosis and clinically related disorders. Clin Exp Immunol. (1991). Mar;, 83(3), 379-86.

[74] Griffith, M. E, Coulthart, A, & Pusey, C. D. T cell responses to myeloperoxidase (MPO) and proteinase 3 (PR3) in patients with systemic vasculitis. Clin Exp Immunol. (1996). Feb;, 103(2), 253-8.

[75] Marinaki, S, Kalsch, A. I, Grimminger, P, Breedijk, A, Birck, R, Schmitt, W. H, Weiss, C, Van Der Woude, F. J, & Yard, B. A. Persistent T-cell activation and clinical correlations in patients with ANCA-associated systemic vasculitis. Nephrol Dial Transplant. (2006). Jul;, 21(7), 1825-32.

[76] Popa, E. R, Stegeman, C. A, Bos, N. A, Kallenberg, C. G, Tervaert, J. W, & Differential, B. and T-cell activation in Wegener's granulomatosis. J Allergy Clin Immunol. (1999). May;103(5 Pt 1):885-94.

[77] Schmitt, W. H, Hagen, E. C, Neumann, I, Nowack, R, Flores-suarez, L. F, & Van Der Woude, F. J. Treatment of refractory Wegener's granulomatosis with antithymocyte globulin (ATG): an open study in 15 patients. Kidney Int. (2004). Apr;, 65(4), 1440-8.

[78] Yoshida, M, Iwahori, T, Nakabayashi, I, Akashi, M, Watanabe, T, & Yoshikawa, N. In vitro production of myeloperoxidase anti-neutrophil cytoplasmic antibody and establishment of Th1-type T cell lines from peripheral blood lymphocytes of patients. Clin Exp Rheumatol. (2005). Mar-Apr;, 23(2), 227-30.

[79] Park, H, Li, Z, Yang, X. O, Chang, S. H, Nurieva, R, Wang, Y. H, Wang, Y, Hood, L, Zhu, Z, Tian, Q, & Dong, C. A distinct lineage of CD4 T cells regulates tissue inflammation by producing interleukin 17. Nat Immunol. (2005). Nov;, 6(11), 1133-41.

[80] Abdulahad, W. H, Stegeman, C. A, Limburg, P. C, & Kallenberg, C. G. Skewed distribution of Th17 lymphocytes in patients with Wegener's granulomatosis in remission. Arthritis Rheum. (2008). Jul;, 58(7), 2196-205.

[81] Velden, J, Paust, H. J, Hoxha, E, Turner, J. E, Steinmetz, O. M, Wolf, G, Jabs, W. J, Ozcan, F, Beige, J, Heering, P. J, Schroder, S, Kneissler, U, Disteldorf, E, Mittrucker, H. W, Stahl, R. A, Helmchen, U, Panzer, U, & Renal, I. L. expression in human ANCA-associated glomerulonephritis. Am J Physiol Renal Physiol. (2012). Jun 15;302(12):F, 1663-73.

[82] Summers, S. A, Steinmetz, O. M, Gan, P. Y, Ooi, J. D, Odobasic, D, Kitching, A. R, & Holdsworth, S. R. Toll-like receptor 2 induces Th17 myeloperoxidase autoimmunity while Toll-like receptor 9 drives Th1 autoimmunity in murine vasculitis. Arthritis Rheum. (2011). Apr;, 63(4), 1124-35.

[83] Ooi, J. D, Chang, J, Hickey, M. J, Borza, D. B, Fugger, L, Holdsworth, S. R, & Kitching, A. R. The immunodominant myeloperoxidase T-cell epitope induces local cell-mediated injury in antimyeloperoxidase glomerulonephritis. Proc Natl Acad Sci U S A. (2012). Sep 5.

[84] Mosmann, T. R, Coffman, R. L, & Cells, T. H1 a. n. d T. H. different patterns of lymphokine secretion lead to different functional properties. Annu Rev Immunol. (1989)., 7, 145-73.

[85] Yao, Z, Fanslow, W. C, Seldin, M. F, Rousseau, A. M, Painter, S. L, Comeau, M. R, Cohen, J. I, & Spriggs, M. K. Herpesvirus Saimiri encodes a new cytokine, IL-17, which binds to a novel cytokine receptor. Immunity. (1995). Dec;, 3(6), 811-21.

[86] Harrington, L. E, Hatton, R. D, Mangan, P. R, Turner, H, Murphy, T. L, Murphy, K. M, Weaver, C. T, & Interleukin 17-producing, C. D. effector T cells develop via a lineage distinct from the T helper type 1 and 2 lineages. Nat Immunol. (2005). Nov;, 6(11), 1123-32.

[87] Yang, J. Q, Singh, A. K, Wilson, M. T, Satoh, M, Stanic, A. K, Park, J. J, Hong, S, Gadola, S. D, Mizutani, A, Kakumanu, S. R, Reeves, W. H, Cerundolo, V, Joyce, S, Van Kaer, L, & Singh, R. R. Immunoregulatory role of CD1d in the hydrocarbon oil-induced model of lupus nephritis. J Immunol. (2003). Aug 15;, 171(4), 2142-53.

[88] Ivanov, I. I, Mckenzie, B. S, Zhou, L, Tadokoro, C. E, Lepelley, A, Lafaille, J. J, Cua, D. J, & Littman, D. R. The orphan nuclear receptor RORgammat directs the differentiation program of proinflammatory IL-17+ T helper cells. Cell. (2006). Sep 22;, 126(6), 1121-33.

[89] Langrish, C. L, Chen, Y, Blumenschein, W. M, Mattson, J, Basham, B, Sedgwick, J. D, Mcclanahan, T, Kastelein, R. A, Cua, D. J, Drives, I. L, & Pathogenic, a. T cell population that induces autoimmune inflammation. J Exp Med. (2005). Jan 17;, 201(2), 233-40.

[90] Mangan, P. R, Harrington, L. E, Quinn, O, Helms, D. B, Bullard, W. S, Elson, D. C, Hatton, C. O, Wahl, R. D, Schoeb, S. M, & Weaver, T. R. CT. Transforming growth factor-beta induces development of the T(H)17 lineage. Nature. (2006). May 11;, 441(7090), 231-4.

[91] Veldhoen, M, Hocking, R. J, Atkins, C. J, Locksley, R. M, & Stockinger, B. TGFbeta in the context of an inflammatory cytokine milieu supports de novo differentiation of IL-17-producing T cells. Immunity. (2006). Feb;, 24(2), 179-89.

[92] Bettelli, E, Carrier, Y, Gao, W, Korn, T, Strom, T. B, Oukka, M, Weiner, H. L, & Kuchroo, V. K. Reciprocal developmental pathways for the generation of pathogenic effector TH17 and regulatory T cells. Nature. (2006). May 11;, 441(7090), 235-8.

[93] Bettelli, E, Korn, T, Oukka, M, & Kuchroo, V. K. Induction and effector functions of T(H)17 cells. Nature. (2008). Jun 19;, 453(7198), 1051-7.

[94] Korn, T, Bettelli, E, Gao, W, Awasthi, A, Jager, A, Strom, T. B, Oukka, M, & Kuchroo, V. K. IL-21 initiates an alternative pathway to induce proinflammatory T(H)17 cells. Nature. (2007). Jul 26;, 448(7152), 484-7.

[95] Nurieva, R, Yang, X. O, Martinez, G, Zhang, Y, Panopoulos, A. D, Ma, L, Schluns, K, Tian, Q, Watowich, S. S, Jetten, A. M, & Dong, C. Essential autocrine regulation by IL-21 in the generation of inflammatory T cells. Nature. (2007). Jul 26;, 448(7152), 480-3.

[96] Zhou, L, Ivanov, I. I, Spolski, R, Min, R, Shenderov, K, Egawa, T, Levy, D. E, Leonard, W. J, Littman, D. R, & Programs, I. L. T(H)-17 cell differentiation by promoting sequential engagement of the IL-21 and IL-23 pathways. Nat Immunol. (2007). Sep;, 8(9), 967-74.

[97] Becher, B, Durell, B. G, & Noelle, R. J. Experimental autoimmune encephalitis and inflammation in the absence of interleukin-12. J Clin Invest. (2002). Aug;, 110(4), 493-7.

[98] Gran, B, Zhang, G. X, Yu, S, Li, J, Chen, X. H, Ventura, E. S, Kamoun, M, & Rostami, A. IL-12mice are susceptible to experimental autoimmune encephalomyelitis: evidence for redundancy in the IL-12 system in the induction of central nervous system autoimmune demyelination. J Immunol. (2002). Dec 15;169(12):7104-10., 35.

[99] Cua, D. J, Sherlock, J, Chen, Y, Murphy, C. A, Joyce, B, Seymour, B, Lucian, L, To, W, Kwan, S, Churakova, T, Zurawski, S, Wiekowski, M, Lira, S. A, Gorman, D, Kastelein, R. A, & Sedgwick, J. D. Interleukin-23 rather than interleukin-12 is the critical cytokine for autoimmune inflammation of the brain. Nature. (2003). Feb 13;, 421(6924), 744-8.

[100] Komiyama, Y, Nakae, S, Matsuki, T, Nambu, A, Ishigame, H, Kakuta, S, Sudo, K, & Iwakura, Y. IL-17 plays an important role in the development of experimental autoimmune encephalomyelitis. J Immunol. (2006). Jul 1;, 177(1), 566-73.

[101] Lock, C. B, & Heller, R. A. Gene microarray analysis of multiple sclerosis lesions. Trends Mol Med. (2003). Dec;, 9(12), 535-41.

[102] Chabaud, M, Durand, J. M, Buchs, N, Fossiez, F, Page, G, Frappart, L, & Miossec, P. Human interleukin-17: A T cell-derived proinflammatory cytokine produced by the rheumatoid synovium. Arthritis Rheum. (1999). May;, 42(5), 963-70.

[103] Murphy, C. A, Langrish, C. L, Chen, Y, Blumenschein, W, Mcclanahan, T, Kastelein, R. A, Sedgwick, J. D, & Cua, D. J. Divergent pro- and antiinflammatory roles for IL-23 and IL-12 in joint autoimmune inflammation. J Exp Med. (2003). Dec 15;, 198(12), 1951-7.

[104] Nakae, S, Nambu, A, Sudo, K, & Iwakura, Y. Suppression of immune induction of collagen-induced arthritis in IL-17-deficient mice. J Immunol. (2003). Dec 1;, 171(11), 6173-7.

[105] Elson, C. O, Cong, Y, Weaver, C. T, Schoeb, T. R, Mcclanahan, T. K, Fick, R. B, & Kastelein, R. A. Monoclonal anti-interleukin 23 reverses active colitis in a T cell-mediated model in mice. Gastroenterology. (2007). Jun;, 132(7), 2359-70.

[106] Duerr, R. H, Taylor, K. D, Brant, S. R, Rioux, J. D, Silverberg, M. S, Daly, M. J, Steinhart, A. H, Abraham, C, Regueiro, M, Griffiths, A, Dassopoulos, T, Bitton, A, Yang, H, Targan, S, Datta, L. W, Kistner, E. O, Schumm, L. P, Lee, A. T, Gregersen, P. K, Barmada, M. M, Rotter, J. I, Nicolae, D. L, & Cho, J. H. A genome-wide association study identifies IL23R as an inflammatory bowel disease gene. Science. (2006). Dec 1;, 314(5804), 1461-3.

[107] Krueger, G. G, Langley, R. G, Leonardi, C, Yeilding, N, Guzzo, C, Wang, Y, Dooley, L. T, & Lebwohl, M. A human interleukin-12/23 monoclonal antibody for the treatment of psoriasis. N Engl J Med. (2007). Feb 8;, 356(6), 580-92.

[108] Wilson, N. J, Boniface, K, Chan, J. R, Mckenzie, B. S, Blumenschein, W. M, Mattson, J. D, Basham, B, Smith, K, Chen, T, Morel, F, Lecron, J. C, Kastelein, R. A, Cua, D. J, Mcclanahan, T. K, & Bowman, E. P. de Waal Malefyt R. Development, cytokine profile and function of human interleukin 17-producing helper T cells. Nat Immunol. (2007). Sep;, 8(9), 950-7.

[109] Ooi, J. D, Phoon, R. K, Holdsworth, S. R, Kitching, A. R, & Not, I. L. IL-12, directs autoimmunity to the Goodpasture antigen. J Am Soc Nephrol. (2009). May;, 20(5), 980-9.

[110] Paust, H. J, Turner, J. E, Steinmetz, O. M, Peters, A, Heymann, F, Holscher, C, Wolf, G, Kurts, C, Mittrucker, H. W, Stahl, R. A, Panzer, U, & The, I. L. Th17 axis contributes to renal injury in experimental glomerulonephritis. J Am Soc Nephrol. (2009). May;, 20(5), 969-79.

[111] Steinmetz, O. M, Summers, S. A, Gan, P. Y, Semple, T, Holdsworth, S. R, & Kitching, A. R. The Th17-Defining Transcription Factor ROR{gamma}t Promotes Glomerulonephritis. J Am Soc Nephrol. (2011). Mar;, 22(3), 472-83.

[112] Summers, S. A, Steinmetz, O. M, Li, M, Kausman, J. Y, Semple, T, Edgtton, K. L, Borza, D. B, Braley, H, Holdsworth, S. R, & Kitching, A. R. Th1 and Th17 cells induce proliferative glomerulonephritis. J Am Soc Nephrol. (2009). Dec;, 20(12), 2518-24.

[113] Kitching, A. R, & Holdsworth, S. R. The emergence of TH17 cells as effectors of renal injury. J Am Soc Nephrol. (2011). Feb;, 22(2), 235-8.

[114] Turner, J. E, Paust, H. J, Steinmetz, O. M, & Panzer, U. The Th17 immune response in renal inflammation. Kidney Int. (2010). Jun;, 77(12), 1070-5.

[115] Etanercept plus standard therapy for Wegener's granulomatosisN Engl J Med. (2005). Jan 27;, 352(4), 351-61.

[116] Abdulahad, W. H, Kallenberg, C. G, Limburg, P. C, Stegeman, C. A, & Urinary, C. D. effector memory T cells reflect renal disease activity in antineutrophil cytoplasmic antibody-associated vasculitis. Arthritis Rheum. (2009). Sep;, 60(9), 2830-8.

[117] De Menthon, M, Lambert, M, Guiard, E, Tognarelli, S, Bienvenu, B, Karras, A, Guillevin, L, & Caillat-zucman, S. Excessive interleukin-15 transpresentation endows NKG2D +CD4+ T cells with innate-like capacity to lyse vascular endothelium in granulomatosis with polyangiitis (Wegener's). Arthritis Rheum. (2011). Jul;, 63(7), 2116-26.

[118] Mckinney, E. F, Lyons, P. A, Carr, E. J, Hollis, J. L, Jayne, D. R, Willcocks, L. C, Koukoulaki, M, Brazma, A, Jovanovic, V, Kemeny, D. M, Pollard, A. J, Macary, P. A, Chaudhry, A. N, & Smith, K. G. A CD8+ T cell transcription signature predicts prognosis in autoimmune disease. Nat Med. (2010). May;p following 91., 16(5), 586-91.

[119] Salama, A. D, Chaudhry, A. N, Holthaus, K. A, Mosley, K, Kalluri, R, Sayegh, M. H, Lechler, R. I, Pusey, C. D, & Lightstone, L. Regulation by CD25+ lymphocytes of autoantigen-specific T-cell responses in Goodpasture's (anti-GBM) disease. Kidney Int. (2003). Nov;, 64(5), 1685-94.

[120] Abdulahad, W. H, Stegeman, C. A, & Van Der Geld, Y. M. Doornbos-van der Meer B, Limburg PC, Kallenberg CG. Functional defect of circulating regulatory CD4+ T cells in patients with Wegener's granulomatosis in remission. Arthritis Rheum. (2007). Jun;, 56(6), 2080-91.

[121] Chavele, K. M, Shukla, D, Keteepe-arachi, T, Seidel, J. A, Fuchs, D, Pusey, C. D, & Salama, A. D. Regulation of myeloperoxidase-specific T cell responses during disease remission in antineutrophil cytoplasmic antibody-associated vasculitis: the role of Treg cells and tryptophan degradation. Arthritis Rheum. (2010). May;, 62(5), 1539-48.

[122] Gilligan, H. M, Bredy, B, Brady, H. R, Hebert, M. J, Slayter, H. S, Xu, Y, Rauch, J, Shia, M. A, Koh, J. S, & Levine, J. S. Antineutrophil cytoplasmic autoantibodies interact with primary granule constituents on the surface of apoptotic neutrophils in the absence of neutrophil priming. J Exp Med. (1996). Dec 1;, 184(6), 2231-41.

[123] Yang, J. J, Tuttle, R. H, Hogan, S. L, Taylor, J. G, Phillips, B. D, Falk, R. J, & Jennette, J. C. Target antigens for anti-neutrophil cytoplasmic autoantibodies (ANCA) are on the surface of primed and apoptotic but not unstimulated neutrophils. Clin Exp Immunol. (2000). Jul;, 121(1), 165-72.

[124] Brinkmann, V, Reichard, U, Goosmann, C, Fauler, B, Uhlemann, Y, Weiss, D. S, Weinrauch, Y, & Zychlinsky, A. Neutrophil extracellular traps kill bacteria. Science. (2004). Mar 5;, 303(5663), 1532-5.

[125] Lande, R, Ganguly, D, Facchinetti, V, Frasca, L, Conrad, C, Gregorio, J, Meller, S, Chamilos, G, Sebasigari, R, Riccieri, V, Bassett, R, Amuro, H, Fukuhara, S, Ito, T, Liu, Y. J, & Gilliet, M. Neutrophils activate plasmacytoid dendritic cells by releasing self-

DNA-peptide complexes in systemic lupus erythematosus. Sci Transl Med. (2011). Mar 9;3(73):73ra19.

[126] Garcia-romo, G. S, Caielli, S, Vega, B, Connolly, J, Allantaz, F, Xu, Z, Punaro, M, Baisch, J, Guiducci, C, Coffman, R. L, Barrat, F. J, Banchereau, J, & Pascual, V. Netting neutrophils are major inducers of type I IFN production in pediatric systemic lupus erythematosus. Sci Transl Med. (2011). Mar 9;3(73):73ra20.

[127] Villanueva, E, Yalavarthi, S, Berthier, C. C, Hodgin, J. B, Khandpur, R, Lin, A. M, Rubin, C. J, Zhao, W, Olsen, S. H, Klinker, M, Shealy, D, Denny, M. F, Plumas, J, Chaperot, L, Kretzler, M, Bruce, A. T, & Kaplan, M. J. Netting neutrophils induce endothelial damage, infiltrate tissues, and expose immunostimulatory molecules in systemic lupus erythematosus. J Immunol. (2011). Jul 1;, 187(1), 538-52.

[128] Sangaletti, S, Tripodo, C, Chiodoni, C, Guarnotta, C, Cappetti, B, Casalini, P, Piconese, S, Parenza, M, Guiducci, C, Vitali, C, & Colombo, M. P. Neutrophil extracellular traps mediate transfer of cytoplasmic neutrophil antigens to myeloid dendritic cells towards ANCA induction and associated autoimmunity. Blood. (2012). Aug 29.

[129] Mulder, A. H, Heeringa, P, Brouwer, E, Limburg, P. C, & Kallenberg, C. G. Activation of granulocytes by anti-neutrophil cytoplasmic antibodies (ANCA): a Fc gamma RII-dependent process. Clin Exp Immunol. (1994). Nov;, 98(2), 270-8.

[130] Little, M. A, Bhangal, G, Smyth, C. L, Nakada, M. T, Cook, H. T, Nourshargh, S, & Pusey, C. D. Therapeutic effect of anti-TNF-alpha antibodies in an experimental model of anti-neutrophil cytoplasm antibody-associated systemic vasculitis. J Am Soc Nephrol. (2006). Jan;, 17(1), 160-9.

[131] Lamprecht, P, Voswinkel, J, Lilienthal, T, Nolle, B, Heller, M, Gross, W. L, & Gause, A. Effectiveness of TNF-alpha blockade with infliximab in refractory Wegener's granulomatosis. Rheumatology (Oxford). (2002). Nov;, 41(11), 1303-7.

[132] Bartolucci, P, Ramanoelina, J, Cohen, P, Mahr, A, & Godmer, P. Le Hello C, Guillevin L. Efficacy of the anti-TNF-alpha antibody infliximab against refractory systemic vasculitides: an open pilot study on 10 patients. Rheumatology (Oxford). (2002). Oct;, 41(10), 1126-32.

[133] Morgan, M. D, Drayson, M. T, Savage, C. O, & Harper, L. Addition of infliximab to standard therapy for ANCA-associated vasculitis. Nephron Clin Pract. (2011). c, 89-97.

[134] Laurino, S, Chaudhry, A, Booth, A, Conte, G, & Jayne, D. Prospective study of TNFalpha blockade with adalimumab in ANCA-associated systemic vasculitis with renal involvement. Nephrol Dial Transplant. (2010). Oct;, 25(10), 3307-14.

[135] Brooks, C. J, King, W. J, Radford, D. J, Adu, D, Mcgrath, M, & Savage, C. O. IL-1 beta production by human polymorphonuclear leucocytes stimulated by anti-neutrophil cytoplasmic autoantibodies: relevance to systemic vasculitis. Clin Exp Immunol. (1996). Nov;, 106(2), 273-9.

[136] Lachmann, H. J, Kone-paut, I, Kuemmerle-deschner, J. B, Leslie, K. S, Hachulla, E, Quartier, P, Gitton, X, Widmer, A, Patel, N, & Hawkins, P. N. Use of canakinumab in the cryopyrin-associated periodic syndrome. N Engl J Med. (2009). Jun 4;, 360(23), 2416-25.

[137] Hewins, P, Williams, J. M, Wakelam, M. J, & Savage, C. O. Activation of Syk in neutrophils by antineutrophil cytoplasm antibodies occurs via Fcgamma receptors and CD18. J Am Soc Nephrol. (2004). Mar;, 15(3), 796-808.

[138] Kettritz, R, Choi, M, Butt, W, Rane, M, Rolle, S, Luft, F. C, & Klein, J. B. Phosphatidylinositol 3-kinase controls antineutrophil cytoplasmic antibodies-induced respiratory burst in human neutrophils. J Am Soc Nephrol. (2002). Jul;, 13(7), 1740-9.

[139] Williams, J. M, & Savage, C. O. Characterization of the regulation and functional consequences of activation in neutrophils by antineutrophil cytoplasm antibodies. J Am Soc Nephrol. (2005). Jan;16(1):90-6., 21ras.

[140] Flight, M. H. Deal watch: high hopes for oral SYK inhibitor in rheumatoid arthritis. Nat Rev Drug Discov. (2012). Jan;11(1):10.

[141] Katzav, A, Kloog, Y, Korczyn, A. D, Niv, H, Karussis, D. M, Wang, N, Rabinowitz, R, Blank, M, Shoenfeld, Y, & Chapman, J. Treatment of MRL/lpr mice, a genetic autoimmune model, with the Ras inhibitor, farnesylthiosalicylate (FTS). Clin Exp Immunol. (2001). Dec;, 126(3), 570-7.

[142] Halbwachs, L, & Lesavre, P. Endothelium-Neutrophil Interactions in ANCA-Associated Diseases. J Am Soc Nephrol. (2012). Sep;, 23(9), 1449-61.

[143] Keogan, M. T, Rifkin, I, Ronda, N, Lockwood, C. M, & Brown, D. L. Anti-neutrophil cytoplasm antibodies (ANCA) increase neutrophil adhesion to cultured human endothelium. Adv Exp Med Biol. (1993). , 336, 115-9.

[144] Ewert, B. H, Becker, M. E, Jennette, J. C, & Falk, R. J. Antimyeloperoxidase antibodies induce neutrophil adherence to cultured human endothelial cells. Ren Fail. (1995). Mar;, 17(2), 125-33.

[145] Johnson, P. A, Alexander, H. D, Mcmillan, S. A, & Maxwell, A. P. Up-regulation of the granulocyte adhesion molecule Mac-1 by autoantibodies in autoimmune vasculitis. Clin Exp Immunol. (1997). Mar;, 107(3), 513-9.

[146] Calderwood, J. W, Williams, J. M, Morgan, M. D, Nash, G. B, & Savage, C. O. ANCA induces beta2 integrin and CXC chemokine-dependent neutrophil-endothelial cell interactions that mimic those of highly cytokine-activated endothelium. J Leukoc Biol. (2005). Jan;, 77(1), 33-43.

[147] Haller, H, Eichhorn, J, Pieper, K, Gobel, U, & Luft, F. C. Circulating leukocyte integrin expression in Wegener's granulomatosis. J Am Soc Nephrol. (1996). Jan;, 7(1), 40-8.

[148] Arrizabalaga, P, Sole, M, Abellana, R, & Ascaso, C. Renal expression of adhesion molecules in anca-associated disease. J Clin Immunol. (2008). Sep;, 28(5), 411-9.

[149] Ewert, B. H, Jennette, J. C, & Falk, R. J. Anti-myeloperoxidase antibodies stimulate neutrophils to damage human endothelial cells. Kidney Int. (1992). Feb;, 41(2), 375-83.

[150] Savage, C. O, Pottinger, B. E, Gaskin, G, Pusey, C. D, & Pearson, J. D. Autoantibodies developing to myeloperoxidase and proteinase 3 in systemic vasculitis stimulate neutrophil cytotoxicity toward cultured endothelial cells. Am J Pathol. (1992). Aug;, 141(2), 335-42.

[151] Porges, A. J, Redecha, P. B, Kimberly, W. T, Csernok, E, Gross, W. L, & Kimberly, R. P. Anti-neutrophil cytoplasmic antibodies engage and activate human neutrophils via Fc gamma RIIa. J Immunol. (1994). Aug 1;, 153(3), 1271-80.

[152] Reumaux, D, Vossebeld, P. J, Roos, D, & Verhoeven, A. J. Effect of tumor necrosis factor-induced integrin activation on Fc gamma receptor II-mediated signal transduction: relevance for activation of neutrophils by anti-proteinase 3 or anti-myeloperoxidase antibodies. Blood. (1995). Oct 15;, 86(8), 3189-95.

[153] Erdbruegger, U, Grossheim, M, Hertel, B, Wyss, K, Kirsch, T, Woywodt, A, Haller, H, & Haubitz, M. Diagnostic role of endothelial microparticles in vasculitis. Rheumatology (Oxford). (2008). Dec;, 47(12), 1820-5.

[154] Kumpers, P, Hellpap, J, David, S, Horn, R, Leitolf, H, Haller, H, & Haubitz, M. Circulating angiopoietin-2 is a marker and potential mediator of endothelial cell detachment in ANCA-associated vasculitis with renal involvement. Nephrol Dial Transplant. (2009). Jun;, 24(6), 1845-50.

[155] De Groot, K, Goldberg, C, Bahlmann, F. H, Woywodt, A, Haller, H, Fliser, D, & Haubitz, M. Vascular endothelial damage and repair in antineutrophil cytoplasmic antibody-associated vasculitis. Arthritis Rheum. (2007). Nov;, 56(11), 3847-53.

[156] Zavada, J, Kideryova, L, Pytlik, R, Vankova, Z, & Tesar, V. Circulating endothelial progenitor cells in patients with ANCA-associated vasculitis. Kidney Blood Press Res. (2008). , 31(4), 247-54.

[157] Yang, J. J, Preston, G. A, Pendergraft, W. F, Segelmark, M, Heeringa, P, Hogan, S. L, Jennette, J. C, & Falk, R. J. Internalization of proteinase 3 is concomitant with endothelial cell apoptosis and internalization of myeloperoxidase with generation of intracellular oxidants. Am J Pathol. (2001). Feb;, 158(2), 581-92.

[158] Kuligowski, M. P, Kitching, A. R, & Hickey, M. J. Leukocyte recruitment to the inflamed glomerulus: a critical role for platelet-derived P-selectin in the absence of rolling. J Immunol. (2006). Jun 1;, 176(11), 6991-9.

[159] Devi, S, Kuligowski, M. P, Kwan, R. Y, Westein, E, Jackson, S. P, Kitching, A. R, & Hickey, M. J. Platelet recruitment to the inflamed glomerulus occurs via an alphaIIb-beta3/GPVI-dependent pathway. Am J Pathol. (2010). Sep;, 177(3), 1131-42.

[160] Radford, D. J, Savage, C. O, & Nash, G. B. Treatment of rolling neutrophils with antineutrophil cytoplasmic antibodies causes conversion to firm integrin-mediated adhesion. Arthritis Rheum. (2000). Jun;, 43(6), 1337-45.

[161] Nolan, S. L, Kalia, N, Nash, G. B, Kamel, D, Heeringa, P, & Savage, C. O. Mechanisms of ANCA-mediated leukocyte-endothelial cell interactions in vivo. J Am Soc Nephrol. (2008). May;, 19(5), 973-84.

[162] Gasser, O, Hess, C, Miot, S, Deon, C, Sanchez, J. C, & Schifferli, J. A. Characterisation and properties of ectosomes released by human polymorphonuclear neutrophils. Exp Cell Res. (2003). May 1;, 285(2), 243-57.

[163] Hong, Y, Eleftheriou, D, Hussain, A. A, Price-kuehne, F. E, Savage, C. O, Jayne, D, Little, M. A, Salama, A. D, Klein, N. J, & Brogan, P. A. Anti-neutrophil cytoplasmic antibodies stimulate release of neutrophil microparticles. J Am Soc Nephrol. (2012). Jan;, 23(1), 49-62.

[164] Medzhitov, R, & Janeway, C. Jr. Innate immune recognition: mechanisms and pathways. Immunol Rev. (2000). Feb;, 173, 89-97.

[165] Li, M, Zhou, Y, Feng, G, & Su, S. B. The critical role of Toll-like receptor signaling pathways in the induction and progression of autoimmune diseases. Curr Mol Med. (2009). Apr;, 9(3), 365-74.

[166] Shirali, A. C, & Goldstein, D. R. Tracking the toll of kidney disease. J Am Soc Nephrol. (2008). Aug;, 19(8), 1444-50.

[167] Wu, H, Chen, G, Wyburn, K. R, Yin, J, Bertolino, P, Eris, J. M, Alexander, S. I, Sharland, A. F, & Chadban, S. J. TLR4 activation mediates kidney ischemia/reperfusion injury. J Clin Invest. (2007). Oct;, 117(10), 2847-59.

[168] Summers, S. A, Hoi, A, Steinmetz, O. M, Sullivan, O, Ooi, K. M, Odobasic, J. D, Akira, D, Kitching, S, Holdsworth, A. R, & Tlr, S. R. and TLR4 are required for the development of autoimmunity and lupus nephritis in pristane nephropathy. J Autoimmun. (2010). Dec;, 35(4), 291-8.

[169] Summers, S. A, Steinmetz, O. M, Kitching, A. R, & Holdsworth, S. R. Toll Like Receptor 9 Ligation Enhances Experimental Crescentic Glomerulonephritis J Am Soc Nephrol Abstracts TH-PO824. (2009). (20)

[170] Hurtado, P. R, Jeffs, L, Nitschke, J, Patel, M, Sarvestani, G, Cassidy, J, Hissaria, P, Gillis, D, & Peh, C. A. CpG oligodeoxynucleotide stimulates production of anti-neutrophil cytoplasmic antibodies in ANCA associated vasculitis. BMC Immunol. (2008).

[171] Tadema, H, Abdulahad, W. H, Lepse, N, Stegeman, C. A, Kallenberg, C. G, & Heeringa, P. Bacterial DNA motifs trigger ANCA production in ANCA-associated vasculitis in remission. Rheumatology (Oxford). (2010). Dec 11.

[172] Tadema, H, Abdulahad, W. H, Stegeman, C. A, Kallenberg, C. G, & Heeringa, P. Increased expression of Toll-like receptors by monocytes and natural killer cells in ANCA-associated vasculitis. PLoS One. (2011). e24315.

[173] Papadimitraki, E. D, Tzardi, M, Bertsias, G, Sotsiou, E, & Boumpas, D. T. Glomerular expression of toll-like receptor-9 in lupus nephritis but not in normal kidneys: impli-

cations for the amplification of the inflammatory response. Lupus. (2009). Aug;, 18(9), 831-5.

[174] Machida, H, Ito, S, Hirose, T, Takeshita, F, Oshiro, H, Nakamura, T, Mori, M, Inayama, Y, Yan, K, Kobayashi, N, & Yokota, S. Expression of Toll-like receptor 9 in renal podocytes in childhood-onset active and inactive lupus nephritis. Nephrol Dial Transplant. (2010). Aug;, 25(8), 2530-537.

[175] Batsford, S, Duermueller, U, Seemayer, C, Mueller, C, Hopfer, H, & Mihatsch, M. Protein level expression of Toll-like receptors 2, 4 and 9 in renal disease. Nephrol Dial Transplant. (2011). Apr;, 26(4), 1413-6.

[176] Uehara, A, Hirabayashi, Y, & Takada, H. Antibodies to proteinase 3 prime human oral, lung, and kidney epithelial cells to secrete proinflammatory cytokines upon stimulation with agonists to various Toll-like receptors, NOD1, and NOD2. Clin Vaccine Immunol. (2008). Jul;, 15(7), 1060-6.

[177] Zipfel, P. F, & Skerka, C. Complement regulators and inhibitory proteins. Nat Rev Immunol. (2009). Oct;, 9(10), 729-40.

[178] Botto, M, Kirschfink, M, Macor, P, Pickering, M. C, Wurzner, R, & Tedesco, F. Complement in human diseases: Lessons from complement deficiencies. Mol Immunol. (2009). Sep;, 46(14), 2774-83.

[179] Amara, U, Flierl, M. A, Rittirsch, D, Klos, A, Chen, H, Acker, B, Bruckner, U. B, Nilsson, B, Gebhard, F, Lambris, J. D, & Huber-lang, M. Molecular intercommunication between the complement and coagulation systems. J Immunol. (2010). Nov 1;, 185(9), 5628-36.

[180] Haas, M, & Eustace, J. A. Immune complex deposits in ANCA-associated crescentic glomerulonephritis: a study of 126 cases. Kidney Int. (2004). Jun;, 65(6), 2145-52.

[181] Brons, R. H, De Jong, M. C, De Boer, N. K, Stegeman, C. A, Kallenberg, C. G, & Tervaert, J. W. Detection of immune deposits in skin lesions of patients with Wegener's granulomatosis. Ann Rheum Dis. (2001). Dec;, 60(12), 1097-102.

[182] Pinching, A. J, Lockwood, C. M, Pussell, B. A, Rees, A. J, Sweny, P, Evans, D. J, Bowley, N, & Peters, D. K. Wegener's granulomatosis: observations on 18 patients with severe renal disease. Q J Med. (1983). Autumn;, 52(208), 435-60.

[183] Xiao, H, Schreiber, A, Heeringa, P, Falk, R. J, & Jennette, J. C. Alternative complement pathway in the pathogenesis of disease mediated by anti-neutrophil cytoplasmic autoantibodies. Am J Pathol. (2007). Jan;, 170(1), 52-64.

[184] Schreiber, A, Xiao, H, Jennette, J. C, Schneider, W, Luft, F. C, & Kettritz, R. C. a receptor mediates neutrophil activation and ANCA-induced glomerulonephritis. J Am Soc Nephrol. (2009). Feb;, 20(2), 289-98.

[185] Hao, J, Meng, L. Q, Xu, P. C, Chen, M, & Zhao, M. H. p. MAPK, ERK and PI3K signaling pathways are involved in C5a-primed neutrophils for ANCA-mediated activation. PLoS One. (2012). e38317.

[186] Yuan, J, Gou, S. J, Huang, J, Hao, J, Chen, M, & Zhao, M. H. C. a and its receptors in human anti-neutrophil cytoplasmic antibody (ANCA)-associated vasculitis. Arthritis Res Ther. (2012). Jun 12;14(3):R140.

[187] Ludewig, B, Odermatt, B, Landmann, S, Hengartner, H, & Zinkernagel, R. M. Dendritic cells induce autoimmune diabetes and maintain disease via de novo formation of local lymphoid tissue. J Exp Med. (1998). Oct 19;, 188(8), 1493-501.

[188] Zinkernagel, R. M, & Hengartner, H. Regulation of the immune response by antigen. Science. (2001). Jul 13;, 293(5528), 251-3.

[189] Csernok, E, Ai, M, Gross, W. L, Wicklein, D, Petersen, A, Lindner, B, Lamprecht, P, Holle, J. U, & Hellmich, B. Wegener autoantigen induces maturation of dendritic cells and licenses them for Th1 priming via the protease-activated receptor-2 pathway. Blood. (2006). Jun 1;, 107(11), 4440-8.

[190] Chan, V. S, Nie, Y. J, Shen, N, Yan, S, Mok, M. Y, & Lau, C. S. Distinct roles of myeloid and plasmacytoid dendritic cells in systemic lupus erythematosus. Autoimmun Rev. (2012). Mar 20.

[191] Wilde, B, Van Paassen, P, Damoiseaux, J, Heerings-rewinkel, P, Van Rie, H, Witzke, O, & Tervaert, J. W. Dendritic cells in renal biopsies of patients with ANCA-associated vasculitis. Nephrol Dial Transplant. (2009). Jul;, 24(7), 2151-6.

[192] Polzer, K, Soleiman, A, Baum, W, Axmann, R, Distler, J, Redlich, K, Kilian, A, Kronke, G, Schett, G, Zwerina, J, & Selective, p. MAPK isoform expression and activation in antineutrophil cytoplasmatic antibody-associated crescentic glomerulonephritis: role of Ann Rheum Dis. (2008). May;67(5):602-8., 38MAPKalpha.

[193] de Lind van Wijngaarden RAHauer HA, Wolterbeek R, Jayne DR, Gaskin G, Rasmussen N, Noel LH, Ferrario F, Waldherr R, Hagen EC, Bruijn JA, Bajema IM. Clinical and histologic determinants of renal outcome in ANCA-associated vasculitis: A prospective analysis of 100 patients with severe renal involvement. J Am Soc Nephrol. (2006). Aug;, 17(8), 2264-74.

[194] Bonventre, J. V, & Yang, L. Cellular pathophysiology of ischemic acute kidney injury. J Clin Invest. (2011). Nov;, 121(11), 4210-21.

[195] Segerer, S, Regele, H, Mac, K. M, Kain, R, Cartron, J. P, Colin, Y, Kerjaschki, D, & Schlondorff, D. The Duffy antigen receptor for chemokines is up-regulated during acute renal transplant rejection and crescentic glomerulonephritis. Kidney Int. (2000). Oct;, 58(4), 1546-56.

[196] Takaeda, M, Yokoyama, H, Segawa-takaeda, C, Wada, T, & Kobayashi, K. High endothelial venule-like vessels in the interstitial lesions of human glomerulonephritis. Am J Nephrol. (2002). Jan-Feb;, 22(1), 48-57.

Chapter 3

Immunological Mechanisms and Clinical Aspects in Pulmonary-Renal Syndrome: A Review

N. Lukán

Additional information is available at the end of the chapter

http://dx.doi.org/10.5772/55181

1. Introduction

McGraw-Hill Concise Dictionary of Modern Medicine [1] defines pulmonary-renal syndrome (PRS) as an idiopathic condition characterized by pulmonary hemorrhage, rapid progressive glomerulonephritis, and positive autoantibodies. Pulmonary-renal syndrome may be also defined as a heterogeneous group of multisystem diseases – e.g. Goodpasture syndrome, Wegener's granulomatosis, collagen vascular disease – in particular systemic lupus erythematosus, polyarteritis nodosa, Henoch-Schönlein purpura, and various other conditions, which all have prominent pulmonary and renal components. According to Sanders [2] the strict definition of pulmonary-renal syndrome is the combined clinical picture of rapid progressive glomerulonephritis and pulmonary capillaritis requiring histological confirmation.

If we translate the definition into pathological nomenclature, pulmonary-renal syndrome is defined as combination of diffuse alveolar hemorrhage (DAH) and immune crescent glomerulonephritis. The essential substrate of all these changes is vasculitis, which is according to contemporary nomenclature based mostly on morphological and histopathological criteria. These criteria for the most common forms of vasculitides were introduced in 1994 by Jennette et al. at the Chapel Hill Consensus Conference organized by the American College of Rheumatology [3]. The inflammation of small vessels (microangiopathic vasculitis) restricts blood flow to various organs and damages them. If correct diagnosis and appropriate treatment are delayed the condition can be fatal. Prognosis is good when treatment begins before onset of respiratory and renal failure. Because of the similarity in clinical picture, differential diagnosis of these diseases at the bedside can be challenging.

The pathophysiology of the vasculitides is based on immunologic mechanisms. These appear to play an active role in mediating the inflammatory response, but their exact mechanisms still remain poorly understood. Although the primary events that initiate this process remain largely unknown, recent investigations have brought us closer to understanding some of the critical pathways involved in disease and provided a rationale for the study of novel therapeutic agents [4].

2. Historical sense of the term „pulmonary - renal syndrome"

The first mention on pulmonary-renal syndrome is dated to year 1919 when the „father of viral pathology" in the United States Dr. Ernest William Goodpasture (1886 – 1960) published his work "The Significance of Certain Pulmonary Lesions in Relation to the Etiology of Influenza in American Journal of the Medical Sciences [5]. He described two cases from more than fifty autopsies where in patients dying in the great flu pandemic (Spanish flu) no bacterial etiology was confirmed. In one of the two patients massive alveolar hemorrhage and fulminant glomerulonephritis were present. It was never discovered what underlying disease other than influenza this patient may have had. Human influenza virus was described fourteen years later by Laidlaw and coworkers [6]. In 1958 two Australian scientists Stanton and Tange in the discussion of their paper analyzed Goodpasture´s old finding and associated pulmonary hemorrhage with glomerulonephritis with the name of Dr. Goodpasture, as Goodpasture syndrome [7]. According to the biography written by Collins (2010), E. Goodpasture did not approve the association of his name with this syndrome [8]. In 1967 the discovery of anti-GBM antibodies were associated with Goodpasture nephritis [9].

At present pulmonary-renal syndrome broadened the family of diseases, where diffuse alveolar hemorrhage and immune crescent glomerulonephritis are participating. Therefore, it is not possible to say only glomerular basement membrane (Goodpasture) disease means pulmonary-renal syndrome. The term pulmonary-renal syndrome should be associated with the term pulmonary-renal vasculitic syndromes [10].

3. Histopathology

Pathological expressions of vasculitis are not usually specific for a particular diagnostic category of vasculitis. The primary pathology in the majority of pulmonary-renal syndrome is inflammation and necrosis of vessel wall classified according to the Chapel Hill Consensus Conference classification [3] as medium/small vessel vasculitis. Generally, inflammation affects arterioles, capillaries and venules with two basic types of necrosis – fibrinoid and granulomatous. In the very early stage of inflammation there is a massive influx of polymorphonuclear leukocytes and monocytes accumulating in the capillary space. Later the condition is accompanied by proteinacous exudate. Damage of the capillaries and disruption of basal membranes with leakage of erythrocytes is followed by an influx of macrophages. Fibrinoid depositions cause the formation of extracapillary (crescent) cell proliferation in the glomerulus [11]. Changes in lungs give rise to isolated necrotic pulmonary capillaritis where damaged red blood cells migrate directly into alveolar tissue resulting in alveolar haemorrhage [12].

Jennette et al. [13] described pathologic features of different necrotizing vasculitis types indicating various pathogenic mechanisms causing the injury. In anti-GBM disease or immune complex disease the pathogenic complexes between antibodies and antigens are located exclusively or predominantly in vessel walls. In patients with ANCA vasculitis, these autoantibodies are in the interstitial fluid and also in the blood. ANCA activate neutrophils and monocytes in blood vessels, as well as in interstitial tissue. Activation in the vessels causes necrotizing vasculitis and activation in the tissues necrotizing tissue inflammation. Clinical association of dominating organs in pulmonary-renal syndrome is shown in table 1.

Organ	MPA	GPA (WG)	CSS	GPS
Kidney	90	80	45	75
Lung	50	90	70	60

Table 1. Approximate frequency of organ system involvement (%)

Interstitial inflammation is accompanied by capillary trombosis, disintegration of blood vessel wall, loss of integrity of tissue structures, epithelial cell hyperplasia, accumulation of red cells (and later hemosiderin), depositions of proteins (immunoglobulins, immune-complex proteins), interstitial fibrosis and atrophy. The actual picture is dependent on different organ structure of lungs and kidneys, as well as on primary stimulus.

Presence of specific granulomatous inflammation is typical for granulomatosis with polyangiitis (GPA, formerly Wegener´s granulomatosis) described and defined by Wegener in 1939 [14] and Former in 1950 [15] respectively. Morphological detected recruitment of inflammatory cells, as well as immune competent cells (T-cells, B, cells, macrophages) and sometimes also giant-cells are confirmed by immunostaining of autoantibodies, detection of cytokine release and oxygen-free radical formation.

Pulmonary-renal syndrome has a wide spectrum of organ histopathological changes. Severe renal vascular damage can be accomapnied by absent or mild pulmonary changes. On the other hand severe pulmonary injury can be followed by mild renal destruction or normal renal histology.

3.1. Renal pathology

Renal pathology is expressed by various forms of glomerulonephritis (anti-GBM, immunocomplex, necrotizing pauci immune). In rare cases sequential development supposed to be of pathogenic importance: injury caused by ANCA may uncover the Goodpasture antigen. The concept that only one antigen may trigger another one requires further support [16].

Immunohistochemical classification of renal capillary vasculitides [17] based on renal biopsies is characterized by the presence of:

1. anti GBM antibodies – type I crescentic GN
2. immune complexes – type II crescentic GN

3. pauci-immune (only circulating ANCA) – type III crescentic GN

3.2. Pulmonary pathology

The underlying pulmonary lesions (necrotic pulmonary capillaritis) are clinically expressed as diffuse alveolar haemorrhage. Disruption and degradation of the pulmonary capillary wall and interstitial matrix results in vessel wall destruction and necrosis. Cordier and Cottin [18] found capillaritis as the most common pathological finding (60%) in ANCA-related vasculitides with pulmonary complications. However, capillaritis was not observed in all patients. It is likely that vessel inflammations may be overlooked in some cases if not specifically searched [19].

According to recommendations of Jennette and Falk [20] an accurate precise clinical diagnosis usually requires the integration of many different types of data, including clinical signs and symptoms, associated diseases, histological pattern of inflammation (eg, granulomatous versus necrotizing), immunopathological features (e.g. presence and composition of vascular immunoglobulin deposits), and serological findings (cryoglobulins, hypocomplementemia, hepatitis B antibodies, hepatitis C antibodies, ANCAs, anti–GBM antibodies, ANA). Specific diagnosis of a vasculitis is very important because the prognosis and appropriate therapy vary substantially among different types of vasculitis. Many attempts to re-evaluate and to refine the present nomenclature of vasculitis were done, however the complexity of vasculitic syndromes, as well as of pulmonary-renal syndrome complicates not only the estimation of appropriate diagnosis, differential diagnosis but also hampers effective treatment.

4. Immunopathogenesis

Potentially accepted immunopathological mechanisms of pulmonary-renal syndrome involve antiglomerular basement membrane antibodies, antineutrophil cytoplasm antibodies, generation of immunocomplexes, activation of complement and haemocoagulation. Due to different pathogenesis of pulmonary-renal syndrome in various clinical diagnoses, common immunopathological features (except systemic inflammation) could not be specified. As seen in most inflammatory diseases, the systemic response to insult may be as important as the initial stimulus.

4.1. Genetical and environmental influence

The current understanding of autoimmune disorders suggests that some environmental factors initiate disease in a genetically susceptible individual. The importance of genetic factors, especially the genes of major histocompatibility complex has been increasingly recognized in determining susceptibility to autoimmune diseases. Because of the low incidence of all nosological entities of pulmonary-renal syndrome, it is not possible to examine the inheritance of genes within affected families predisposing to this disease.

In pulmonary-renal syndrome, as in most autoimmune disorders, the precise initiating events are not known. Exposure to hydrocarbons is known to cause damage to pulmonary/renal endothelial cells and so could expose components of the alveolar basement membrane to cells of the immune system, initiating an immune response [21]. The induction of vasculitis seems multifactorial, with interplay of environmental factors and genetic predisposition creating the environment for development of disease [22].

4.2. Kidney-lung crosstalk

New experimental data have emerged in recent years focusing on the interactive effects of kidney and lung dysfunction, and these studies have highlighted the pathophysiological importance of proinflammatory and other immunologic pathways as well as the complex nature of interorgan crosstalk. Because pulmonary and renal dysfunction frequently coexist, the effects of failure of either organ are particularly relevant to the function of the other. Evidence suggests that deleterious kidney-lung interactions or crosstalk rise, at least in part, due to the loss of the normal balance of immune, inflammatory and soluble mediator metabolism. These processes occur after severe insults and cause induction of organ injury [23]. Organ crosstalk is a consequence of both direct loss of normal function and inflammatory dysregulation resulting from both organ failure. Cellular (e.g. neutrophils) as well as soluble mediators (cytokines) contribute to the inflammatory dysregulation under these circumstances [24].

4.3. Immunology of inflammation

Interactions between inflammatory cells and damaged endothelium end in vessel inflammation (vasculitis), the major manifestation of all clinical entities. Cytokines, chemokines (such as IL-8) complement components, circulating immune complexes, and antibodies can be primary determinants of initiators of endothelial cell damage. When focusing on two basic clinical representatives – Goodpasture disease and granulomatosis with polyangiitis, damage of the vessel wall of glomeruli and alveolar capillaries are caused by antigen-stimulated white blood cells, anti-GBM antibodies and ANCA, respectively. In anti-GBM and ANCA vasculitis, the pathologic finding of focal, lytic necrotizing injury suggests highly effective local activation of neutrophils and monocytes with release of oxidants and proteases that are neutralized beyond the site of injury [13].

Concurrent ANCA and anti-GBM antibody production can be seen in selected patients, but reasonable explanation is unknown. It is possible that ANCA-related proteases damage or expose the nephritogenic epitopes in cr3 (IV) collagen in GBM, and this in turn leads to anti-GBM antibody production. It is unlikely that the crossreactivity between p-ANCA and anti-GBM antibodies is derived from the same autoantibody repertoire, because there does not appear to be a structural relationship between c-ANCA and a3 (IV) NC 1 collagen [25]. It is currently unclear whether there is any structural cross-reactivity between c-ANCA and anti-GBM antibodies [26].

4.4. Cellular and humoral mechanisms

Immunological mechanisms involved in initiation and prolongation of inflammatory state could be divided to two groups: cellular mechanisms (activity of immune-competent cells) and humoral mechanisms (proteins, mediators). Inflammation is tightly connected also to oxidative stress either through increased formation of ROS and/or the decreased activity of antioxidant systems.

It should be postulated in the view of common association in all disease entities that the damage is caused by free radical formation of injured tissues. Local release of inflammatory cytokines and chemokines further activate endothelial cells to upregulate soluble adhesion molecules, enhanced activation of neutrophils and generation of reactive oxygen species which serve to amplify the initial inflammation leading to dysregulated apoptosis, secondary necrosis and overt vascular injury.

The immune system may target the tissues due to structural alterations in proteins or cell surfaces. Finally, the production of necessary anti-inflammatory factors may be impaired after hypoxia. Initiating signals – triggers of inflammation can activate the inflammatory process by several mechanisms that may occur simultaneously [27]:

1. Passively released factors from injured or exposed cells due to breakdown of cellular barriers.
2. Stress or injury (hypoxia) can induce the active synthesis of pro-inflammatory signals.
3. Immune system receptors (cellular, humoral) may recognize altered or exposed surface structures.
4. Damaged cells have decreased expression of inhibitory (anti-inflammatory) factors permitting uncontrolled activation of inflammatory cells or systems.

Binding of ANCA to neutrophil membranes activates the cells leading to the release of lytic enzymes, chemoatractant interleukin-8 and oxygen free radicals. Neutrophils subsequently aggregate on endothelium causing inflammation and damage to the vasculature. Still, it remains unclear in many diseases whether or not ANCAs are simply playing a bystander role in the inflammatory cascade or directly driving vasculitic inflammation [28].

Gröne [29] describes except of the role of ANCAs, other immunopathogenetic factors important in vasculitides. They include innate immunity factors, transcription factors such as NFkB, endothelial cytoprotective agents such as NO. In summary:

1. ANCA may be directed against several antigens, in the majority of cases against proteinase-3 and myeloperoxidase. The complex of proteinase-3 and ANCA leads to an increased expression of CD14, CD18 and an elevated synthesis of cytokines and chemokines such as interleukin 1, interleukin 8 in monocytes. In addition granulocytes generate reactive oxygen species, ANCA may also bind to a surface glycoprotein (gp130) expressed on glomerular and peritubular endothelia in the kidney. Thus the activation of granulocytes, monocytes and endothelial cells by ANCA may be a critical step in the initiation phases of vasculitis, ultimately leading to apoptosis.
2. NO is cytoprotective for endothelial cells in low concentrations.
3. The transcription factor complex NFkB is a key regulatory transcription factor for the expression of genes and proteins associated with acute inflammatory processes and

"endothelialitis". Inhibition of NFkB activity by a decoy-oligonucleotide prevented activation of endothelial cells in reperfusion injury and vascular rejection.

4. The complement system probably plays an essential role in the initiation and propagation phases of vasculitis. Specifically the pneumococcal C-polysaccharide-reactive protein (CRP), synthesized after trauma and infection, can potently activate the complement cascade leading to activation of endothelial cells with increased expression of adhesion molecules.

Above mentioned pathogenetic mechanisms of vasculitides seem to be important and common factors for the generation and maintenance of vascular inflammation; nevertheless these factors are only part of the spectrum of different humoral and cellular responses in vasculitis [29].

4.5. Ischemic/reperfusion injury

Acute onset of severe pulmonary-renal syndrome is closely connected with ischemia-reperfusion injury when both innate and adaptive immunity contribute to their pathogenesis. Kidney resident cells promote inflammation after ischemic/reperfusion injury by increasing endothelial cell adhesion molecule expression and vascular permeability. Kidney epithelial cells bind complement and express toll-like receptors and resident and infiltrating cells produce cytokines/chemokines. Early activation of kidney dendritic cells initiates a cascade of events leading to accumulation of interferon-γ-producing neutrophils, infiltrating macrophages, CD4+ T cells, B cells and invariant natural killer T cells. Bajwa et al. [30] recently implicated the IL23/IL17 pathway in kidney ischemic/reperfusion injury, as well as the importance that T-regulatory cells can directly suppress the early innate inflammation, induced by ischemia/reperfusion, in an IL-10 dependent manner. Following the initial early phase of inflammation, the late phase involves infiltration of anti-inflammatory cells including regulatory T cells, alternatively activated macrophages and stem cells leading to attenuation of inflammation and initiation of repair.

4.6. TNFalfa – proinflammatory cytokine

Another possible connection between kidney and lung inflammation as a part of the systemic inflammatory pathway describe Campanholle et al. [31]. They concluded that pro-inflammatory mediators, TNF-alfa, IL-1β and MCP-1, released by the ischemic kidney might reach the lungs, induce inflammation, up-regulate COX-2 and iNOS expressions, and ultimately contribute to the accumulation and to activation of neutrophils and mononuclear cells.

TNF-alpha, a potent pro-inflammatory cytokine belongs to the group of mediators that activate leukocytes and endothelial cells. Neutrophils, other leukocytes, and platelets adhere via cognate receptors to the pulmonary endothelium. Activated neutrophils release proteases, leukotrienes, reactive oxygen intermediates, and other inflammatory molecules that amplify the inflammatory response. ROS and proteases can directly damage alveolar–capillary membrane integrity [32]. On the other side the lectin-like domain of TNF-alpha has positive effects on permeability of the epithelial-endothelial barrier in the lungs. This domain is able to blunt ROS production in pulmonary artery endothelial cells under hypoxia and reoxygenation, and reduce ROS content in inflammatory conditions [33].

TNF-alpha - an important cytokine involved in pathogenesis of inflammation, is an example of a "moonlighting protein", with differential activities mediated by its receptor-binding versus its lectin-like domains, which opens the possibility to design and develop more sophisticated therapeutic regimens for patients with increased permeability of the epithelial-endothelial barrier of the lung, which in pulmonary-renal syndrome can occur. However, in the future, more research is needed in order to reveal the underlying mechanisms of TNF's protective versus deleterious effects [34].

4.7. Reactive oxygen species and nitric oxide engagement

Among enzymes incorporated in the free radical formation, eNOS (NOS3) has been shown to inhibit vascular inflammation in many different model systems, but its role in the pathogenesis of vasculitis has not been elucidated yet. According to Schoeb et al. [35] eNOS serves as a negative regulator of vasculitis in experimental (mice) model of pulmonary-renal syndrome and they further suggest that nitric oxide produced by this enzyme may be critical for inhibiting lesion formation and vascular damage in human vasculitides. Derangements in the key oxidative stress enzymes, nitric oxide synthase and heme oxygenase may also facilitate distant organ dysfunction. Disordered NO metabolism in the setting of inflammation is well established. While the cause of this dysregulation is not entirely clear, asymmetric dimethyarginine seems to play a significant role [36, 37]. Asymmetric dimethyarginine is an inhibitor of endothelial NO synthase and shifts NO metabolism toward production of oxygen-based free radicals [38]. MPO released from activated neutrophils are involved in the formation of NO-derived reactive oxygen species [39]. ROS produced by macrophages in combination with reactive nitrogen intermediates cause protein nitration in endothelial cells [40]. This could be related to activation of cytokines produced by macrophages to elicit proinflammatory and prothrombotic responses in endothelial cells [41]. MPO produces a highly deleterious reactive oxygen species, the hypochlorous acid (HOCl). Anti-MPO antibodies from patients with small vessel vasculitis (MPA) can trigger the release of MPO by neutrophils and monocytes. Anti-MPO antibodies can activate MPO to generate an oxidative stress deleterious for the endothelium.

Guilpain et al. [42] recently demonstrated that MPA sera with anti-MPO antibodies activated MPO in vitro, and generated free radicals (hypochlorous acid), whereas sera from MPA patients with no anti-MPO antibodies or healthy individuals did not. Free oxygen radical production and endothelial lysis were abrogated by N-acetylcysteine (NAC), an antioxidant molecule through the augmentation of glutathione biosynthesis. N-acetylcysteine significantly reduced the activation of myeloperoxidase and improved the survival of endothelial cells exposed to byproducts of myeloperoxidase activation. Thus, anti-MPO antibodies could play a pathogenic role in vivo by triggering an oxidative burst leading to severe endothelial damages.

http://dx.doi.org/10.5772/55181

During early stage of human septic shock Spapen et al. [43] founded massive decrease of IL-8 after N-acetylcystein (NAC) administration. According to that finding, Park et al. [44] supposes another possible mechanism of NAC effect - through inhibition of IL-8.

In Goodpasture´s syndrome normal exposure of epitopes by self-limited generation of ROS is not itself sufficient to launch a fatal autoimmune response. ROS can be produced in response to various normal stimuli such as mediators of inflammation, environmental toxins, de-novo respiratory bursts. Excessive ROS may influence GBM degradation by proteolytic enzymes [45]. Therefore, the presence of ROS in the microenvironment around the GBM can likely activate several pathways of protein modification in renal, as well as in pulmonary tissue in Goodpasture´s syndrome. Kalluri et al. [46] suggest that ROS can alter the hexameric structure of type IV collagen to expose or destroy selectively immunologic epitopes embedded in basement membrane. The reasons for autoimmunity in Goodpasture syndrome may lie in an age-dependent deterioration in inhibitor function modulating oxidative damage to structural molecules. ROS therefore may play an important role in shaping post-translational epitope diversity or neoantigen formation in organ tissues.

4.8. Natural antibodies

Natural antibodies produced by B-cells may play a role in prevention of pathological autoimmune reactions by binding to microbial epitopes that are similar or identical to self-antigens [47].

Bacterial superantigens trigger the activation of autoreactive cells such as toxic shock syndrome toxin 1 and Staphylococcal enterotoxins. These superantigens are generally considered to be the triggers of exacerbation in Wegener´s granulomatosis [48, 49].

4.9. Role of Th 17

Under certain conditions, T helper type cells can differentiate into regulatory T cells producing immunosuppressive cytokines such as transforming growth factor-ß and IL-10. These regulatory T cells representing about 5% to 10% of CD4+ T cells in the steady state, play a central role in immune homeostasis and in preventing autoimmune diseases in general [50, 51]. Regulatory T cells exist naturally and are called natural regulatory T cells expressing CD25 and Foxp3. T cells can also convert into regulatory T cells upon certain antigen recognition and are called antigen-specific regulatory T cells that secrete IL-10 and/or transforming growth factor-β. Indeed, regulatory T cells are required to control infection-induced immunity in a host, including autoimmunity inhibition [52].

Recently discovered regulatory Th17-cells and cell-derived cytokines play an important role in the pathogenesis of several autoimmune/inflammatory diseases including vasculitides. In Wegener´s granulomatosis, regulatory T-cells display impaired suppressor activity potentially favouring inflammation and break of tolerance [53]. Th17-cells produce several cytokines such as IL-17, IL-21, IL-22, CCL-20 which induce massive inflammatory tissue reactions and these cytokines also stimulate nonimmune cells (fibroblasts, endothelial and epithelial cells) to the production of proinflammatory mediators (IL-6, TNF-alfa, prostaglandins, NO, MMP and chemokines [54]. New results, showing the possibility that regulatory Th17 cells and corresponding cytokines (IL-17, IL-23) involved in the pathogenesis of GPS as well in WG might be used for the directed therapy of pulmonary-renal syndrome in the future.

Vasculitis (especially Wegener´s granulomatosis) is associated with bacterial infection, in particular nasal occurence of Staphylococcus aureus. Infection may play a role in the induction of autoimmunity as well as in the effector phase of the disease. In this relation Tadema et al. [55] emphasize the role of innate immunity that is involved in the development of a Th17-driven immune response, consistent with skewing towards a Th17 T cell phenotype that has been observed in Wegener's granulomatosis. Their findings shed new light on the potential role of γ/δ T cells in host defense and inflammatory diseases, provide important new information on the pathogenic role of IL-23 and IL-1β, and underline the importance of targeting these cytokines in the development of new therapeutic interventions against many autoimmune diseases.

Sutton et al. [56] demonstrated that γ/δ T cells activated by IL-1β and IL-23 are an important source of innate IL-17 and IL-21 and provide an alternative mechanism whereby IL-1 and IL-23 may mediate autoimmune inflammation.

In other study Ooi et al. [57] suggested the importance of IL-23, a key cytokine in the induction and maintenance of autoimmune responses, in Th1 responses that could play a role in some forms of glomerulonephritis especially in anti-GBM (Goodpasture) disease. This experimental work emphasizes potential mechanisms in the treatment of several forms of glomerulonephritis.

Accumulating data from animal models support a role for Th17 cells and their cytokines in various autoimmune and inflammatory processes. Emerging data from running clinical trials indicate the importance of Th17 cells in such immunological processes, too. Future studies will allow us to evaluate the role of each cytokine independently in contributing to human diseases with immune-mediated pathologies and to design optimal cytokine-targeted therapies for these diseases [58].

4.10. Perspectives of treatment – modulation of inflammation

After careful analysis of numerous animal studies demonstrating the importance of inflammation in the pathogenesis of pulmonary-renal syndrome, as well as the clinical correlates demonstrating activation of the same systems in patients with systemic autoimmunity, there is a reason to hope that different modalities of anti-inflammatory treatment could ameliorate the course of the disease. The inflammatory process is however extremely complex due to its multifactorial etiology and considering also in the context of differences among systems [59]. For example renal failure involves complex host-kidney interactions in which the inflammatory state of the host contributes to the development of renal failure and injury of the inflamed tissue further modulates the inflammatory state of the host. One of the greatest obstacles to effective treatment is establishing the diagnosis as early as possible based on all available diagnostic procedures, including invasive ones. Earlier and more reliable identification of clinical signs and laboratory markers has become an important tool in relation to establish effective treatment modalities. Once the inflammatory response has been set in motion, treatment may be ineffective and could conceivably delay recovery. Strategies that prevent the initiation of inflammation by targeting the earliest signals or recognition of the injured tissue may be of particular therapeutic benefit in these conditions [25].

5. Semi-systemic (pathologic/clinical) classification

The etiology of pulmonary-renal syndrome could be associated with variety of diseases. A possible classification based on clinical symptomatology and histopathology is described in Table 2.

	Etiology of pulmonary-renal syndrome
Cause	**Disease**
Systemic vasculitides	Wegener's granulomatosis Churg-Strauss syndrome Cryoglobulinemia Henoch-Schönlein purpura Behçet's syndrome Microscopic polyarteritis
Connective tissue disorders	Polymyositis or dermatomyositis Progressive systemic sclerosis RA SLE MCTD "Catastrophic" APS
Renal disorders	Goodpasture´s disease Idiopathic immune complex glomerulonephritis IgA nephropathy Rapidly progressive glomerulonephritis with heart failure
Other	Drugs (D-penicillamine, propylthiouracil, carbimazole, cocaine, ...) Post-renal transplation failure Idiopathic pulmonary-renal syndrome Infection Coagulopathy Heart failure

Table 2. Etiology of pulmonary-renal syndrome

6. Clinical involvement

It is very important to establish an early diagnosis based on clinical vigilance, contemporary diagnostic laboratory support (immunology and biopsy) for the pulmonary-renal syndrome in order to avoid the severe consequences of rapid and irreversible loss of renal function or from severe pulmonary hemorrhage. Both can be avoided by appropriate initial immunosuppressive treatment [60]. In pulmonary-renal syndrome better understanding of interorgan-crosstalk is of utmost importance, as current clinical care is many times limited to preventive and supportive measures [24].

In main clinical entities (Goodpasture´s disease, ANCA associated vasculitis, SLE-associated vasculitis) induction and maintenance immunosupression is achieved by steroids and cyclophosphamide. Intensive plasma exchange to remove pathological antibodies, proinflammatory cytokines, complement compounds and factors of coagulation from circulation is beneficial for patients with pulmonary hemorrhage and severe kidney disease. Except of antibody removal, plasma exchange may have also other immunoregulatory effects and could potentiate the effects of immunosuppressive drugs [61]. Exchange procedures have beneficial effect on long-term renal recovery [62, 63]. Severe renal function impairment requires haemodialysis and progression to end stage renal failure renal replacement therapy is required [17]. In case of inevitable ICU admission supportive care is important as well.

During immunosuppressive regimes nosocomial infection used to be a common complication associated with high mortality [64]. Therefore minimizing the risk of infection has the highest of high priority. Patients with pulmonary-renal syndrome are often hypotensive because of a combination of dehydration, haemorrhage and systemic inflammatory response and may therefore require inotropic support [28]. Endotracheal intubation, tracheostomy, lung protective ventilation, transfusion and anticoagulation may be also necessary.

Antioxidant effect of N-acetylcystein published by Fernández-Fernández and Sesma [65] in one patient with WG and also our unpublished experience suggests clinical improvement of systemic inflammation. Administration of NAC is based on two significant studies: the IFIGENIA trial in 2005 [66] (Idiopathic Pulmonary Fibrosis International Group Exploring N-acetylcysteine I Annual study) and the study by Guilpain et al. [42]. Both studies have reported that NAC significantly reduced the activation of MPO and improved the survival of endothelial cells. In a recent experimental study by Lee et al. [67] continuous infusion of NAC attenuated inflammatory response and acute lung and kidney injury after hemorrhagic shock in rats. This result supports the clinical experience.

Some recent studies are focused on anti-TNF molecules, anti-B-cells blockers [68], anti-BlyS [69], anti-IL5 molecules [70], antithymocyte globulin [71], blockers of costimulatory molecules [72], tyrosine-kinase inhibitors [73] and proteasome inhibitors [74]. The results of these studies are sometimes controversial but there is a real hope that they will provide useful knowledge in the near future.

Many questions still remain unanswered also in the use of intravenous immunoglobulins (IVIG). Such treatment should be considered as an effective regimen in many "off label" indications particularly in cases where standard immunosuppressive regimes fail or could be harmful. Despite some evidence of efficacy, dosage and timing of IVIG therapy, as well as the question of its costs/benefit ratio still remain insufficiently documented and controlled trials with definitive conclusions for clinical indications are needed.

The basic immunomodulatory mechanisms of IVIG in autoimmune and inflammatory diseases are twofold. One is its action on humoral immunity and the second involves mechanisms of cell-mediated immunity. Both mechanisms interdependently involve modulation of expression and function of Fc receptors, interference with complement activation and the cytokine network, provision of antiidiotypic antibodies, modulation of dendritic cells, T and B-cell activation and differentiation and their effector functions [75]. Analogous to normal circulating immunoglobulins intravenous immunoglobulins have also anti-inflammatory properties modulating systemic inflammation during various inflammatory states.

According to BSR guidelines [76] IVIG may be considered as an alternative therapy in patients with refractory disease or in patients for whom conventional therapy is contraindicated, for example, in the presence of infection, in severely ill patients or in pregnancy (grade of recommendation B). In the management of refractory vasculitis it is important to identify causes of the vasculitis, such as, intercurrent infection or malignancy. In many European countries use of IVIG is limited for treatment of primary immune deficiencies where such treatment has been known to be life saving. Even though use of intravenous immunoglobulins in inflammatory diseases has been increased and a recent literature search revealed more than 150 off-label usages of IVIG, which included 6781 patients in clinical trials and 362 patients in case reports [77].

Until present immunological mechanisms of immunomodulatory effect of IVIG are not clearly known. In such context a question of adequate dosage appears in the relation of cost/benefits of unlabeled treatment. It is supposed that patients who respond to high-dose IVIG therapy would probably also respond to much lower doses, in many rheumatological indications vasculitides not excluded. In addition to economic reasons, low-dose regimen would likely help to reduce treatment related side effects. The lack of validated and generally accepted outcome measures as well as prospective clinical studies makes it difficult to compare the effect of different interventions in different cases [78].

7. Conclusions

Pulmonary-renal syndrome is a complex and heterogenous clinical picture involving rapid progressive glomerulonephritis and pulmonary capillaritis based on inflammation and necrosis of vessel wall. Morphological changes of pulmonary-renal syndrome are consequences of immunologically mediated processes and the unconctrolled derangement of the immune system could cause multiorgan dysfunction and fatal outcome.

The diagnostic procedure should focus on recognizing the earliest phases of the initiation and progression of the inflammation through a reliable panel of immunological and organ specific functional markers. In the near future novel diagnostic tools should be introduced in the diagnosis and differential diagnosis of pulmonary-renal syndrome, including gene expression profiles, cytokine profiles, markers of oxidative stress and many others.

Traditional clinical approach to treat pulmonary-renal syndrome was divided among rheumatologists, nephrologist and pneumologists but the improving knowledge of its pathogenesis clearly indicates the need of an interdisciplinary team work incorporating intensive care specialists and immunologists as well. This integrative approach could pave the way toward the introduction of more efficient novel treatment regimes. Another challenge is the high risk of relapses in these condition occurring up to 50 %, of the patients. Early establishment of the exact diagnosis and effective etiology oriented treatment in such cases is rather difficult task requiring further experimental and clinical research and cooperation of different specialists.

Perspective therapeutic approaches based on contemporary immunological knowledge (B-cell depletion, costimulatory molecule blockers, siRNAs controlling intracellular processes, cytokine treatment) supported by clinical experience will bring benefits for induction and maintenance of remission or also excluding the menacing catastrophic scenario of the disease.

Abbreviations

ANCA – anti-neutrophil cytoplasmic antibody, APS – antiphospholipid syndrome, CSS – Churg-Strauss syndrome, DAH – diffuse alveolar hemorrhage, GBM – glomerular basement membrane, GN - glomerulonephritis, GPA – granulomatosis with polyangiitis, GPS – Goodpasture´s syndrome, ICU – intensive care unit, IVIG – intravenous immunoglobulin, MCTD – mixed connective tissue disease, MPA – microscopic polyangiitis, MPO - myeloperoxidase, NAC – N-acetylcystein, NO –nitric oxide, eNOS – endothelial nitric oxide synthase, iNOS – inducible nitric oxide synthase, PRS – pulmonary-renal syndrome, RA – rheumatoid arthritis, siRNA - small interfering ribonucleic acids, ROS – reactive oxygen species, SLE – systemic lupus erythematosus, WG – Wegener´s granulomatosis

Author details

N. Lukán

4th Internal Department Medical Faculty, Safarik University, Košice, Slovak Republic

References

[1] Segen JC., editor. Concise Dictionary of Modern Medicine. New York: McGraw-Hill Companies; 2002.

[2] Sanders JS, Rutgers A, Stegeman CA, Kallenberg CG. Pulmonary-renal syndrome with a focus on anti-GBM disease. Semin Respir Crit Care Med 2011;32(3):328-34.

[3] Jennette JC, Falk RJ, Andrassy K, Bacon PA, Churg J, Gross WL, Hagen EC, Hoffman GS, Hunder GG, Kallenberg CG et al.Nomenclature of systemic vasculitides.Proposal of an international consensus conference. Arthritis Rheum 1994;37(2):187-192.

[4] Langford CA.Vasculitis. J Allergy Clin Immunol 2010;125(2)Suppl.2:S216-S225.

[5] Goodpasture EW.The significance of certain pulmonary lesions in relation to the aetiology of pneumonia. Am J Med Sci 1919;158:863-70.

[6] Smith W, Andrewes CH, Laidlaw PP.A virus obtained from influenza patients. Lancet 1933;2 (5732):66–68.

[7] Stanton MC, Tange JD. Goodpasture's syndrome (pulmonary haemorrhage associated with glomerulonephritis). Australas Ann Med 1958;7:132-44.

[8] Collins RD. Dr. Goodpasture: "I was not aware of such a connection between lung and kidney disease". Ann Diagn Pathol 2010;14(3):194-8.

[9] Lerner RA, Glassock RJ, Dixon FJ.The role of anti-glomerular basement membrane antibody in the pathogenesis of human glomerulonephritis. The Journal of experimental medicine 1967;126(6):989-1004.

[10] Lee RW, D'Cruz DP. Pulmonary renal vasculitis syndromes. Autoimmun Rev. 2010; 9 (10):657-60.

[11] Salant, DJ. Immunopathogenesis of crescentic glomerulonephritis and lung purpura. Kidney Int 1987; 32:408-425.

[12] Schwarz MI, Zamora MR, Hodges TN, Chan ED, Bowler RP, Tuder RM. Isolated pulmonary capillaritis and diffuse alveolar hemorrhage in rheumatoid arthritis and mixed connective tissue disease. Chest June 1998;113(6):1609-15.

[13] Jennette JC. Implications for pathogenesis of patterns of injury in small- and medium-sized vessel vasculitis. Cleve Clin J Med 2002;69(Suppl 2):SII33-38.

[14] Wegener F. Uber die eigenartige Rhinogene Granulomatose mit besonderer Beteiligung des Arteriensystems un der Nieren. Beitr Pathol Anat 1939;102:36-68.

[15] Former F. Uber die granulomatose Periglomerulitis. Schweiz Zeitschrift allgemeine Pathol Bakteriol 1950;13:42-59.

[16] Rutgers A, Slot M, van Paassen P, van Breda Vriesman P, Heeringa P, Tervaert JW. Coexistence of anti-glomerular basement membrane antibodies and myeloperoxidase-ANCAs in crescentic glomerulonephritis. Am J Kidney Dis 2005;46(2):253-62.

[17] Kambham N. Crescentic Glomerulonephritis: an update on Pauci-immune and Anti-GBM diseases. Adv Anat Pathol 2012;19(2):111-24.

[18] Cordier JF, Cottin V. Alveolar hemorrhage in vasculitis: primary and secondary. Semin Respir Crit Care Med 2012;32(3):310-21.

[19] Miller LR, Greenberg SD, McLarty JW. Lupus lung. Chest 1985;88(2):265-9.

[20] Jennette JC, Falk RJ.Vasculitis (Polyarteritis Nodosa, Microscopic Polyangitis, Wegener´s Granulomatosis, Henoch-Schönlein Purpura). In: Schrier RW. (ed.): Atlas of Diseases of the Kidney. Systemic Diseases and the Kidney. Volume IV. New Jersey: Wiley&Sons; 1999, pp. 22 – 34. Available from www.scribd.com/doc/70966728/Atlas-of-Diseases-of-the-Kidney-Vol-IV.

[21] Alenzi FQ, Salem ML, Alenazi FA, Wyse RK. Cellular and molecular aspects of Goodpasture syndrome. Iran J Kidney Dis 2012;6(1):1-8.

[22] de Lind van Wijngaarden RA, van Rijn L, Hagen EC, Watts RA, Gregorini G, Tervaert JW, Mahr AD, Niles JL, de Heer E, Bruijn JA, Bajema IM. Hypotheses on the etiology of antineutrophil cytoplasmic autoantibody associated vasculitis: the cause is hidden, but the result is known. Clin J Am Soc Nephrol 2008;3(1):237-52.

[23] Ko GJ, Rabb H, Hassoun HT. Kidney-lung crosstalk in the critically ill patient. Blood Purif 2009;28(2):75-83.

[24] Singbartl K. Renal-pulmonary crosstalk. Contrib Nephrol 2011;174:65-70.

[25] Short AK, Esnault VL, Lockwood CM. Anti-neutrophil cytoplasm antibodies and anti-glomerular basement membrane antibodies: two coexisting distinct autoreactivities detectable in patients with rapidly progressive glomerulonephritis. Am J Kidney Dis 1995;26(3):439-45.

[26] Kalluri R, Meyers K, Mogyorosi A, Madaio MP, Neilson EG. Goodpasture syndrome involving overlap with Wegener's granulomatosis and anti-glomerular basement membrane disease. J Am Soc Nephrol 1997;8(11):1795-800.

[27] Thurman JM. Triggers of inflammation after renal ischemia/reperfusion. Clin Immunol 2007;123(1):7-13.

[28] McCabe C, Jones Q, Nikolopoulou A, Wathen C, Luqmani R. Pulmonary-renal syndromes: an update for respiratory physicians. Respir Med 2011;105(10):1413-1421.

[29] Gröne HJ. Vasculitis - aspect of cellular and molecular pathogenesis. (German) Verh Dtsch Ges Pathol 2001;85:142-52.

[30] Bajwa A, Kinsey GR, Okusa MD. Immune mechanisms and novel pharmacological therapies of acute kidney injury. Curr Drug Targets 2009;10(12):1196-204.

[31] Campanholle G, Landgraf RG, Gonçalves GM, Paiva VN, Martins JO, Wang PH, Monteiro RM, Silva RC, Cenedeze MA, Teixeira VP, Reis MA, Pacheco-Silva A, Jancar S, Camara NO. Lung inflammation is induced by renal ischemia and reperfusion injury as part of the systemic inflammatory syndrome. Inflamm Res 2010;59(10): 861-9.

[32] Groshaus HE, Manocha S, Walley KR, Russell JA. Mechanisms of beta-receptor stimulation induced improvement of acute lung injury and pulmonary edema. Crit Care 2004; 8(4): 234-42.

[33] Hamacher J, Stammberger U, Roux J, Kumar S, Yang G, Xiong C, Schmid RA, Fakin RM, Chakraborty T, Hossain HM, Pittet JF, Wendel A, Black SM, Lucas R. The lectin-like domain of tumor necrosis factor improves lung function after rat lung transplantation - potential role for a reduction in reactive oxygen species generation. Crit Care Med 2010;38(3):871-8.

[34] Yang G, Hamacher J, Gorshkov B, White R, Sridhar S, Verin A, Chakraborty T, Lucas R. The Dual Role of TNF in Pulmonary Edema. J Cardiovasc Dis Res 2010;1(1):29-36.

[35] Schoeb TR, Jarmi T, Hicks MJ, Henke S, Zarjou A, Suzuki H, Kramer P, Novak J, Agarwal A, Bullard DC. eNOS inhibits the development of autoimmune-mediated vasculitis. Arthritis Rheum. 2012 Aug 29. doi: 10.1002/art.37683. [Epub ahead of print].

[36] Wever R, Boer P, Hijmering M, Stroes E, Verhaar M, Kastelein J, Versluis K, Lagerwerf F, van Rijn H, Koomans H, Rabelink T. Nitric oxide production is reduced in patients with chronic renal failure. Arterioscler Thromb Vasc Biol 1999;19(5):1168-72.

[37] Vaziri ND, Ni Z, Oveisi F, Liang K, Pandian R. Enhanced nitric oxide inactivation and protein nitration by reactive oxygen species in renal insufficiency. Hypertension 2002;39(1):135-41.

[38] Druhan LJ, Forbes SP, Pope AJ, Chen CA, Zweier JL, Cardounel AJ. Regulation of eNOS derived superoxide by endogenous methylarginines. Biochemistry 2008;47(27): 7256-63.

[39] Eiserich JP, Hristova M, Cross CE, Jones AD, Freeman BA, Halliwell B, van der Vliet A. Formation of nitric oxide-derived inflammatory oxidants by myeloperoxidase in neutrophils. Nature 1998;391(6665):393-7.

[40] Weyand CM, Goronzy JJ. Pathogenic mechanisms in giant cell arteritis. Cleve Clin J Med 2002;69(Suppl 2):SII28-32.

[41] Bratt J, Palmblad J. Cytokine-induced neutrophil-mediated injury of human endothelial cells. J Immunol 1997;159(2):912-8.

[42] Guilpain P, Servettaz A, Batteux F, Guillevin L, Mouthon L. Natural and disease associated anti-myeloperoxidase (MPO) autoantibodies. Autoimmun Rev 2008;7(6): 421-5.

[43] Spapen H, Zhang H, Demanet C, Vleminckx W, Vincent JL, Huyghens L. Does N-acetyl-L-cysteine influence cytokine response during early human septic shock? Chest 1998;113(6):1616-24.

[44] Park SJ, Pai KS, Kim JH, Shin JI. Beneficial effect of N-acetylcysteine on antineutrophil cytoplasmic antibody-associated vasculitis. J Rheumatol 2012;39(1):186.

[45] Shah SV, Baricos WH, Basci A. Degradation of human glomerular basement membrane by stimulated neutrophils. Activation of a metalloproteinase(s) by reactive oxygen metabolites. J Clin Invest 1987;79(1):25-31.

[46] Kalluri R, Cantley LG, Kerjaschki D, Neilson EG. Reactive oxygen species expose cryptic epitopes associated with autoimmune Goodpasture syndrome. J Biol Chem 2000;275(26):20027-32.

[47] Cohen IR, Cooke A. Natural autoantibodies might prevent autoimmune disease. Immunol Today 1986;7(12):363-364.

[48] Stegeman CA, Cohen-Tervaert JW, Sluiter WJ, Manson WL, de Jong PE, Kallenberg CGM. Association of chronic nasal carriage of staphylococcus aureus and higher relapse rates in Wegener granulomatosis. Ann Intern Med 1994;120(1):12-17.

[49] Boros P, Gondolesi G, Bromberg JS. High dose intravenous immunoglobulin treatment: mechanisms of action. Liver Transpl 2005;11(12):1469-1480.

[50] Sakaguchi S, Sakaguchi N, Asano M, Itoh M, Toda M. Immunologic self-tolerance maintained by activated T cells expressing IL-2 receptor alpha-chains (CD25). Breakdown of a single mechanism of self-tolerance causes various autoimmune diseases. J Immunol 1995;155(3):1151-64.

[51] Taams LS, Akbar AN. Peripheral generation and function of CD4+CD25+ regulatory T cells. Curr Top Microbiol Immunol 2005;293:115-31.

[52] Mills KH, McGuirk P. Antigen-specific regulatory T cells - their induction and role in infection. Semin Immunol 2004;16(2):107-17.

[53] Abdulahad WH, Stegeman CA, van der Geld YM, Doornbos-van der Meer B, Limburg PC, Kallenberg CG. Functional defect of circulating regulatory CD4+ T cells in patients with Wegener's granulomatosis in remission. Arthritis Rheum 2007;56(6): 2080-2091.

[54] Miossec P, Korn T, Kuchroo VK. Interleukin-17 and type 17 helper T cells. N Engl J Med 2009;361(9):888-898.

[55] Tadema H, Heeringa P, Kallenberg CG. Bacterial infections in Wegener's granulomatosis: mechanisms potentially involved in autoimmune pathogenesis. Curr Opin Rheumatol 2011;23(4):366-71.

[56] Sutton CE, Lalor SJ, Sweeney CM, Brereton CF, Lavelle EC, Mills KH. Interleukin-1 and IL 23 induce innate IL-17 production from gammadelta T cells, amplifying Th17 responses and autoimmunity. Immunity 2009;31(2):331-41.

[57] Ooi JD, Phoon RK, Holdsworth SR, Kitching AR. IL-23, not IL-12, directs autoimmunity to the Goodpasture antigen. J Am Soc Nephrol 2009;20(5):980-9.

[58] Fouser LA, Wright JF, Dunussi-Joannopoulos K, Collins M: Th17 cytokines and their emerging roles in inflammation and autoimmunity. Immunol Rev 2008;226:87-102.

[59] Thadhani R, Pascual M, Bonventre JV.Acute renal failure. N Engl J Med 1996 ; 334:1448-1460.

[60] Niles JL et al. The syndrome of lung hemorrhage and nephritis is usually an ANCA-associated condition. Arch Intern Med 1996;156:440-445.

[61] Peters DK, Rees AJ, Lockwood CM, Pusey CD. Treatment and prognosis in antibasement membrane antibody-mediated nephritis. Transplant Proc 1982;14(3):513-21.

[62] Gaskin G, Pusey CD. Plasmapheresis in antineutrophil cytoplasmic antibody-associated systemic vasculitis. Ther Apher 2001;5(3):176-81.

[63] Levy JB, Turner AN, Rees AJ, Pusey CD. Long term outcome of anti-glomerular basement membrane antibody disease treated with plasma exchange and immunosuppression. Ann Intern Med 2001;134:1033-42.

[64] Griffiths M, Brett S. The pulmonary physician in critical care illustrative care 3: pulmonary vasculitis. Thorax 2003;58:543-6.

[65] Fernández-Fernández FJ, Sesma P. Acetylcysteine as adjuvant therapy for vasculitis associated with antineutrophil cytoplasmic antibody. J Rheumatol 2011;38(4):785.

[66] Demedts M, Behr J, Buhl R, Costabel U, Dekhuijzen R, Jansen HM, MacNee W, Thomeer M, Wallaert B, Laurent F, Nicholson AG, Verbeken EK, Verschakelen J, Flower CD, Capron F, Petruzzelli S, De Vuyst P, van den Bosch JM, Rodriguez-Becerra E, Corvasce G, Lankhorst I, Sardina M, Montanari M; IFIGENIA Study Group. High-dose acetylcysteine in idiopathic pulmonary fibrosis. N Engl J Med 2005;353(21): 2229-42.

[67] Lee JH, Jo YH, Kim K, Lee JH, Rim KP, Kwon WY, Suh GJ, Rhee JE. Effect of N acetylcysteine (NAC) on acute lung injury and acute kidney injury in hemorrhagic shock. Resuscitation 2012 Jun 1. [Epub ahead of print].

[68] Dharmapalaiah C, Watts RA. The role of biologics in treatment of ANCA-associated vasculitis. Mod Rheumatol 2012;3:319-26.

[69] Manzi S, Sánchez-Guerrero J, Merrill JT, Furie R, Gladman D, Navarra SV, Ginzler EM, D'Cruz DP, Doria A, Cooper S, Zhong ZJ, Hough D, Freimuth W, Petri MA; on behalf of the BLISS-52 and BLISS-76 Study Groups. Effects of belimumab, a B lymphocyte stimulator-specific inhibitor, on disease activity across multiple organ domains in patients with systemic lupus erythematosus: combined results from two phase III trials. Ann Rheum Dis 2012;71(11):1833-1838.

[70] Walsh GM, Reslizumab. A humanized anti-IL-5 mAb for the treatment of eosinophil-mediated inflammatory conditions. Curr Opin Mol Ther 2009;11:329–36.

[71] Schmitt WH, Hagen EC, Neumann I, Nowack R, Flores-Suárez LF, Van der Woude FJ, European Vasculitis Study Gro up. Treatment of refractory Wegener's granuloma-

tosis with antithymocyte globulin (ATG): an open study in 15 patients. Kidney Int 2004;65:1440–8.

[72] Podojil JR, Miller SD. Molecular mechanisms of T-cell receptor and costimulatory molecule ligation/blockade in autoimmune disease therapy. Immunol Rev 2009;229(1):337-55.

[73] Kälsch AI, Soboletzki M, Schmitt WH, van der Woude FJ, Hochhaus A, Yard BA, Birck R. Imatinib mesylate, a new kid on the block for the treatment of anti-neutrophil cytoplasmic autoantibodies-associated vasculitis? Clin Exp Immunol 2008;3:391-8.

[74] Bontscho J, Schreiber A, Manz RA, Schneider W, Luft FC, Kettritz R. Myeloperoxidase-specific plasma cell depletion by bortezomib protects from anti-neutrophil cytoplasmic autoantibodies-induced glomerulonephritis. J Am Soc Nephrol 2011;22(2): 336-48.

[75] Negi VS, Elluru S, Siberil S, Graff-Dubois S, Mouthon L, Kazatchkine MD, Lacroix-Desmazes S, Bayry J, Kaveri SV. Intravenous immunoglobulin: an update on the clinical use and mechanisms of action. J Clin Immunol 2007;27(3):233-245.

[76] Lapraik C, Watts R, Bacon P, Carruthers D, Chakravarty K, D'Cruz D, Guillevin L, Harper L, Jayne D, Luqmani R, Mooney J, Scott D.BSR and BHPR Standards, Guidelines and Audit Working Group. BSR and BHPR guidelines for the management of adults with ANCA associated vasculitis. Rheumatology (Oxford) 2007;46(10): 1615-1626.

[77] Leong H, Stachnik J, Bonk ME, Matuszewski KA.Unlabeled uses of intravenous immune globulin. Am J Health Syst Pharm 2008;65(19):1815-1824.

[78] Yu Z, Lennon VA.Mechanism of intravenous immune globulin therapy in antibody-mediated autoimmune diseases. N Engl J Med 1999;340(3):227-228.

Chapter 4

Immunopathophysiology of Large Vessel Involvement in Giant Cell Arteritis — Implications on Disease Phenotype and Response to Treatment

Panagiota Boura, Konstantinos Tselios,
Ioannis Gkougkourelas and
Alexandros Sarantopoulos

Additional information is available at the end of the chapter

http://dx.doi.org/10.5772/55222

1. Introduction

Giant cell arteritis (GCA) or temporal arteritis or Horton's disease is classified amongst the primary large-vessel vasculitides, according to the 2012 revision of the Chapel-Hill classification criteria. The disease develops almost exclusively in patients older than 50 years (prevalence of 1 in 500 individuals in this age spectrum) and represents the most common vasculitis in Western countries. [1] Incidence rates are progressively increased and estimated to range between 10-30 new cases per 100000 persons beyond the age of 50, while the highest frequency is reported in Scandinavian and North American populations. [2]

The disease affects, mainly, the large- and medium-sized extracranial branches of the carotid artery and, classical clinical features, such as headache, jaw claudication, scalp tenderness and visual impairment, are closely related to this marked cranial tropism of GCA. [3]

On a histopathological basis, GCA involves all layers of the arterial wall, including the adventitia. Inflammatory lesions consist of activated T cells, dendritic cells (DCs) and macrophages. These lesions are believed to be the histopathologic hallmark of GCA and are characterized by a predominance of mononuclear infiltrates or granulomas, usually with multinucleated giant cells. [4]

Besides the inflammation of the carotid branches, involvement of the great arteries, such as the aorta and its main tributaries, was initially recognized in the late 1930s and reported sporadically thereafter in necropsy or histopathologic studies of surgically resected tissues. [5,

6] The prevalence of aortic inflammation, in unselected patients with GCA, has not been fully estimated, although in a systematic necropsy study of 13 patients, large artery involvement was demonstrated in over 90% of them. [7] In more recent studies, an increased prevalence of aortic aneurysm (compared to the general population), was observed in GCA patients. [8]

Retrospective surveys, over extended time periods (20-50 years), confirmed that aortic aneurysm occurs in 9.5-22.5% of these patients and, particularly, in the first 5 years of follow up. [9, 10] These findings indicate that large vessel involvement in GCA may be more frequent than anticipated. Based on these data, a recent prospective study from Prieto-Gonzalez et al, using non-invasive techniques (CT angiography), concluded that large vessel vasculitis occurs in two thirds of patients with GCA, while aortic dilatation is already present in 15% of them at the time of diagnosis. [11]

Large vessel involvement represents a significant cause of death in GCA and it may be asymptomatic and lead to aortic dissection and/or rupture. [12] These findings underline the importance of elucidating the pathophysiologic basis of the disease, in which the immune system seems to play a central role.

In this chapter, a thorough review of the current evidence for disease immunopathophysiology, in regard to disease phenotype and response to treatment, is presented.

2. The pathophysiologic basis of GCA

In accordance with the pathophysiology of many immune-mediated diseases, GCA is believed to represent the final result of the complex interactions between three distinct factors, namely the host (by means of the individual genetic background), the environment (pathogens, physicochemical exposures etc.) and the unique immune system response. However, the exact etiology of the disease remains unknown.

3. Genetic predisposition

Several studies have demonstrated that GCA is a complex disease, where multiple genes confer susceptibility. In most surveys, the allele HLA-DRB1*04 has been shown to be related to disease and its severity. [13] More recent studies have implied the role of genetic variants in the evolution of the immune and inflammatory pathways in GCA and its clinical expression. Polymorphisms include the rs20541 (R130Q) polymorphism of the IL-13 gene [14], the rs2779251 in the NOS2 gene, the rs1885657 and the rs2010963 in the VEGF gene [15] and, also, the TLR-4 (+896A/G) gene. [16]

http://dx.doi.org/10.5772/55222

4. Environmental factors

Several experimental studies, using DNA analysis, have shown a possible relation of GCA with certain infectious agents, such as the human papilloma virus (HPV) [17], *Chlamydia spp,* herpes viruses and PARVO B19 among others. [18] Older epidemiological studies have also demonstrated that increased incidence of GCA was observed in close relation to two independent epidemics of *Mycoplasma pneumoniae* infection. [19] However, not all studies confirmed these associations and GCA initiation is not definitely considered to be triggered by infectious agents. [20]

5. The immune system in GCA

Although evidence regarding the genetic background of GCA and the possible influence of external factors, such as viruses and bacteria, have not elucidated disease pathogenesis, it is now well understood that the immune system plays a central role in the disease process. GCA is a complex systematic disorder and it is believed to represent the result of the breakdown of immunologic tolerance, resulting from interactions between the immune system and poorly defined components of the arterial wall.

A single triggering factor, initiating the inflammatory process, has not been yet identified. The initial insult may lead to a foreign-body giant cell attack on calcified internal elastic membrane in arteries and calcified atrophic parts of the medium layer of the aorta. [21] The prerequisite for a calcified artery explains why GCA almost exclusively occurs in older people.

Recent studies have raised the possibility that, in GCA, both the innate and the adaptive arms of the immune system are activated and may lead to vessel wall injury through, at least two, distinct pathophysiological mechanisms. [22]

6. Innate immunity abnormalities in GCA

Immune responses are initiated by the recognition of foreign molecular structures, such as invading pathogens, by the antigen presenting cells (APCs) of the innate immune system. Tissue macrophages and dendritic cells (DCs) represent the main classes of professional APCs and are characterized by the membrane expression of germ-line receptors (pattern recognition receptors, PRRs). These receptors are able to recognize specific molecular patterns of exogenous and/or endogenous foreign proteins, known as pathogen associated molecular patterns (PAMPs) and damage associated molecular patterns (DAMPs).

Upon recognition of a certain PAMP or DAMP, dendritic cells become differentiated and activated and produce cytokines, which are able to recruit neutrophils and macrophages, activate the adaptive immune system and trigger the complement cascade. The physiological goal of early innate immune response is to control and demarcate infection and prevent microbe spreading and further tissue damage.

Recently, DCs were shown to initiate the immune response in GCA. [23] These cells lay dormant, in a ring-like structure around the adventitia-media border. It is suggested that, in normal arteries, DCs are sentinels that form a part of the first line immune defense of the vessel wall. [24]

The population of the immune cells in the adventitia of the large-vessel wall is mainly consisted of immature myeloid DCs, with a characteristically high threshold of activation. [25] In contrast to mature APCs that induce adaptive immunity, immature DCs do not express co-stimulatory molecules on their surface, such as CD80 and CD86. This condition is primarily responsible for maintaining an anergic state for T cells. In normal arteries, immature APCs are tolerogenic, thus supporting T-cell unresponsiveness. [21] They have been found to be positive for the S-100 protein and express the chemokine receptor CCR6. [26] As guardians of the immunoprivileged arterial wall, DCs are committed to protect the structural integrity of these vital and non-regenerative tissue structures.

However, in susceptible individuals, such as those bearing the HLA-DR4 allele or in older persons (immune-aging), an unknown instigator or a persistent stimulus activates DCs and initiates an innate immune response. In this context, certain antigens (derived from pathogens or locally formatted by tissue calcification) are considered to infiltrate the vessel wall adventitia, through vasa vasorum, and activate immature DCs.

Physiologically, dendritic cells subsequently migrate to the local lymph nodes and clear the antigens, without triggering inflammation. [26] In GCA, however, for yet ill-defined reasons, the activated DCs remain *in situ* and mature in the vessel wall. [27] Existing evidence supports that the maturation of DCs is a very early step in the initiation of the vasculitic process and occurs long before the chronic phase of wall inflammation. In biopsy studies from patients with polymyalgia rheumatica (PMR), mature DCs, already expressing co-stimulatory molecules, were found in their temporal arteries, despite the absence of any clinically apparent sign of inflammation. [25] These observations are closely correlated with the fact that a great proportion of PMR patients will eventually develop giant cell arteritis.

The principal role of DCs in GCA pathogenesis lies, not only in initiating the inflammatory process, but, also, in perpetuating immune reactions. Dendritic cells, found in vasculitic lesions, are able to produce high amounts of IL-12 and IL-18 and up-regulate the release of IFN-γ from T cells. [22] In addition, dendritic cells, in inflamed arteries, can release the homing chemokines CCL19 and CCL21, which bind to the receptor CCR7. The expression of CCR7 results in the local arrest of activated DCs, which are no longer able to leave the tissue. Instead, they are trapped in the arterial wall and enforce an aberrant T-cell response. [28] Furthermore,

http://dx.doi.org/10.5772/55222

it has been shown that DCs' depletion abrogates vasculitis, thus confirming the critical role of activated DCs in sustaining wall inflammation. [29]

The activation of vascular DCs is mediated via the ligation of their TLRs. It has been shown that certain infectious agents are able to legate to specific Toll-like receptors, such as TLR-4 (LPS) or TLR-5 (flagellin). The ligation of a PAMP (or DAMP), such as LPS or flagellin, to the extracellular portion of the TLR provokes the activation of the intracellular TRAM motif and the consequent activation of an intracellular phosphorylation cascade (second message). The final result is the activation of the NfKB, which enters the nucleus and induces certain genes. This mechanism leads to the translation of pro-inflammatory molecules with autocrine or paracrine actions, expression of co-stimulatory receptors on cell surface and production of antimicrobial substances. [26]

Additional research, in regard to the role of TLRs in GCA pathogenesis, led to some very interesting results. It is well known that GCA shows an impressive, yet unexplained, predilection for specific sites of the vasculature, such as the 2nd to 5th aortic branches. [1] Histopathologic studies demonstrated that DCs express different type of TLRs in different arteries. [30]

The distribution of TRLs in the vessel wall is highly determined by the embryological origin of the tissue. The aortic arch and its branches derive from the ectoderma, whereas the descending aorta derives from mesodermal cells. The heterogeneity of the immune response in GCA is believed to be strongly influenced by the specific type of TLRs, whose expression varies in the different blood vessels. Indeed, in an experimental study, Pryshchep et al showed that the distribution of TLRs, in various sites of the vascular tree, determine the extent and profile of the inflammatory reactions. [30] DCs, with differential surface expression of TLRs, display a marked heterogeneity in their immune-regulatory functions, providing a possible clue toward the tissue tropism of GCA. Furthermore, the immunological identity of blood vessels, as defined by the expression of a vessel-specific profile of TLRs, has been considered to determine the nature of the inflammatory reaction in various types of vasculitides. [21]

In this context, it has been shown that TLR-4, abundantly expressed on adventitial DCs, recognize LPS from bacterial pathogens. Upon recognition, IFN-γ is produced in large amounts and leads the subsequent mononuclear infiltration in all layers of the arterial wall. This all-layer inflammation characterizes panarteritis, with granuloma formation, which is typically found in biopsies of the temporal artery in GCA. [31]

On the contrary, when TLR-5 recognizes flagellin, the elicited inflammatory response is characterized by the sole infiltration of the adventitia (periarteritis). In this case, disruption of the elastic lamina and subsequent luminal occlusion is typically lacking. [31] Clinical observations have suggested that periarteritis rarely accompanies systematic inflammatory processes, such as aneurysm formation. Subtle alterations in inflammatory reactions guided by DCs with TLR-4 and/or TLR-5 overexpression may explain the differences in the clinical phenotype of giant cell arteritis.

Nevertheless, independently of the mode of the initial stimulation, DCs become activated and subsequently produce cytokines with redundant and pleiotropic actions. In inflamed temporal arteries, DCs secrete pro-inflammatory cytokines, mainly IL-2, IL-6 and IFN-γ, which, in turn, mediate the recruitment of inflammatory cells, inhibition of cell migration, enhancement of T cell proliferation and stimulation of T and B cells. [32] The net result is further amplification of the immune response, through positive feedback loops.

7. Adaptive immunity abnormalities in GCA

The differentiation and activation of DCs (following stimulation via their TLRs) induces the subsequent recruitment of T cells into the vessel wall. Indeed, several studies on activation patterns and inflammatory mediators in GCA, have confirmed that the progression of the immune response is totally dependent on CD4+ T cells. [33] These cells are able to orchestrate the stimulation of macrophages that lead to vessel response to injury, resulting in luminal stenosis or wall destruction and aneurysm formation.

Upon antigen recognition, CD4+ T cells are activated and differentiated into effector and memory T cells, while the antigen-specific subpopulation is 10 to 100-fold expanded. Under physiological conditions, only a few antigen-specific memory T cells are capable to persist indefinitely and provide life-long protection against pathogens. In parallel, these memory cells comprise the main barrier against the elimination of T-cell mediated autoimmune responses.

In GCA, several efforts to recognize a single antigen that may initiate the pathogenic specific immune response have not been fruitful. [20] In accordance, attempts to isolate the T cell clone, which is responsible for the vascular pathology in the disease, have suggested more heterogeneity than expected. Studies focusing on T cell receptor V genes in the arterial wall and the peripheral blood of GCA patients have arrived at the conclusion that the T cell repertoire is significantly biased. [34, 35] Sequence analysis of the CD4+ T cells isolated from the inflamed temporal arteries has strongly supported local T cell activation and expansion of only a few selected T cell specificities. Notably, T cells isolated from the right and left temporal arteries of the same patient utilized identical T cell receptors. [36]

More recent studies confirmed that multiple T cell lineages contribute to the disease process. Histopathologic analyses from temporal arteries, both prior to therapy and on therapy, convincingly proved that two cell lineages, Th1 and Th17, infiltrate the vessel wall prior to therapy. [37] The concurrent presence of the two T cell lineages coincided closely with the stimulation of two distinct immune axes, an IL-12-IFN-γ axis and an IL-1-IL-23 axis. It seems that different APC signals are able to recruit either the IFN-γ-dependent or the IL-17-dependent arm of the adaptive immunity, thus raising the possibility that more than one instigator is involved in GCA. [21]

8. Th1 cells in GCA

Th1 cells represent the dominant cell population in the intramural lesions and the periphery of patients with untreated GCA. [37] These cells produce IFN-γ, as their signature cytokine, which, physiologically, has a critical role against viral and intracellular bacterial infections. Once called macrophage activating factor, IFN-γ target macrophages and provide a substantial pro-inflammatory environment.

IFN-γ committed T cells are considered to account for >20% of circulating CD4+ T cells, an almost 100% increase compared to age-matched healthy controls. [38] Corticosteroid therapy cannot affect the expansion of this subpopulation, indicating continuous signaling from the respective DCs. The underlying mechanism of this resistance involves the triggering of APCs that continue to release IL-12. Actually, both in the blood and the temporal arteries of GCA patients, IL-12 production continued unabated during the chronic phase of the disease in treated patients. [38]

At the tissue level, cytokine profiling in GCA temporal arteries has demonstrated robust expression of IFN-γ and an association with a defined disease phenotype. [32] In particular, high tissue IFN-γ levels are typical for patients with ischaemic complications, implicating its crucial participation in the process leading to luminal occlusion. Pathophysiological studies have correlated increased IFN-γ levels with the production of vascular endothelial growth factor (VEGF) and platelet derived growth factor (PDGF), which are molecules implicated in the intimal response that leads to lumen stenosis. [39, 40] VEGF may, in turn, promote IFN-γ production, thus leading to a vicious cycle of inflammation and structural stenosis. [39]

It is currently unknown which aspects of the granulomatous inflammation depend upon IFN-γ. The ability of this cytokine to activate monocytes and macrophages certainly has a role in promoting the differentiation of lesional histiocytes. However, the profound differences in the clinical presentation of treated and untreated GCA patients suggest that IFN-γ is less relevant to the systemic manifestations of the disease and, instead, the major mediator of vessel wall destruction. [21]

9. Th17 cells in GCA

Th17 cells play an important role in antimicrobial immunity where they regulate the recruitment of neutrophils and facilitate protection against extracellular bacteria and fungi. Far beyond their role in host defense, Th17 cells have been implicated in the pathogenesis of several autoimmune and inflammatory disorders, such as rheumatoid arthritis, multiple sclerosis and inflammatory bowel disease. [41]

In untreated GCA patients, the frequency of Th17 cells is 10-fold elevated in the peripheral blood and they accumulate in the vascular infiltrates. [37] In healthy individuals, Th17 cells are infrequent and account for less than 0.3% of the circulating CD4+ T cells. In newly diagnosed GCA patients, an average of 2.2% of circulating CD4+ T cells were found to be IL-17 producers, while in some patients these cells were >5%.

In contrast to the Th1 lineage, Th17 cells displayed a totally different sensitivity to corticosteroid therapy. Prednisone therapies led to a fast and, almost, complete reduction of both circulating and lesional Th17 cells, as, in treated patients, only 0.4% of the circulating CD4+ T cells were capable of producing IL-17. [38] Taking into account that the systemic manifestations of GCA, such as fever and PMR, are the most responsive to steroid therapy and coincide with the normalization of Th17 cells, it can be speculated that these features are pathophysiologically related to the Th17 response. In addition, corticosteroid therapy was shown to suppress the entire IL-1 – IL-6 – IL-17 axis. [38]

The specific circumstances under which the Th17 response is amplified are not well understood, but studies, in untreated patients, showed that circulating monocytes (primed by IFN-γ) produce significant amounts of Th17-polarizing cytokines, such as IL-6 and IL-23. Of note, IL-6 may represent a reliable biomarker for assessing disease activity over time.

Latest studies showed that Th17 cells posses a substantial plasticity and they are able to transform into Th1 cells and release IFN-γ. [22] It is possible that, at least partially, Th17 represent the precursor cells that will progress to Th1 cells in a chronic disease process. On the other hand, one could expect that the successful suppression of Th17 cells (after steroid therapy) would eventually lead to the reduction of the Th1 cells, but this was not confirmed in experimental studies. Furthermore, there is evidence that there may be a small proportion of CD4+ T cells that are able to secrete both IL-17 and IFN-γ. The presence of these double producers was confirmed in atherosclerosis, although in GCA, these cells behave like the Th17 cells, in terms of steroid responsiveness. [22, 42] These findings suggest that these cells are not important in promoting the chronic phase of the disease.

10. The final common pathway: Mechanisms of arterial wall destruction in GCA

After the expansion of the Th1 and Th17 cells, the production of their related cytokines is capable to drive the inflammatory reaction in the vessel wall. IFN-γ induces macrophages towards their effector functions, mainly, the formation of multinucleated giant cells and granulomatous inflammation. [29] Granuloma formation may lead to lumen stenosis and, thus to the ischemic complications of GCA. It is interesting that PMR patients share some clinical features with GCA, although they do not develop ischemic complications. [3] This is possibly related to the lack of IFN-γ from resected arteries of PMR patients. [22] Unsuppressed actions of IFN-γ on macrophages could explain why patients, under corticosteroid treatment, may still develop devastating occlusive vasculitis.

The pro-inflammatory environment, shaped by IL-1, IL-6, IL-17, IL-23 and IFN-γ, promotes the infiltration of the arterial wall adventitia by activated monocytes and neutrophils, via the vasa vasorum. The endothelial cells of these small capillaries in the vessel wall upregulate the expression of certain adhesion molecules, which attract and restrain inflammatory cells. Within the vessel wall, altered macrophage function enhances IFN-γ production (through IL-12 release) and the subsequent recruitment of additional macrophages and lymphocytes, thus creating a vicious cycle. Intimal macrophages also express nitric oxide (NO) synthetase, which augments the capillary permeability and peroxynitrite, which has been associated with endothelial dysfunction. [29]

Additionally, reactive oxygen species (ROS) are secreted by macrophages into the surrounding tissues and degrade the proteins of the extracellular matrix. Oxygen-derived free radicals and their metabolites promote tissue injury through multiple mechanisms, the most important being oxidation of membrane lipids, resulting in structural disintegration and cell death. Reactive oxygen intermediates are not only directly cytotoxic; they can also alter cellular function by disrupting intracellular signaling cascades. The net result is the degradation of the media and the weakening of the arterial wall.

Additionally, metalloproteases (MMPs) that are released by macrophages and vascular smooth muscle cells are associated with matrix degeneration, intimal hyperplasia and luminal narrowing. In particular, matrix metalloproteases MMP-2 and MMP-9, which possess gelatinase activity, have both been detected in the infiltrates of the arterial wall in patients with GCA. [43] Due to their ability to destroy elastin, MMP-2 and MMP-9 have been suggested to play a primary role in the internal elastic lamina degradation, a characteristic pathologic finding in GCA. These metalloproteases are able to differentially regulate vascular smooth muscle cell migration and cell-mediated collagen organization. [44]

In parallel, the inflammatory milieu provokes the apoptosis of smooth muscle cells, which are primarily responsible for the compliance of the arterial wall. Aneurysms can eventually be formed in these hemodynamically non-compliant sites of the vasculature. [29]

Although the pathophysiologic mechanism underlying aneurysm formation in GCA is well understood, the pathophysiologic basis of lumen stenosis is not equally clear. It has been shown that IFN-γ may produce endothelial hyperplasia and subsequent narrowing of the vascular lumen. [22] Interestingly, it was demonstrated that the extent of platelet-derived growth factor (PDGF) production, in the vascular lesions, correlates with the degree of luminal occlusion and the severity of the ischaemic manifestations. [40] In accordance, VEGF derived from activated macrophages deregulate the endothelial functions. Eventually, anatomical alterations will ensue, leading to the remodeling of inflamed arteries. The physiologic basis of these findings may rely on the increased needs of the hyperplastic arterial wall in means of oxygen and nutrients. Neoangiogenesis, provoked by these factors, may supply the needed nutrients in the hyperplastic wall but, also, effectively supports the destructive inflammatory reaction. [45] Nonetheless, thrombotic occlusions are rare complications of giant cell arteritis.

The outline of GCA immunopathogenesis is displayed in Figure 1.

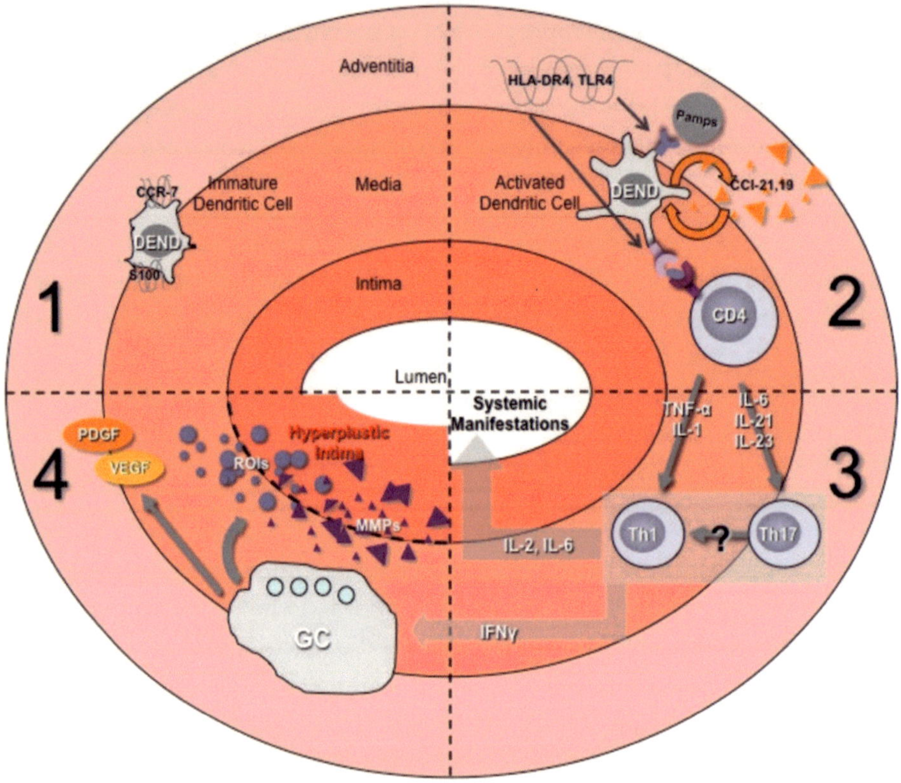

Figure 1. The immunopathophysiologic basis of giant cell arteritis. 1. In normal arteries, immature DCs, in the adventitia-media border, are the immune sentinels of the vessel wall. 2. In GCA, their maturation and activation (by an unknown instigator) leads to the recruitment of CD4+ T cells into the vessel wall. 3. CD4+ T cells are able to differentiate into either the Th17 arm of the immune response, which is responsible for the systemic manifestations of the disease, or the Th1 arm. 4. Th1 cells along with IFN-γ are able to drive the activation of macrophages, the formation of granuloma and the destruction of the structural integrity of the vessel wall via the secretion of MMPs and ROS.

11. Newer concepts in GCA pathogenesis: Immune and vascular aging

According to the 1990 ACR criteria for the diagnosis of GCA, age above 50 is considered a major criterion for disease diagnosis. [46] Susceptibility of elder persons for GCA is considered to be the result of two separate degenerative processes.

Firstly, immunesenescence is characterized by the shrinkage of the naïve T-cell pool, loss of immune-regulation and impairment of innate immunity. [47] More specifically, alterations in innate immunity functions, such as impairment of DC trafficking and prolonged maintenance of TLR expression raise the possibility of uncontrolled inflammatory reactions in immunopriviliged sites. Furthermore, the immune aging process results in an increase in basal cytokine production by macrophages, dendritic cells, endothelial cells and fibroblasts.

http://dx.doi.org/10.5772/55222

Secondly, biochemical modifications in vessel wall extracellular structures, such as the disorganization of the elastic fibers, render the vessel wall extremely compliant. Vascular smooth muscle cells decrease in number and function. The media becomes thinner and deposition of calcium is not unusual. Beyond the alterations observed in biomechanical parameters, the "old" artery seems to provide a distinct micro-environment that potentially increases the risk for the formation of a novel spectrum of neoantigens and the persistence of inflammatory reactions. [48]

12. Clinical phenotype and response to treatment are dependent on pathophysiology

Aneurysm formation in GCA is reported in 3% of the patients with 3 months disease duration and 18-27 % of patients with 6 months duration. [49, 50] Cumulatively, the relative risk for aneurysm formation is estimated to be 17.3. [51]

Disease diagnosis is straightforward in typical cases with headache, temporal tenderness, non palpable temporal arteries, jaw claudication and systemic symptoms (fever, malaise, weight loss) in an individual beyond 50 years of age. Unfortunately, a considerable proportion of patients presents with minor or no symptoms from the cranial arteries, which is presumably the hallmark of GCA.

Temporal artery biopsy represents the diagnostic gold standard, as its sensitivity is reported to exceed 85%. It should be mentioned that negative biopsy does not exclude GCA, as the lesions are skipped and long tissue specimens (>20mm) are required. Common causes of false negative results are the incomplete technique (sampling error) and the lack of sensitive pathologic criteria. Thus, in highly suspected cases, a second, contralateral, biopsy is recommended. Recent studies suggest ultrasonography-guided biopsy to precisely locate the patchy lesions of vessel wall inflammation. [52]

Another advanced technique to detect vascular inflammatory sites is FDG-PET (fluorodeoxyglucose positron emission tomography) imaging, which is currently incorporated in diagnostic algorithms. [53]

Immune system abnormalities play a critical role in GCA pathogenesis and are able to drive, not only clinical phenotype, but, also, response to treatment. DCs have been shown to initiate the immune response, as the number of myeloid DCs significantly increases in the adventitia of affected arteries and they appear to be activated via ligation of their TLR-4 (LPS) or TLR-5 (flagellin). [31] Stimulation of DCs via these TLRs induces the subsequent recruitment of T cells into the vessel wall, where they undergo local proliferation and activation. T cells produce pro-inflammatory cytokines to regulate the functions of macrophages, vascular smooth muscle cells and endothelial cells, while they were proved to belong to either Th1 or Th17 lineage. [22]

Th17 cells secrete IL-17 and provide the early immune response in GCA, where these cells are reported to be 10-fold elevated in initial phases. Furthermore, in untreated patients, circulating monocytes (primed by IFN-γ) produce significant amounts of Th17-polarizing cytokines, such as IL-6 and IL-23. Th17 response is considerably sensitive to steroids and is related to the inflammatory phenotype of GCA, like fever and PMR. [37] The most common clinical manifestations of the disease include constitutional symptoms (anorexia, weight loss), fever (in some cases fever of unknown origin), headache (usually localized in the temporal region), and polymyalgia rheumatica. This cluster of symptoms is attributed to the initial Th17 response and has been shown to respond adequately to steroids. [38]

Th1 cells represent the dominant cellular population at the tissue level and the periphery of patients with untreated GCA. These cells produce IFN-γ, target macrophages and provide a substantial pro-inflammatory environment. Additionally, IFN-γ is strongly related to elevated levels of metalloproteases (MMP-2, MMP-9), which lead to vessel wall destruction and aneurysm formation. Th1 response is believed to be steroid resistant (in usual doses), as IFN-γ committed T cells and soluble IFN-γ are not affected even after months of steroid therapy. [38] The late clinical manifestations in the disease course, such as jaw claudication, tongue claudication, scalp necrosis and visual impairment, represent ischemic complications resulting from this Th1-IFN-γ driven process.

On the other hand, thoracic and abdominal aortic aneurysms comprise the most dreaded complications of GCA. These manifestations are mediated through an intense Th1 response that leads to IFN-γ secretion, macrophage activation and release of metalloproteases into the aortic wall. This leads eventually to internal elastic lamina rupture, intimal hyperplasia and lumen stenosis or aneurysm formation. [21] This sequela has been shown to be steroid-resistant even if used in high doses.

Glucocorticoids, while the mainstay of therapy in GCA, do not exert the expected efficacy in Th1-driven aneurysmal disease. [38] Based on these data, glucocorticoids should be instituted promptly once the diagnosis of GCA is suspected. The optimal dose for remission induction in GCA remains uncertain. An initial daily dose of 40 to 60 mg of prednisone or its equivalent is reported to be adequate in almost all cases. [54] In severe, life threatening cases or, when the visual loss is considered imminent, intravenous methylprednisolone is recommended, while tapering can begin once the disease has been adequately controlled, with a rate of 3-4 mg/week. Most patients require medium doses of steroids for at least two years, since relapse risk is high.

Adjuvant therapy is usually needed to avoid chronic side effects, but no agent (methotrexate, IVIGs or other cytotoxic agents) has so far proven satisfactory efficacy. [55-57] Recent advances in GCA pathophysiology may lead to alternative treatments, like those which interrupt Th17 differentiation, such as tocilizumab. [58]

In conclusion, large vessel involvement in GCA is characterized by a biphasic pathophysiologic process. Initial Th17 response will lead to the steroid-sensitive systemic inflammatory features of the disease, while, in late phases, Th1 response is responsible for the steroid-resistant aneurysmal disease. Given the fact that these complications may be life-threatening, it is reasonable to be thoroughly evaluated and managed promptly, either by surgical or by pharmaceutical means or both.

http://dx.doi.org/10.5772/55222

Author details

Panagiota Boura*, Konstantinos Tselios, Ioannis Gkougkourelas and Alexandros Sarantopoulos

Clinical Immunology Unit, 2nd Department of Internal Medicine, Hippokration General Hospital, Aristotle University of Thessaloniki, Thessaloniki, Greece

References

[1] Salvarani C, Cantini F, Hunder GG. Polymyalgia rheumatica and giant cell arteritis. Lancet 2008; 372: 234-45

[2] Gonzalez-Gay MA, Martinez-Dubois C, Agudo M, Pompei O, Blanco R, Llorca J. Giant cell arteritis: epidemiology, diagnosis, and management. Curr Rheumatol Rep 2010; 12(6): 436-42

[3] Salvarani C, Pipitone N, Versari A, Hunder GG. Clinical features of polymyalgia rheumatica and giant cell arteritis. Nat Rev Rheumatol 2012 Jul 24 doi: 10.1038/nrrheum.201.97 (Epub ahead of print)

[4] Stacy RC, Rizzo JF, Cestari DM. Subtleties in the histopathology of giant cell arteritis. Semin Ophthalmol 2011; 26: 342-8

[5] Hunder GG. The early history of giant cell arteritis and polymyalgia rheumatica: first descriptions to 1970. Mayo Clin Proc 2006; 81: 1071-83

[6] Homme JL, Aubry MC, Edwards WD et al. Surgical pathology of the ascending aorta: a clinicopathologic study of 513 cases. Am J Surg Pathol 2006; 30: 1159-68

[7] Ostberg G. Morphological changes in the large arteries in polymyalgia rheumatica. Acta Med Scand Suppl 1972; 533: 135-59

[8] Evans JM, O'Fallon WM, Hunder GG. Increased incidence of aortic aneurysm and dissection in giant cell (temporal) arteritis. A population-based study. Ann Intern Med 1995; 122: 502-7

[9] Nuenninghoff DM, Hunder GG, Christianson TJ et al. Incidence and predictors of large-artery complication (aortic aneurysm, aortic dissection and/or large artery stenosis) in patients with giant cell arteritis: a population-based study over 50 years. Arthritis Rheum 2003; 48: 3522-31

[10] Garcia-Martinez A, Hernandez-Rodriguez J, Arguis P et al. Development of aortic aneurysm/dilatation during the follow-up of patients with giant cell arteritis: a cross-sectional screening of fifty-four prospectively followed patients. Arthritis Rheum 2008; 59: 422-30

[11] Pietro-Gonzalez S, Arguis P, Garcia-Martinez A, Espigol-Frigole G, Tavera-Bahilo I, Butjosa M et al. Large vessel involvement in biopsy-proven giant cell arteritis: prospective study in 40 newly diagnosed patients using CT angiography. Ann Rheum Dis 2012; 71: 1170-6

[12] Nuenninghoff DM, Hunder GG, Christianson TJ et al. Mortality of large-artery complication (aortic aneurysm, aortic dissection and/or large artery stenosis) in patients with giant cell arteritis: a population-based study over 50 years. Arthritis Rheum 2003; 48: 3532-7

[13] Gonzalez-Gay MA, Amoli MM, Garcia-Porrua C, Ollier WE. Genetic markers of disease susceptibility and severity in giant cell arteritis and polymyalgia rheumatica. Semin Arthritis Rheum 2003; 33: 38-48

[14] Alvarez-Rodriguez L, Lopez-Hoyos M, Carrasco-Marin E, Mata C, Calvo-Alen J, Aurrecoechea E et al. Analysis of the rs20541 (R130Q) polymorphism in the IL-13 gene in patients with elderly-associated chronic inflammatory diseases. Rheumatol Clin 2012 Jun 27 (Epub ahead of print)

[15] Enjuanes A, Benavente Y, Hernandez-Rodriguez J, Queralt C, Yaque J, Jares P et al. Association of NOS2 and potential effect of VEGF, IL-6, CCL2 and IL-1rn polymorphisms and haplotyoes on susceptibility to GCA. A simultaneous study of 130 potentially functional SNPs in 14 candidate genes. Rheumatology 2012; 51: 841-51

[16] Palomino-Morales R, Torres O, Vazquez-Rodriguez TR, Morado IC, Castaneda S, Callejas-Rubio JL et al. Association between toll-like receptor 4 gene polymorphism and biopsy-proven giant cell arteritis. J Rheumatol 2009; 36: 1501-6

[17] Mohammadi A, Pfeifer JD, Lewis JS Jr. Association between human papilloma virus DNA and temporal arteritis. BMC Musculoskelet Disord 2012; 13: 132

[18] Cooper RJ, D'Arcy S, Kirby M, Al-Buhtori M, Rahman MJ, Proctor L et al. Infection and temporal arteritis: a PCR-based study to detect pathogens in temporal artery biopsy specimens. J Med Virol 2008; 80: 501-5

[19] Elling P, Olsson AT, Elling H. Synchronous variations in the incidence of temporal arteritis and polymyalgia rheumatica in Danish countries. Association with epidemics of Mycoplasma pneumoniae infection. Ugeskr Laeger 1997; 159: 4123-8

[20] Duhaut P, Bosshard S, Ducroix JP. Is giant cell arteritis an infectious disease? Biological and epidemiological evidence. Presse Med 2004; 33: 1403-8

[21] Mohan SV, Liao J, Kim JW, Goronzy JJ, Weyand CM. Giant cell arteritis: immune and vascular aging as disease risk factors. Arthritis Res Ther 2011; 13: 231

[22] Weyand CM, Younge BR, Goronzy JJ. IFN-γ and IL-17: The two faces of T cell pathology in giant cell arteritis. Curr Opin Rheumatol 2011; 23: 43-9

[23] Yilmaz A, Arditi M. Giant cell arteritis: DCs take two T's to tango. Circ Res 2009; 104: 425-7

[24] Ma-Krupa W, Dewan M, Jeon MS, Kurtin PJ, Younge BR, Goronzy JJ et al. Trapping of misdirected dendritic cells in the granulomatous lesions of giant cell arteritis. Am J Pathol 2002; 161: 1815-23

[25] Ma-Krupa W, Jeon MS, Spoerl S, Tedder TF, Goronzy JJ, Weyand CM. Activation of the arterial wall dendritic cells and breakdown of self-tolerance in giant cell arteritis. J Exp Med 2004; 199: 173-83

[26] Caux C, Ait-Yahia S, Chemin K, De Bouteiller O, Dieu-Nosjean MC, Homey B et al. Dendritic cell biology and regulation of dendritic cell trafficking by chemokines. Springer Semin Immunopathol 2000; 22: 345-69

[27] Han JW, Shimada K, Ma-Krupa W, Johnson TL, Nerem RM, Goronzy JJ et al. Vessel-wall embedded dendritic cells induce T-cell autoreactivity and initiate vascular inflammation. Circ Res 2008; 102: 546-53

[28] Weyand CM, Ma-Krupa W, Pryschep O, Groschel S, Bernardino R, Goronzy JJ. Vascular dendritic cells in giant cell arteritis. Ann N Y Acad Sci 2005; 1062: 195-208

[29] Chang K, Rizzo F. Recent advances in the immunopathology of giant cell arteritis. Int Ophthalmol Clin 2009; 49: 99-109

[30] Pryschep O, Ma-Krupa W, Younge BR, Goronzy JJ, Weyand CM. Vessel specific Toll-like receptor profiles in human medium and large arteries. Circulation 2008; 118: 1276-84

[31] Deng J, Ma-Krupa W, Gewirtz AT, Younge BR, Goronzy JJ, Weyand CM. TLR4 and TLR5 induce distinct types of vasculitis. Circ Res 2009; 104(4): 488-95

[32] Weyand CM, Tetzlaff N, Bjornsson J, Brack A, Younge BR, Goronzy JJ. Disease patterns and tissue cytokine profiles in giant cell arteritis. Arthritis Rheum 1997; 40: 19-26

[33] Brack A, Geisler A, Martinez-Taboada VM, Younge BR, Goronzy JJ, Weyand CM. Giant cell vasculitis is a T cell-dependent disease. Mol Med 1997; 3: 530-43

[34] Grunewald J, Andersson R, Rydberg L, Gigliotti D, Schaufelberger C, Hansson GK et al. CD4+ and CD8+ T cell expansions using selected TCR V and J gene segments at the onset of giant cell arteritis. Arthritis Rheum 1994; 37: 1221-7

[35] Schaufelberger C, Andersson R, Nordborg E, Hansson GK, Nordborg C, Wahlstrom J. An uneven expression of T cell receptor V genes in the arterial wall and peripheral blood in giant cell arteritis. Inflammation 2008; 31: 372-83

[36] Weyand CM, Schonberger J, Oppitz U, Hunder NN, Hicok KC, Goronzy JJ. Distinct vascular lesions in giant cell arteritis share identical T cell clonotypes. J Exp Med 1994; 179: 951-60

[37] Deng J, Younge BR, Olshen RA, Goronzy JJ, Weyand CM. Th17 and Th1 T-cell responses in giant cell arteritis. N Engl J Med 2009; 361: 1114-6

[38] Deng J, Younge BR, Olshen RA, Goronzy JJ, Weyand CM. Th17- and Th1-cell responses in giant cell arteritis. Circulation 2010; 121: 906-15

[39] Basu A, Hoerning A, Datta D, Edelbauer M, Stack MP, Calzadilla K et al. Cutting edge: Vascular endothelial growth factor-mediated signalling in human CD45RO +CD4+ T cells promotes Akt and ERK activation and costimulates IFN-gamma production. J Immunol 2010; 184: 545-9

[40] Kaiser M, Weyand CM, Bjornsson J, Goronzy JJ. Platelet-derived growth factor, intimal hyperplasia and ischemic complications in giant cell arteritis. Arthritis Rheum 1998; 41: 623-33

[41] Mesquita D, Cruvinel WM, Camara NOS, Kallas EG, Andrade LEC. Autoimmune diseases in the Th17 era. Braz J Med Biol Res 2009; 42: 47-86

[42] Eid RE, Rao DA, Zhou J, Lo SF, Ranjbaran H, Gallo A et al. Interleukin-17 and interferon-gamma are produced concomitantly by human coronary artery-infiltrating T cells and act synergistically on vascular smooth muscle cells. Circulation 2009; 119: 1424-32

[43] Rodriguez-Pla A, Bosch-Gil JA, Rosello-Urgell J, Huguet-Redecilla P, Stone JH, Vilardell-Tarres M. Metalloproteinase-2 and -9 in giant cell arteritis: involvement in vascular remodelling. Circulation 2005; 112: 264-9

[44] Johnson C, Galis ZS. Matrix metalloproteinase -2 and -9 differentially regulate smooth muscle cell migration and cell-mediated collagen organization. Arterioscler Thromb Vasc Biol 2004; 24: 54-60

[45] Kaiser M, Younge BR, Bjornsson J, Goronzy JJ, Weyand CM. Formation of new vasa vasorum in vasculitis. Production of angiogenic cytokines by multinucleated giant cells. Am J Pathol 1999; 155: 765-74

[46] Hunder GG, Bloch DA, Michel BA, Stevens MB, Arend WB, Calabrese LH et al. The American College of Rheumatology 1990 criteria fort he classification of giant cell arteritis. Arthritis Rheum 1990; 33: 1122-8

[47] Campisi J, d'Adda di Fagagna F. Cellular senescence: when bad things happen to good cells. Nat Rev Mol Cell Biol 2007; 8: 729-40

[48] Wang M, Monticone RE, Lakatta EG. Arterial aging: a journey into subclinical arterial disease. Curr Opin Nephrol Hypertens 2010; 19: 201-7

[49] Bossert M, Prati C, Balblanc JC, Lohse A, Wendling D. Aortic involvement in giant cell arteritis: Current data. Joint Bone Spine 2011; 78(3): 246-51

http://dx.doi.org/10.5772/55222

[50] Ghinoi A, Pipitone N, Nicolini A, Boiardi L, Silingardi M, Germano G et al. Large-vessel involvement in recent-onset giant cell arteritis: a case-control colour-Doppler sonography study. Rheumatology 2012; 51(4): 730-4

[51] Evans JK, Bowles CA, Bjornsson J, Mullany CJ, Hunder GG. Thoracic aortic aneurysm and rupture in giant cell arteritis. A descriptive study of 41 cases. Arthritis Rheum 1994; 37(10): 1539-47

[52] Noel B. An easy and safe procedure for temporal artery biopsy. J Cutan Med 2006; 10(3): 147-50

[53] Lehmann P, Buchtala S, Achajew N, Haerle P, Ehrenstein B, Lighvani H et al. 18F-FDG PET as a diagnostic procedure in large vessel vasculitis-a controlled, blinded re-examination of routine PET scans. Clin Rheumatol 2011; 30(1): 37-42

[54] Chan M, Lugmani R. Pharmacotherapy of vasculitis. Expert Opin Pharmacother 2009; 10(8): 1273-89

[55] Hoffman GS, Cid MC. A multicenter, randomized, double-blind, placebo-controlled trial of adjuvant methotrexate treatment for giant cell arteritis. Arthritis Rheum 2002; 46(5): 1309-18

[56] Jover A. Combined treatment of giant-cell arteritis with methotrexate and prednisone. A randomized, double-blind, placebo-controlled trial. Ann Intern Med 2001; 134(2): 106-14

[57] Langford CA. Drug insight: anti-tumor necrosis factor therapies for the vasculitic diseases. Nat Clin Pract Rheumatol. 2008; 4(7): 364-70

[58] Seitz M, Reichenbach S, Bonel HM, Adler S, Wermelinger F, Villiger PM. Rapid induction of remission in large vessel vasculitis by IL-6 blockade. A case series. Swiss Med Wkly 2011; 141: w13156

Chapter 5

Giant Cell Arteritis and Arteritic Anterior Ischemic Optic Neuropathies

Dragos Catalin Jianu and Silviana Nina Jianu

Additional information is available at the end of the chapter

http://dx.doi.org/10.5772/55345

1. Introduction

Ischemic optic neuropathies (IONs) are a major cause of blindness or seriously impaired vision in the middle-aged and elderly population, although they can occur at any age. ION is of two types: anterior (AION) and posterior (PION), the first involving the anterior part of the optic nerve (also called the optic nerve head, ONH) and the second, the rest of the optic nerve. Pathogenetically AION and PION are very different diseases. AION represents an acute ischemic disorder (a segmental infarction) of the ONH supplied by the posterior ciliary arteries (PCAs), while PION has no specific location in the posterior part of the optic nerve and does not represent ischemia in a specific artery [1].

Blood supply blockage can occur with or without arterial inflammation. For this reason, AION is of two types: non-arteritic AION (NA-AION) and arteritic AION (A-AION). The former is far more common than the latter, and they are distinct entities etiologically, pathogenetically, clinically and from the management point of view [1, 2].

A-AION is an ocular emergency and requires immediate treatment with systemic corticosteroids to prevent further visual loss. This is almost invariably due to giant cell arteritis (GCA), which is a primary vasculitis that affects extracranial medium (especially external carotid artery-ECA-branches) and sometimes large arteries (aorta and its major branches)-large-vessel GCA [3, 4]. The diagnosis of GCA requires age more than 50 years at disease onset, new headache in the temporal area, temporal artery tenderness, and/or reduced pulse, jaw claudication, systemic symptoms, erythrocyte sedimentation rate (ESR) exceeding 50 mm/hr, and typical histologic findings (granulomatous involvement) in temporal artery biopsy (TAB) [5]. Approximately 40-50% of patients with GCA have ophthalmologic complications, including visual loss secondary to A-AION, central retinal artery occlusion, homonymous hemianopsia or cortical blindness (uni- or bilateral occipital infarction) [6].

NA-AION is a multifactorial disease with multiple risk factors that contribute to its development: the nocturnal arterial hypotension is the most important risk factor. Often, NA-AION patients have an anatomical predisposition: small discs, where structural crowding of nerve fibers (crowded disk), and reduction of the vascular supply, which may combine to impair perfusion to a critical degree [1, 2].

2. Arterial blood supply of the anterior part of the optic nerve

Arterial blood supply of the anterior part of the ONH is presented in figure 1.

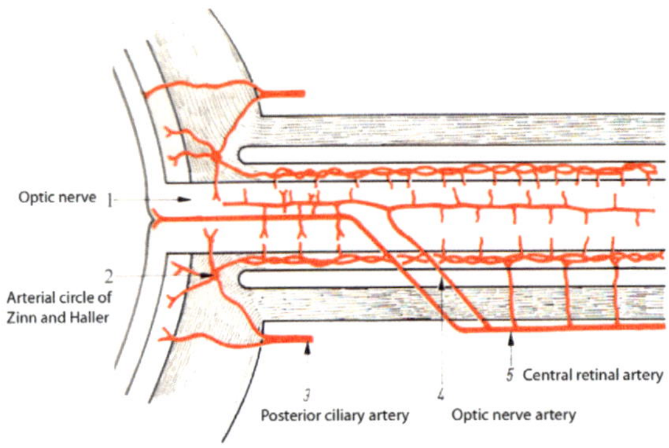

Figure 1. Arterial blood supply of the anterior part of the optic nerve.

The ONH consists of, from front to back: a). surface nerve fiber layer, b). prelaminar region, c). lamina cribrosa region, and d). retrolaminar region.

a. The surface nerve fiber layer is mostly supplied by the retinal arterioles. The cilioretinal artery, when present, usually irrigates the corresponding sector of the surface layer [1, 2].

b. The prelaminar region is situated in front of the lamina cribrosa. It is supplied by centripetal branches from the peripapillary choroid [1, 2].

c. The region of the lamina cribrosa is irrigated by centripetal branches from the PCAs, either directly or by the so-called arterial circle of Zinn and Haller, when that is present [1, 2].

d. The retrolaminar region is the part of the ONH that lies immediately behind the lamina cribrosa. It is supplied by two vascular systems: the peripheral centripetal and the axial centrifugal systems. The former represents the major source of irrigation to this part. It is formed by recurrent pial branches arising from the peripapillary choroid and the circle of Zinn and Haller (when present, or the PCAs instead). In addition, pial branches from the central retinal artery (CRA) also supply this part. The latter is not present in all eyes. When present, it is formed by inconstant branches arising from the intraneural part of the CRA. From the account of the arterial irrigation of the ONH given above, it is evident that the PCAs are the main source of blood supply to the ONH [1, 2].

http://dx.doi.org/10.5772/55345

3. Pathophysiology of factors controlling blood flow in the optic nerve head

The blood flow in the ONH depends upon: a). resistance to blood flow, b). arterial blood pressure (BP), and c). intraocular pressure (IOP) [1, 2].

a. resistance to blood flow. It depends upon the state and calibre of the vessels supplying the ONH, which in turn are influenced by: the efficiency of autoregulation of the ONH blood flow, the vascular changes in the arteries feeding the ONH circulation, and the rheological properties of the blood.

b. arterial blood pressure (BP). Both arterial hypertension and hypotension can influence the ONH blood flow in a number of ways. In an ONH, a fall of blood pressure below a critical level of autoregulation would decrease its blood flow. Fall of BP in the ONH may be due to systemic (nocturnal arterial hypotension during sleep, intensive antihypertensive medication, etc.) or local hypotension.

c. intraocular pressure (IOP). There is an inverse relationship between IOP and perfusion pressure in the ONH.

The blood flow in the ONH is calculated by using the following formula [1]:

Perfusion pressure = Mean BP minus intraocular pressure (IOP). Mean BP = Diastolic BP + 1/3 (systolic BP- diastolic BP).

AION cases can be broadly classified into two groups [1, 2]:

1. AION due to thrombotic or embolic lesions of the arteries/arterioles feeding the ONH:

   a. thrombotic lesions: Occlusion of the PCAs is most commonly caused by GCA (resulting in infarction of the ONH and A-AION) and less commonly by other types of vasculitis.

   b. embolic lesions: Multiple emboli in the vessels of the ONH have been demonstrated histopathologically in NA-AION.

2. AION due to transient non-perfusion or hypoperfusion of the nutrient vessels in the ONH (paraoptic branches of PCAs). A transient non-perfusion or hypo-perfusion of the ONH can occur due to a transient fall of perfusion pressure in its vessels, which in turn in susceptible persons would produce NA-AION. Almost all NA-AION cases belong to this group.

4. The major features of arteritic-anterior ischemic optic neuropathies and nonarteritic-anterior ischemic optic neuropathies

For the comparison of major features of A-AION and NA-AION we use a *complex protocol:*

- a detailed history of all previous or current systemic diseases, particularly of arterial hypertension, diabetes mellitus, hyperlipidemia, ischemic heart disease, stroke, transient ischemic attack, and carotid artery disease.
- a physical examination including the temporal arteries (TAs).
- a comprehensive ophthalmic evaluation, including visual acuity with the Snellen visual acuity chart, visual fields with a Goldmann perimeter, relative afferent pupillary defect, intraocular pressure, slit-lamp examination of the anterior segment, lens and vitreous, direct ophthalmoscopy, color fundus photography, and, in acute cases, fluorescein fundus angiography [1].
- color Doppler imaging (CDI) of retrobulbar (orbital) vessels with an ultrasound (US) equipment with a 10MHz linear probe for detecting and measuring orbital vessel blood flow in: the ophthalmic arteries (OAs), the CRAs, the superior ophthalmic veins, and the PCAs [7, 8].

While the patient is supine, the transducer is applied to the closed eyelids using sterile ophthalmic metylcellulose as a coupling gel. During the examination, minimal pressure is applied to the globe to avoid artifacts. The patient is asked to stay still, and not move his eyes.

Blood flow toward the transducer is depicted as red, and flow away from the transducer is colored blue. With the probe resting on the closed eyelids, the US beam is directed posteriorly in the orbit.

After systematic scanning of the orbit, the CRAs, PCAs, and OAs are imaged:

a. the CRA is identified just bellow the optic disc (<1 cm), and has a forward red-coded blood flow;

b. the nasal and temporal trunks of PCA are identified along both sides of the optic nerve. The arteries have a forward red-coded blood flow;

c. the OA is identified deeper in the orbit, usually before crossing the optic nerve. It has a forward red-coded blood flow.

The Doppler sample gate placed on the detected vessel has 1.5 cm. Sometimes, the orbital vessels are not paralel to the US beam. For this reason, we perform an angle correction between 0-60°.

Also, a spectral velocity analysis is performed. The peak systolic velocity (PSV), and end-diastolic velocity (EDV) are calculated for each vessel.

The Resistance Index (RI), also referred to as Pourcelot Index, is automatically calculated according to the following equation:

RI = (PSV-EDV)/PSV.

Absent signals not corresponding to carotid occlusive disease are classified as Doppler sonographic findings typical of GCA of the orbital arteries [9].

- extracranial Duplex sonography is performed with an US equipment with a 7.5-10 MHz linear array transducer.

For the examination of TAs, we use a 10 MHz linear probe. Color box steering and beam steering are maximal, and the color coveres the artery lumen exactly because using these machine adjustments, sensitivities and specificities with regard to clinical diagnosis of temporal arteritis and histology are high [10]. We examine both common superficial TAs and the frontal and parietal rami as completely as possible in longitudinal and transverse planes. Concentric hypoechogenic mural thickening (a so-called halo) is considered to be an ultrasonographic finding typical of GCA. Stenosis is considered to be present if blood-flow velocity is more than twice the rate recorded in the area before the stenosis, perhaps with waveforms demonstrating turbulence and reduced velocity behind the area of stenosis. Acute occlusion is considered to be present if the US image showes hypoechoic material in the former artery lumen with absence of color signals [10].

- fluorescein fundus angiography.

- laboratory findings in the form of a TAB are assessed at 3-7 days when GCA is suspected (based on systemic symptoms, elevated ESR, elevated C-reactive protein-CRP, and suspicion of A-AION). Because of unilateral clinical ocular involvement in all cases, we took a biopsy either from the ipsilateral side (representing 2.5 cm of the tender, swollen segments of the affected artery-"skip lesions") or from the ipsilateral site targeted by the ultrasonographer. Serial sections are examined, as there could be variations in the extent of involvement along the length of the artery [11].

- Cranial computed tomography (CT) scanning is performed for eventual associated stroke.

- CT-Angiography (CT-A) is performed at presentation, after Extracranial Duplex sonography, only in selected cases. It allowes analysis of the arterial wall and the endoluminal part of the aorta and its branches in cases of large-vessel GCA, and/or severe internal carotid artery (ICA) stenosis, or occlusion.

- Transthoracic echocardiography (TTE) is used for eventual cardiac embolic source of NA-AION.

The comparison of major features of A-AION and NA-AION is presented in table I [1-3, 5, 6, 9, 12, 13, 16, 18, 24-26].

4.1. Age and gender distribution

A-AION, like GCA is almost always seen in persons aged older than 50 years (more often women than men), with a mean age of near 70 years (mean age for NA-AION is aproximately 60 years, with no gender predisposition) [1, 2, 6, 12]. In a study of 406 patients with NA-AION [1], the age range was 11-91 years (mean age 60±14 and median 61 years) and 43 (10.5%) of the 406 patients were young (<45 years), 60% were men and 40% women [1].

4.2. Classic clinical symptoms of GCA with A-AION

The majority of GCA patients with A-AION present the classic clinical symptoms of GCA: new moderate bitemporal headache, especially common at night, scalp tenderness (which is first noticed when combing the hair), and abnormal TAs on palpation (tender, nodular, swollen, and thickened arteries) (Figure 2).

A study of Gonzales-Gay aiming to establish the best set of clinical features that may predict a positive TAB in a community hospital disclosed that headache, jaw claudication, and abnormal TAs on palpation were the best positive predictors of positive TAB in patients on whom a biopsy was performed to diagnose GCA [6]. This author established clinical differences between biopsy proven GCA and biopsy-negative GCA patients. Moreover, he observed a non–significantly increased frequency of abnormal palpation of the TA on physical examination in biopsy-proven GCA patients (73.3%) compared with biopsy-negative GCA patients (54.2%). The lack of pulsation is very suggestive of GCA because it is most unusual for the superficial TAs to be non-pulsatile in normal elderly individuals. The jaw claudication is the result of ischemia of the masseter muscles, which causes pain on speaking and chewing [6, 13].

FEATURE	A-AION	NA-AION
Age (mean years)	70	60
Sex ratio	Female > male	Female = male
Associated symptoms	New temporal headache, jaw claudication, abnormal temporal arteries on palpation, with reduced pulse, scalp tenderness	Pain occasionally noted
Visual acuity	Up to 76% < 20/200 (6/60)	Up to 61% > 20/200 (6/60)
Optic disc	Pale edema > hyperemic edema Cup normal	Hyperemic edema > pale edema Cup small
Erythrocyte sedimentation rate (mm/h) C-reactive protein (mg/l)	>50 > 5	<50 < 5
Temporal artery biopsy	Granulomatous inflammation of the media layer	-
Color Doppler Imaging of the retrobulbar (orbital) vessels	Severe diminished blood flow velocities in the posterior ciliary arteries (PCAs), especially on the affected side, and high resistance index (RI) in all retrobulbar vessels, in both orbits.	Blood flow velocities and RI in PCAs are preserved.
Fluorescein fundus angiography	Disc and choroid filling delay	Disc filling delay
Treatment	Corticosteroids	None proved

Table 1. The comparison of major features of arteritic-anterior ischemic optic neuropathies (A-AION) and nonarteritic-anterior ischemic optic neuropathies (NA-AION).

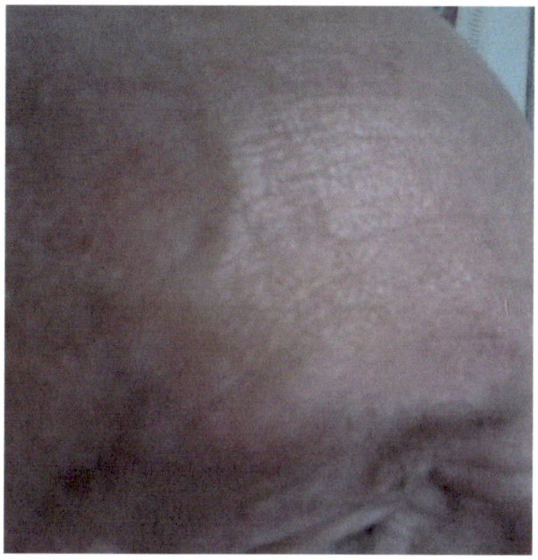

Figure 2. Patient MM with giant cell arteritis. Dilated and nodular right superficial temporal artery.

The classic clinical symptoms of GCA cases with A-AION are absent in NA-AION patients [1].

Large vessel GCA is a subgroup of GCA described in at least 17% of cases. In these patients, inflammation occurs also at the level of the aorta and its branches (especially of the subclavian, the axillary arteries, etc), despite the fact that symptoms of aortic involvement (aortic aneurysm rupture) may appear years after the initial diagnosis of this vasculitis [4, 14, 15, 16].

4.3. Systemic symptoms of GCA with A-AION

The majority of patients with GCA and A-AION present fever, fatigue, malaise, and weight loss. Some patients with GCA develop severe bilateral pain and aching involving the neck, shoulders, and pelvic girdles associated with morning stiffness (polymyalgia rheumatica) [13]. However, a study [17] showed that 21% of the patients with positive TAB for GCA had no systemic symptoms or signs and the only presenting sign was visual loss. This type of GCA is called occult GCA, which is fairly common - a very important fact to be borne in mind when dealing with AION [1].

The systemic symptoms of GCA are absent in NA-AION patients [1].

4.4. Systemic diseases associated with NA-AION

Nocturnal hypotension seems to be an important precipitating factor in the susceptible patients. It is the most important systemic disease associated with NA-AION [1, 2]. In Hayreh series [1, 2] of 544 NA-AION cases, where the patients could give some information on the time of onset of visual loss, 73.3% gave a definite history of discovering the visual loss on waking up in the morning. When antihypertensive drugs were taken at bedtime, they produced a far more marked degree of nocturnal hypotension than when taken in the morning, because they aggravate the naturally occurring fall of BP during sleep. Hayreh's studies [1, 2] suggest that in an ONH already susceptible to ischaemic disorder, nocturnal hypotension may act as "the straw that breaks the camel's back". In a healthy ONH with normal autoregulation, a similar fall of BP during the night may have no deleterious effect at all. All these facts indicate that NA-AION may be occurring as an iatrogenic disease in some persons. A combination of arterial hypertension and associated nocturnal hypotension can play an important role in either the development or the progression of NA-AION.

Hayreh [1] showed that, compared with the prevalence reported in the general population, young (<45 years), middle-aged (45-64 years) and elderly (≥65 years) patients with NA-AION showed a significantly higher prevalence of arterial hypertension, diabetes mellitus, and gastro-intestinal ulcer. Development of NA-AION following massive or recurrent haemorrhages has been know for well over twenty centuries. These usually occur from the gastrointestinal tract or uterus. Also, middle-aged and elderly patients showed a significantly higher prevalence of ischaemic heart disease and thyroid disorders. Following NA-AION, patients with both arterial hypertension and diabetes mellitus had a significantly higher incidence of cerebrovascular disease.

As a part of generalized atherosclerosis and arteriosclerosis, the ICAs, OAs, and PCAs may contribute to the development of NA-AION. ICA disease can contribute to development of NA-AION either by embolism or by lowering the perfusion pressure because of marked stenosis. The most likely mechanism of development of NA-AION in cardiac valvular disease is microembolism to the ONH [1, 2].

Patients with NA-AION may give a history of migraine. Hayreh studies have shown that serotonin released by platelets at the site of atheromatous plaques in the atherosclerotic arteries can also produce vasospasm of the PCAs [1, 2].

NA-AION has been reported in patients with haematologic disorders, including sickle-cell trait, polycythaemia, thrombocytopenic purpura, leukaemia and various types of anaemia [1, 2].

4.5. Ocular conditions associated with NA-AION

The most important ocular conditions associated with NA-AION are: a). absent or small cup in the optic disc, b). raised intraocular pressure, c). marked optic disc edema, d). location of the watershed zone of the PCAs in relation to the ONH, and e). vascular disorders in the nutrient vessels of the ONH [1, 2].

4.5.1. Absent or small cup in the optic disc

Studies have shown that eyes with NA-AION have no cup or only a very small cup in the optic disc. The overcrowding of the nerve fibers in a small scleral canal may be a precipitating factor in the production of NA-AION, although not the primary factor. The ONH in the prelaminar region is surrounded by a firm, non-yielding Bruch's membrane. When the axons swell, they can expand only at the expense of capillaries in the ONH, so the capillaries are compressed, causing impaired blood flow. When BP falls during sleep due to nocturnal arterial hypotension, there may be little or no blood flow in the ONH capillaries, resulting in hypoxia or ischaemia of the axons. The patient discovers the visual loss upon waking. If the optic disc has a large enough cup, the axons have sufficient space to swell without significantly compressing the capillaries; thus the presence of a cup is a protective mechanism [1, 12].

4.6. Laboratory findings in GCA with A-AION

ESR is often very high in GCA, with levels more than 50 mm/hr (fairly suggestive of this disease). In interpreting the ESR it should be emphasized that the levels of 40 mm/hour may be normal in the elderly and cases of biopsy-proven GCA have been reported in patients with ESR levels lower than 30 mm/hr. Approximately 20% of the patients who have a positive TAB for GCA present a normal ESR; hence "normal" ESR does not rule out GCA. CRP is often raised in GCA (the normal range is <5mg/l). It generally runs parallel with ESR, and may be helpful when the ESR is equivocal. However, in some cases there is elevation of ESR but not of CRP. The combination of ESR and CRP together gives the best specificity (97%) for detection of GCA [1, 6, 18].

Patients with NA-AION do not show any of these laboratory abnormalities [1, 6, 18].

4.7. Temporal artery biopsy and the histopathologic picture in GCA with A-AION

A TAB is the gold standard test for the diagnosis of GCA. Because corticosteroid therapy is required in most cases for more than 1 year in GCA with A-AION, the pathologic confirmation of this vasculitis is advisable. A biopsy result may be negative in 9-44% of patients with clinical positive signs of temporal arteritis, because of segmental (discontinous) involvement of TA [10, 19-21]. For this reason, the TAB has to be guided in all cases with clinical suspicion of GCA by Doppler Ultrasonography and typical TAs signs (tender, swollen portions of TAs). In all cases with A-AION due to GCA the histopathologic picture is represented by a granulomatous inflammation of the media layer (chronic inflammatory infiltrate with giant cells) with characteristic fragmentation of the internal limiting lamina and intimal thickening.

4.8. Extracranial Dupplex Sonography in AION patients

4.8.1. Extracranial Dupplex Sonography in A-AION patients

US of the TAs in temporal arteritis has garnered considerable interest as a GCA diagnosis tool. It indicates segmental inflammation of TAs [14, 22]. Schmidt demonstrated that the most specific (almost 100% specificity) and sensitive (73% sensitivity) sign for GCA is a concentric hypoechogenic mural thickening "halo", which was interpreted as vessel wall edema. Other positive findings for GCA are the presence of occlusion and stenoses. US investigation of the TAs must be performed before corticosteroid treatment, or within the first 7 days of treatment, because the halo revealed by TAs US disappears within 2 weeks of corticotherapy [10, 14, 22].

Similar US patterns can be find in other branches of the ECAs, including the facial, internal maxilary, and lingual arteries.

Interestingly, in some cases with large-vessel GCA, the common carotid arteries (CCAs) and the ICAs are also involved [16] (figure 3).

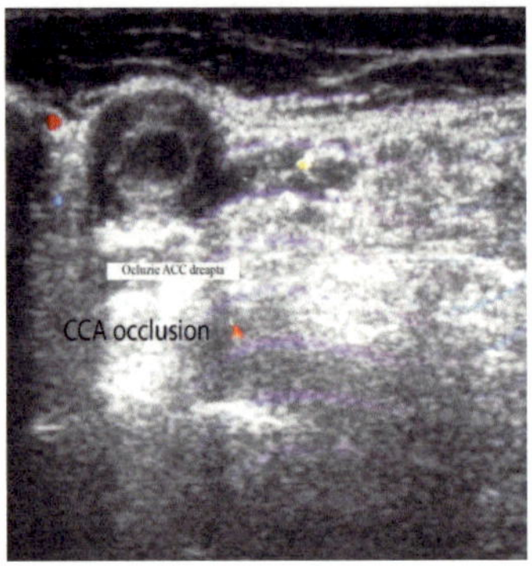

Figure 3. Patient MO - B mode insonation in large vessel giant cell arteritis. Transverse view of the left CCA. Hypoechoic wall swelling with CCA occlusion.

After weeks with corticosteroids treatment, the halo revealed by TAs US disappeares, but the wall swelling of the larger arteries (subclavians, axilars, CCAs, ICAs, etc.) remains in large-vessel GCA cases [16].

Schmidt compared the results of TAs US examinations with the occurrence of visual ischemic complications in 222 consecutive patients with newly diagnosed, active GCA. However, findings of TAs US did not correlate with eye complications [14].

4.8.2. Extracranial Dupplex Sonography in NA-AION patients

Ipsilateral ICA severe stenosis/occlusion can contribute to development of NA-AION either by embolism or by transient nonperfusion or hypoperfusion of the nutrient vessels in the ONH (paraoptic branches of PCAs) (figure 4) [1, 23].

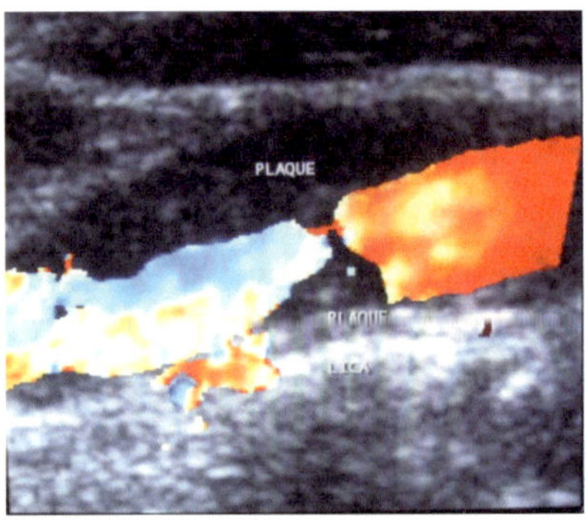

Figure 4. Patient AP- Color Doppler ultrasound. Longitudinal view of the left CCA with severe stenosis.

In Hayreh oppinion [1, 2], embolic occlusion of the PCAs or of the ONH arterioles seems to occur much less frequently than thrombotic occlusion, but this impression may be erroneous because of our inability to see the emboli in these vessels on ophthalmoscope compared to the ease with which they are seen in the retinal arterioles. Embolic etiology of NA-AION can be clinically suspected if the patients presents the following features: a). sudden onset of visual loss, definitely later on in the day, and not related to sleep or any other condition associated with arterial hypotension; b). the optic disc has a large cup; c). evidence of occlusion of a PCA on fluorescein fundus angiography, and on CDI of retrobulbar vessels, but d). no systemic symptoms or signs suggestive of GCA and, e). a negative TAB for GCA [1, 24-26].

4.9. Cranial computed tomography, Computed tomography angiography, and transthoracic echocardiography

CT-scanning identifies associated strokes (including occipital infarction), CT-A confirmes cases of large-vessel GCA associated with A-AION, or patients with ipsilateral occlusion/ severe ICA stenosis associated with NA-AION. TTE represents a part of the embolic evaluation in AION patients. Cardiac embolic source is rarely detected only in NA-AION cases.

4.10. Ocular symptoms

Anterior segment examination of both eyes is generally normal in all AION cases. Simultaneous bilateral AION onset is very rare (during cardio-pulmonary surgery with massive blood loss) [1].

4.10.1. Monocular amaurosis fugax and permanent visual loss

If a patient with AION has a history of amaurosis fugax before the permanent visual loss, it is highly suggestive of GCA associated with A-AION. Other A-AION patients develop permanent visual loss without any warning [1, 12].

However, amaurosis fugax is never found in NA-AION cases [1, 12].

A-AION results from PCAs vasculitis and the consecutive ONH infarction. Human autopsy studies of acute A-AION demonstrated ischemic necrosis of the prelaminar, laminar, and retrolaminar portions of the ONH and infiltration of the PCAs by chronic inflammatory cells. In some cases of these studies, segments of PCAs were occluded by inflammatory thickening and thrombi [12, 23].

In a Hayreh study [1], 54% of patients with A-AION had initial visual acuity ranging from counting fingers to no light perception, as compared to 26% in the NA-AION group, and only light or no light perception in 29% and 4%, respectively. This result shows that sudden, painless, severe permanent deterioration/loss of vision is extremely suggestive of A-AION. However, in Hayreh's series, about 21% of eyes with A-AION had 6/12 or better vision [1]. In NA-AION cases, generally there is progressive visual loss, and the patient usually notices further loss on waking in the morning [1].

4.10.2. Visual fields

Perimetry usually shows relative or absolute visual field defects. The most common visual field defect in NA-AION is an inferior nasal sectoral defect, which is relative or absolute. The next most common visual field defect is the relative or absolute inferior altitudinal; other optic disc-related field defects (central scotoma, etc) are less common (Figure 5). While the disc has edema, the visual fields may improve or deteriorate further, but once the disc edema has resolved completely, the visual field defects tend to stabilize [1, 12].

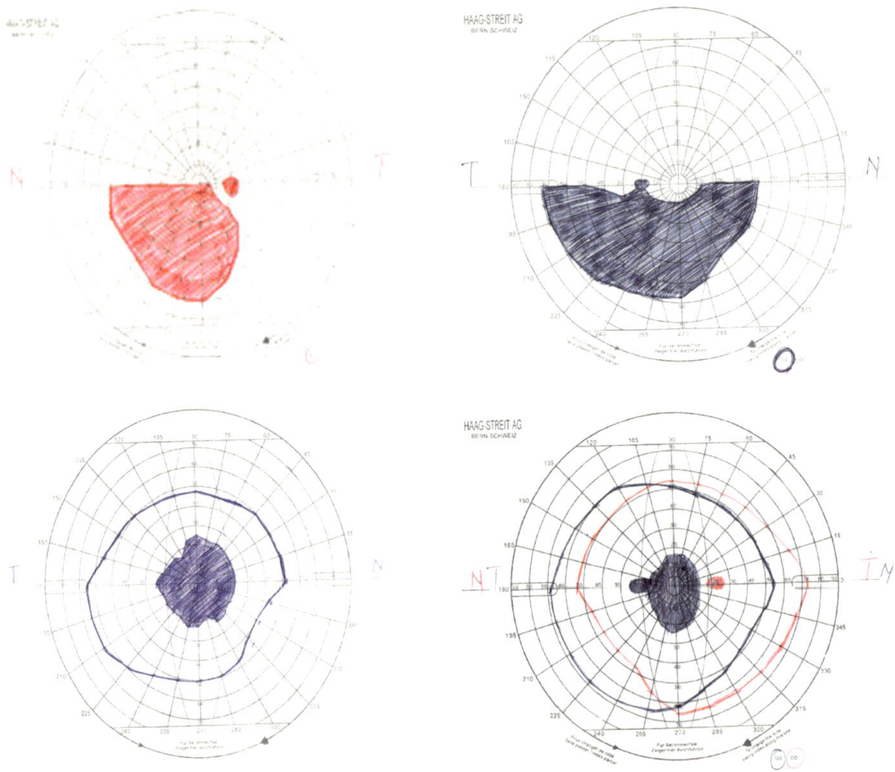

Figure 5. Common visual field defects in patients with nonarteritic-anterior ischemic optic neuropathies.

A relative afferent pupillary defect is invariably present in all cases of monocular AION.

4.11. Ophthalmoscopy

The majority of A-AION cases (69 % in Hayreh study [1]) unlike NA-AION patients have optic disc swelling with a characteristic chalky white color (pallor is associated with the edema of the optic disc) (Figure 6.A.).

http://dx.doi.org/10.5772/55345

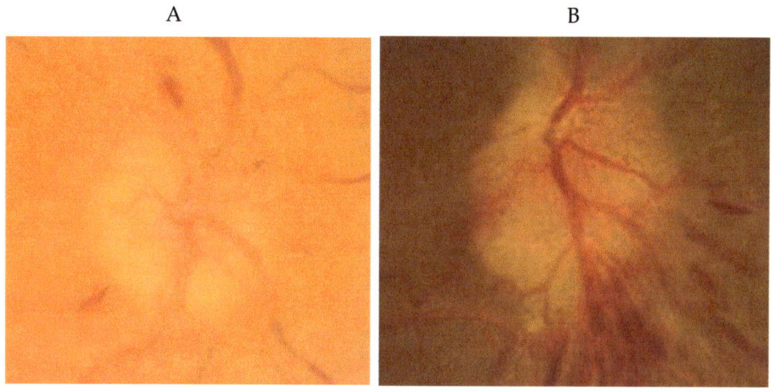

Figure 6. A. Patient TL. Fundus view of the left eye. Arteritic-anterior ischemic optic neuropathy. The optic disc demonstrates pale, diffuse edema. B. Patient AN. Fundus view of the left eye. Nonarteritic-anterior ischemic optic neuropathy. The optic disc demonstrates hyperemic diffuse edema.

Diffuse disc pallor develops 2 weeks after the onset of visual loss. On resolution of optic disc edema within 1-2 months, the optic disc develops cupping in almost all cases. Also unlike NA-AION, all A-AION patients have a contralateral optic disc, with normal diameter/normal physiological cup (absence of "disk at risk").

Initially, the optic disc is edematous in all NA-AION patients. Sometimes, the edema is more prominent in one part of the disc. Frequently, there are associated splinter hemorrhages at the disc margin. Hyperemia is associated with optic disc edema in the majority of cases (Figure 6.B.). The fellow optic disc showes a very small cup in the majority of cases (>75% of NA-AION patients present a contralateral "disk at risk", with associated mild disc elevation, and disc margin blurring without over edema) [1,12].

At 2 months, the optic disc edema resolves spontaneusly, resulting in generalised or sectoral pallor of the optic disc.

Consequently, ophthalmoscopy indicates that optic disc edema is associated more frequently with pallor (a chalky white color) in A-AION patients, and more frequently with hyperemia in NA-AION patients [1, 2, 24, 25].

4.12. Fluorescein fundus angiography

If angiography is performed during the first few days after the onset of A-AION (acute A-AION) there is almost always evidence of PCA thrombotic occlusion, with absence of choroidal and optic disc filling in its distribution in all A-AION patients. However, later, with the establishment of collateral circulation, this information may be lost. In contrast, there is an impaired optic disc perfusion, with relatively conserved choroidal perfusion in all NA-AION cases.

Consequently, extremely delayed or absent filling of the choroid, which was identified in acute A-AION patients, has been suggested as a fluorescein-angiogram characteristic of A-AION. It has been considered as one useful factor to differentiate A-AION from NA-AION [1, 12].

4.13. Color Doppler imaging of the retrobulbar (orbital) vessel features

4.13.1. Spectral Doppler analysis of the retrobulbar vessels in A-AION

In acute stage, blood flow cannot be detected in the PCAs in the clinically affected eye of any of the GCA patients with A-AION. Low EDV and high RI are identified in all other retrobulbar vessels (including the PCAs in the fellow eye) of all A-AION patients.

At one week, CDI examination of retrobulbar vessels reveales blood flow alterations in all A-AION patients despite the treatment with high-dose corticosteroids. Severely diminished blood flow velocities (especially EDV) in the PCAs of the affected eye (both nasal and temporal), compared to the unaffected eye, are noted (Figure 7 A., B., C., D.). An increased RI in the PCAs is noted (the RI is higher on the clinically affected eye as compared to the unaffected eye) (Figure 7 A., B., C., D.).

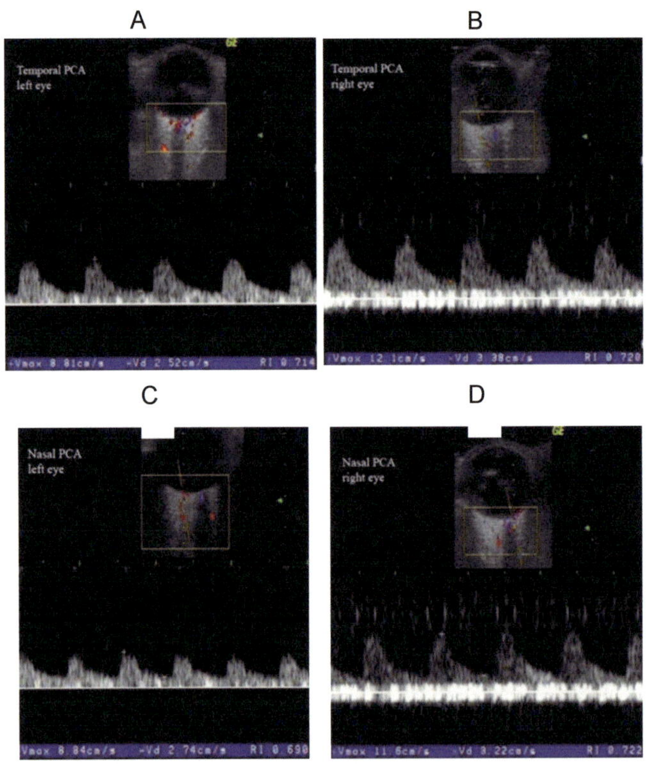

Figure 7. A. B. Pacient TL with arteritic-anterior ischemic optic neuropathy – Color Doppler Imaging of temporal posterior ciliary arteries (PCAs) of both eyes. Diminution of blood flow velocities (especially end-diastolic velocities) in the temporal PCA of the affected left eye, compared to the other side. C. D. Pacient TL with arteritic-anterior ischemic optic neuropathy – Color Doppler Imaging of nasal posterior ciliary arteries (PCAs) of both eyes. Diminution of blood flow velocities (especially end-diastolic velocities) in the nasal PCA of the affected left eye, compared to the other side.

http://dx.doi.org/10.5772/55345

Fewer abnormalities are observed in the CRAs: high RI are measured in both sides, with decreased PSV in the CRA of the clinically affected eye (Figure 8 A., B.).

Similar abnormalities are noted in the OAs: high RI are measured in both sides (Figure 8 C., D.).

At one month, after treatment with high-dose corticosteroids, CDI examinations of orbital blood vessels reveal that blood flow normalization is slow in all A-AION patients.

In conclusion, the Spectral Doppler Analysis of the orbital vessels in A-AION indicates (after a few days of treatment with corticosteroids) low blood velocities, especially EDV, and high RI in all retrobulbar vessels, in both orbits. These signs represent characteristic features of the CDI of the orbital vessels in A-AION.

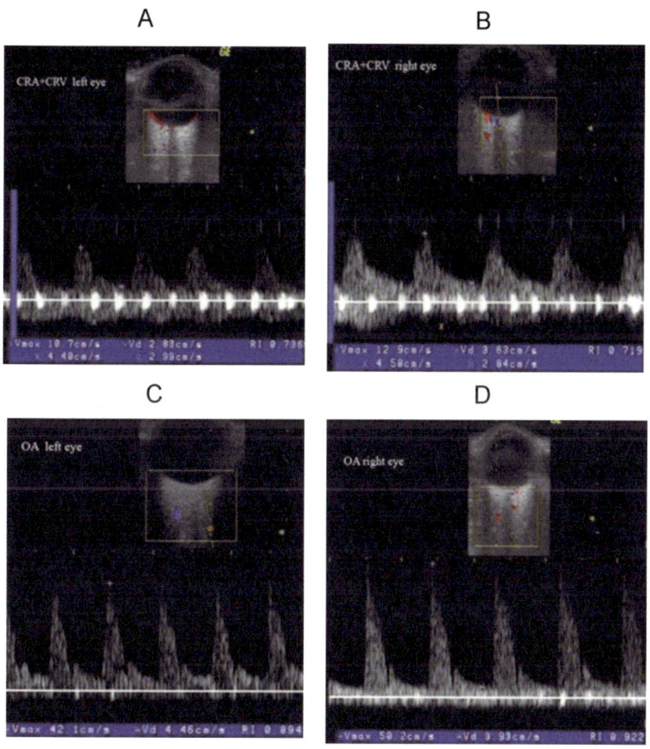

Figure 8. A. B. Pacient TL with arteritic-anterior ischemic optic neuropathy - Color Doppler Imaging of central retinal arteries of both eyes. High RI in both sides. C. D. Pacient TL with arteritic-anterior ischemic optic neuropathy - Color Doppler Imaging of ophthalmic arteries of both eyes. High RI in both sides.

4.13.2. Spectral Doppler analysis of the retrobulbar vessels in NA-AION

In contrast, the patients with NA-AION present the following aspects in acute stage, and at one week of evolution:

a. slight decrease of PSV in PCAs (nasal and temporal) in the affected eye, compared to the unaffected eye (Figure 9 A., B., C., D.);

b. slight decrease of PSV in CRA of the affected eye, due to papillary edema (Figure 9 E., F.);

c. in OAs, PSV are variable: normal to decreased, according to ipsilateral ICAs status. Severe ICA stenosis (>70% of vessel diameter)/occlusion combined with an insufficient Willis polygon led to decreased PSV in ipsilateral OA.

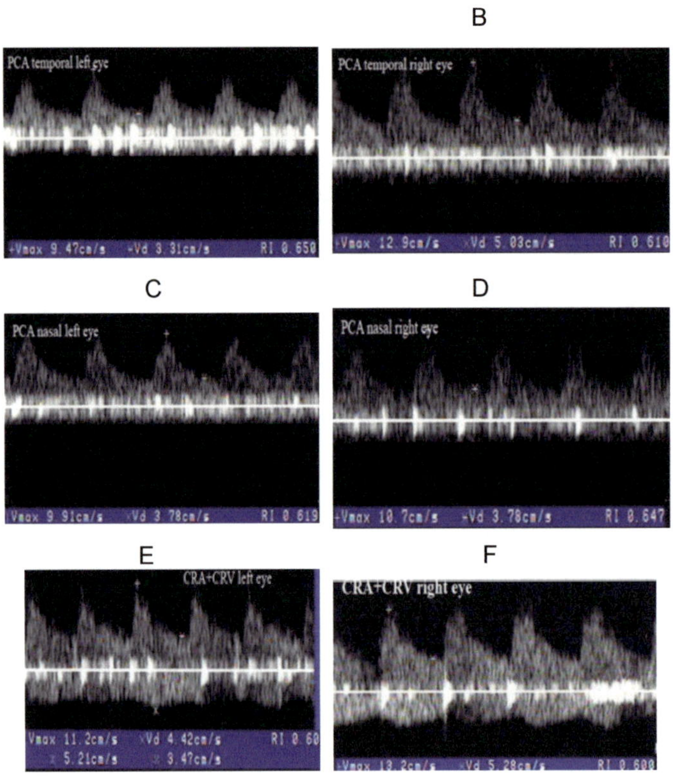

Figure 9. A. B. Pacient AN with nonarteritic-anterior ischemic optic neuropathy - Color Doppler Imaging of temporal posterior ciliary arteries (PCAs) of both eyes. Slight diminution of systolic blood flow velocities in temporal PCA in the affected left eye, compared to the normal side. C.D. Pacient AN with nonarteritic-anterior ischemic optic neuropathy - Color Doppler Imaging of nasal posterior ciliary arteries (PCAs) of both eyes. Slight diminution of systolic blood flow velocities in nasal PCA in the affected left eye, compared to the normal side. E. F. Pacient AN with nonarteritic-anterior ischemic optic neuropathy - Color Doppler Imaging of central retinal arteries of both eyes. Slight diminution of systolic blood flow velocities in CRA of affected left eye, due to papilar edema.

At one month, CDI examinations of orbital blood vessels reveal that blood flow normalization is reached. The exceptions are the cases with severe ipsilateral ICA stenosis/occlusion.

Consequently, in NA-AION, blood velocities and RI in PCAs are preserved. Similar results were obtained in other studies [24-26].

CDI of retrobulbar vessels and fluorescein fundus angiography data support the histopathological evidence of involvement of the entire PCA trunck in A-AION (impaired both ONH and choroidal perfusion in these patients) [12, 24, 25].

In contrast, in NA-AION cases, affected flow to the ONH is distal to the PCA trunck, possibly at the level of the paraoptic branches. These branches directly supply the ONH with only one-third of the flow of the PCAs (impaired optic disc perfusion, with relatively preserved choroidal perfusion in NA-AION patients) [12, 16, 23].

CDI of retrobulbar vessels sustains the involvement of the entire PCA trunk in A-AION in a non-invasive manner and in real time and may rapidly point to an A-AION diagnosis. While CDI of orbital vessels does not eliminate the need for fluorescein fundus angiography, hematologic assessment, carotid US, and echocardiography, it does however enhance the precision of the diagnostic evaluation for patients, because it accurately, reproducibly, and safely assesses the vascular supply of the ONH.

There are certain cases where the differential diagnosis between arteritic and nonarteritic AION is difficult: GCA without systemic/clinical symptoms, even a swollen TA, GCA with a normal ESR, and patients with NA-AION that have high ESR levels due to a neoplasm association. When CDI detects a NA-AION, the patient does not have to be subjected to high-dose corticosteroids until a TAB is performed even if the ESR is elevated. Conversely, patients with clinical evidence of A-AION, who have typical signs on CDI of retrobulbar vessels, should be treated before TAB in order to protect the fellow eye from going blind [16].

In our opinion, the results from CDI of retrobulbar vessels and extracranial duplex US (especially of TAs) can substitute the TAB, which is more inconvenient for the patient, more expensive and has up to 40% false negative error data, because of skip lesions [14].

5. Conclusions

A history of amaurosis fugax before an abrupt, painless, and severe loss of vision of the involved eye, with concomitant diffuse pale optic disc edema is extremely suggestive of A-AION. None of these symptoms are found in NA-AION patients.

Because findings of TAs US does not correlate with eye complications in A-AION patients, CDI of the retrobulbar vessels is of critical importance. It allows the detection and monitoring of alterations in orbital blood flow, especially of the PCAs, which corespond with the clinical features of A-AION.

Patients with clinical evidence of A-AION, who have typical signs on CDI of retrobulbar vessels, should be treated before TAB, with corticosteroids to protect against blindness of the fellow eye.

Although none of all presented criteria is individually infallible and present in one hundred percent of AION cases, the collective information provided by the various parameters is extremely helpful in diagnosis of A-AION or NA-AION.

Author details

Dragos Catalin Jianu[1*] and Silviana Nina Jianu[2]

*Address all correspondence to: dcjianu@yahoo.com

1 University of Medicine and Pharmacy "Victor Babes", County Emergency Hospital Department of Neurology, Timisoara, Romania

2 Military Emergency Hospital Department of Ophthalmology, Timisoara, Romania

References

[1] Hayreh, S S. Ischaemic optic neuropathy. Indian J. Ophthalmol. (2000). , 48, 171-194.

[2] Hayreh, S S. Management of ischemic optic neuropathies. Indian J. Ophthalmol. (2011). , 59(2), 123-136.

[3] Levine, S. M, & Hellmann, D. B. Giant cell arteritis. Curr. Opin. Rheumatol. (2002). , 14, 3-10.

[4] Martínez-Valle, F, Solans-Laqué, R, Bosch-Gil, J, et al. Aortic involvement in giant cell arteritis. Autoimmun. Rev. (2010). , 9, 521-524.

[5] Hunder, G. G, et al. The American College of Reumatology criteria for the classification of giant cell arteritis. Arteritis Rheum. (1990). , 33, 1122-28.

[6] Gonzalez-Gay, M. A, Garcia-Porrua, C, Llorca, J, Hajeer, A. H, Branas, F, Dababneh, A, et al. Visual manifestations of giant cell arteritis: trends and clinical spectrum in 161 patients. Medicine (Baltimore) (2000). , 79, 283-92.

[7] Lieb WE Jr., Cohen SM., Merton DA., et al. Color Dopper imaging of the eye and orbit: Technique and normal vascular anatomy. Arch. Ophthalmol.(1991). , 09, 527-531.

[8] Pichot, O, Gonzalvez, B, Franco, A, & Mouillon, M. Color Doppler ultrasonography in the study of orbital and ocular vascular diseases. J Fr Ophtalmol.(1996). , 19(1), 19-31.

[9] Ghanchi, F. D, Williamson, T. H, Liam, C. S, Butt, Z, Baxter, G. M, Mckillop, G, & Brien, O. C. Color Doppler imaging in giant cell (temporal) arteritis: serial examination and comparison with non-arteritic anterior ischaemic optic neuropathy. Eye (1996). , 10(4), 459-64.

[10] Schmidt, W. A, Kraft, H. E, Vorpahl, K, et al. Color duplex ultrasonography in the diagnosis of temporal arteritis. N. Engl. J. Med. (1997). , 337, 1336-1342.

[11] Taylor-Gjevre, R, Vo, M, Shukla, D, & Resch, L. Temporal artery biopsy for giant cell arteritis, J. Rheumatol. (2005). , 32, 1279-1282.

[12] Arnold, A. C. Ischemic optic neuropathy. In: Ianoff M., Duker JS. (ed.), Ophtalmology, second edition: Mosby; (2004). , 1268-1272.

[13] Gonzalez-Gay, M. The diagnosis and management of patients with giant cell arteritis. J. Rheumatol. (2005). , 32, 1186-1188.

[14] Schmidt, W. A. Takayasu and temporal arteritis. In: Baumgartner RW. (ed.) Handbook on Neurovascular Ultrasound. Front. Neurol. Neurosci. Basel. Karger; (2006). , 96-104.

[15] Pipitone, N, Versari, A, & Salvarani, C. Role of imaging studies in the diagnosis and follow-up of large-vessel vasculitis: an update. Rheumatology (Oxford) (2008). , 47, 403-408.

[16] Jianu, D. C, Jianu, S. N, Petrica, L, & Serpe, M. Large giant cell arteritis with eye involvement. In Amezcua-Guerra. (ed.), Advances in the diagnosis and treatment of vasculitis, Rijeka: InTech; (2011). , 311-330.

[17] Salvarani, C, Cantini, F, & Hunder, G. G. Polymyalgia rheumatica and giant-cell arteritis, Lancet (2008). , 372, 234-245.

[18] Lopez-Diaz, M. J, Llorca, J, Gonzalez-Juanatey, C, et al. The erythrocyte sedimentation rate is associated with the development of visual complications in biopsy-proven giant cell arteritis, Semin. Arthritis Rheum. (2008). , 38, 116-123.

[19] Foroozan, R, Deramo, V. A, Buono, L. M, et al. Recovery of visual function in patients with biopsy-proven giant cell arteritis. Ophthalmology (2003). , 110, 539-542.

[20] Breuer, G. S, Nesher, R, & Nesher, G. Effect of biopsy length on the rate of positive temporal artery biopsies. Clin. Exp. Rheumatol. (2009). Suppl 52):SS13., 10.

[21] Gonzalez-Gay, M. A, Garcia-Porrua, C, Llorca, J, Gonzalez-Louzao, C, & Rodriguez-Ledo, P. Biopsy-negative giant cell arteritis: clinical spectrum and predictive factors for positive temporal artery biopsy. Semin. Arthritis Rheum. (2001). , 30, 249-56.

[22] Arida, A, Kyprianou, M, Kanakis, M, & Sfikakis, P. P. The diagnostic value of ultrasonography-derived edema of the temporal artery wall in giant cell arteritis: a second meta-analysis. BMC Musculoskelet. Disord. (2010).

[23] Collignon-Robe, N. J, Feke, G. T, & Rizzo, J. F. Optic nerve head circulation in nonarteritic anterior ischemic optic neuropathy and optic neuritis. Ophthalmology, (2004). , 111, 1663-72.

[24] Jianu, D. C, & Jianu, S. N. The role of Color Doppler Imaging in the study of optic neuropathies. In: Jianu DC., Jianu SN. (ed.) Color Doppler Imaging. Neuro-ophthalmological correlations, Timisoara: Mirton; (2010). , 125-142.

[25] Jianu, D. C, Jianu, S. N, & Petrica, L. Color Doppler Imaging of retrobulbar vessels findings in large giant cell arteritis with eye involvement. Journal of US-China Medical Science (2011). , 8(2), 99-108.

[26] Tranquart, F, Aubert-urena, A. S, Arsene, S, Audrierie, C, Rossazza, C, & Pourcelot, L. Echo- Doppler couleur des arteres ciliaires posterieures dans la neuropathie optique ischemique anterieure aigue, J.E.M.U., (1997). , 18(1), 68-71.

Chapter 6

Infectious Causes of Vasculitis

Jacques Choucair

Additional information is available at the end of the chapter

http://dx.doi.org/10.5772/55189

1. Introduction

1.1. Infectious vasculitis

The vasculitides are a heterogeneous group of clinicopathological entities that share the common feature of vascular inflammation and injury. There is no universally acceptable classification of this group of disorders. While a number of underlying causes can be identified in some disorders, the aetiology is unknown in many. The pathogenetic mechanisms involved are mainly immunological, immune complex mediated tissue injury being the most commonly incriminated factor.

In 1952, Zeek [1] became the first author to incorporate a clinicopathological assessment based on the size of the vessels involved in the inflammatory process in her classification of necrotizing vasculitis. A number of alternative classification systems were proposed later and a major break was made in the 1990s with the 1990 American College of Rheumatology criteria (ACR 1990 criteria); and the elaboration of a uniform terminology for naming, defining, classifying and diagnosing vasculitic disorders at the Chapel

Hill Conference 1992 (1992 CHC definitions). The 1990 ACR criteria were reviewed in 1996 by Hunder [2]. The 1992 CHC definitions now include immunodiagnostically significant markers [e.g. ANCA in Wegener's granulomatosis (WG) and immunohistological findings (e.g. IgA-dominant immune deposits in Henoch–Schönlein purpura) which are specific for certain diseases and were described by Jennette *et al.* [3]

The major problem with previous classification schemes was the lack of standardized diagnostic terms and definitions. As a consequence, different names had been applied to the same disease and the same name to different diseases. Therefore, the CHC committee—comprised of internists, rheumatologists, nephrologists, immunologists and pathologists who have in common extensive experience with diagnosing vasculitides—proposed the names and definitions given in Table 3.

Large vessel vasculitis[a]	
Giant cell (temporal) arteritis	Granulomatous arteritis of the aorta and its major branches, with a predilection for the extracranial branches of the carotid artery. *Often involves the temporal artery. Usually occurs in patients older than 50 yr and often is associated with polymyalgia rheumatica.*
Takayasu arteritis	Granulomatous inflammation of the aorta and its major branches. *Usually occurs in patients younger than 50 yr.*
Medium-sized vessel vasculitis[a]	
Polyarteritis nodosa[b] (classic polyarteritis nodosa)	Necrotizing inflammation of medium-sized or small arteries without glomerulonephritis or vasculitis in arterioles, capillaries, or venules.
Kawasaki disease	Arteritis involving large-, medium-sized, and small arteries, and associated with mucocutaneous lymph node syndrome. *Coronary arteries are often involved. Aorta and veins may be involved. Usually occurs in children.*
Small vessel vasculitis[a]	
WG[c]	Granulomatous inflammation involving the respiratory tract, and necrotizing vasculitis affecting small- to medium-sized vessels (e.g. capillaries, venules, arterioles, and arteries). *Necrotizing glomerulonephritis is common.*
CSS[c]	Eosinophil-rich and granulomatous inflammation involving the respiratory tract, and necrotizing vasculitis affecting small- to medium-sized vessels, and associated with asthma and eosinophilia.
MPA[b,c] (microscopic polyarteritis)	Necrotizing vasculitis, with few or no immune deposits affecting small vessels (i.e. capillaries, venules, or arterioles). *Necrotizing arteritis involving small- and medium-sized arteries may be present. Necrotizing glomerulonephritis is very common. Pulmonary capillaritis often occurs.*
Henoch-Schönlein purpura	Vasculitis, with IgA-dominant immune deposits, affecting small vessels (i.e. capillaries, venules, or arterioles). *Typically involves skin, gut, and glomeruli, and is associated with arthralgias or arthritis.*
Essential cryoglobulinaemic vasculitis	Vasculitis, with cryoglobulin immune deposits, affecting small vessels (i.e. capillaries, venules, or arterioles), and associated with cryoglobulins in serum. *Skin and glomeruli are often involved.*
Cutaneous leucocytoclastic angiitis	Isolated cutaneous leucocytoclastic angiitis without systemic vasculitis or glomerulonephritis.

[a]Large vessel refers to the aorta and the largest branches directed towards major body regions (e.g. to the extremities and the head and neck); medium-sized vessel refers to the main visceral arteries (e.g. renal, hepatic, coronary, and mesenteric arteries); small veseel refers to venules, capillaries, arterioles, and the intraparenchymal distal arterial radicals that connect with arterioles. Some small and large vessel vasculitides may involve medium-sized arteries,but large- and medium- sized vessel vasculitides do not involve vessels smaller than arteries. Essential components are represented by normal type; italicized type represent usual, but not essential components.

[b]Preffered term.

[c]Strongly associated with ANCA.

Reproduced from [4] with permission.

Table 1. Names and definitions of vasculitides adopted by the Chapel Hill Concensus Conference on the Nomenclature ot Systemic Vasculitis

2. Immunopathogenesis

Most of the vasculitic syndromes are mediated by immunopathogenic mechanisms ('immune vasculitides') and most 'immune vasculitides' are idiopathic (='primary' vasculitis).

The immunopathogenic mechanisms of vasculitides have been classified into the four types of hypersensitivity reaction described by Coombs and Gell [4]; this classification was reviewed recently [5]. Accordingly, clinicopathological and immunohistochemical studies have led to the terms allergic angiitis (I), antibody-mediated angiitis, including the 'new' group of ANCA-associated vasculitides (II), immune complex vasculitis (III), and vasculitis associated with T-cell-mediated hypersensitivity (IV). Eosinophilia and elevated IgE in the blood and tissues (*in situ*) are characteristically associated with allergic angiitis and granulomatosis ('Churg–Strauss syndrome'; CSS); in 'ANCA-associated vasculitides' (AAV) few or no immune deposits are found *in situ* ('pauci-immune vasculitis').

By contrast, immune complex deposits *in situ* are the hallmark of immune complex vasculitis, which is frequently associated with low complement levels. Granulomatous arteritis is characterized by an inflammatory infiltrate induced by Th1 cells. The predominant immune phenomena in systemic vasculitides associated with the major hypersensitivity reaction type are given in Fig. 1.

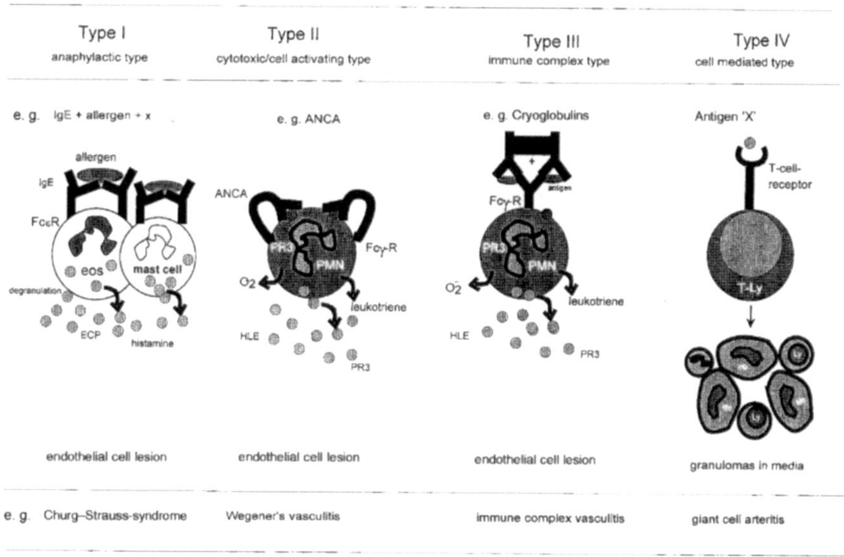

Figure 1. Pease add caption

While some forms of vasculitides may be ascribed to underlying factors like infections, malignancy, drug reactions or connective tissue disorders, the cause may remain undetermined in many vasculitic syndromes. Immunologic damage by immune-complex deposition or cell-mediated hypersensitivity is responsible in the majority of cases.

The possible immunopathologic mechanism in the causation of vasculitis are:

1. **Deposition of circulating antigen-antibody complex** or in -situ formation of immune complex within the vessel wall. This leads to complement activation and chemotactic attraction of neutrophils by complement components. Subsequent phagocytosis of such complexes with liberation of neutrophil granular products leads to vascular damage.

2. **Cell-mediated hypersensitivity**: Antigenic exposure may attract lymphocytes which liberate cytokines causing tissue damage and further activation of macrophages and lymphocytes.

3. Failure to clear the antigen may lead to persistent inflammation and eventual formation of epithelioid cells and giant cells, giving rise to a **granulomatous tissue reaction**.

Whatever the underlying mechanism, vascular inflammation and necrosis ensues which is often accompanied by thrombosis. These pathologic changes result in tissue ischaemia, necrosis and infarction, leading to a variety of clinical manifestations depending on the anatomic structures involved

3. Pathology

Perivascular cellular infiltration is a common histological finding in many disease entities, but for a definitive diagnosis of vasculitis, the presence of vascular damage, particularly in the form of fibrinoid degeneration, is necessary.

Vasculitis may involve blood vessels of varying calibers and this feature forms the basis of a useful pathological classification of vasculitis. An infiltrate, composed of a variety of cell types, like neutrophils, lymphocytes, and histiocytes may invade the vessel wall and the surrounding tissue. Extravasation of red cells is a prominent feature in many vasculitides. Granulomatous inflammation with giant cell formation is a characteristic finding in some types.

4. Classification

Vasculitis is a taxonomist's nightmare. Diseases with diverse causes and pathology may share the same symptomatology. On the other hand, a disease may show different histopathologic features at different periods in its evolution. Many diseases have overlapping features and it is impossible to formulate a classification scheme that unifies clinicopathological, etiological and immunological features of different diseases.

4.1. Immunopathologic classification

i. Immune- complex mediated vasculitis:

- Polyarteritis nodosa
- Microscopic polyangiitis
- Hypersensitivity vasculitis
- (Leukocytoclastic vasculitis)
- Henoch-Schonlein purpura

ii. Vasculitis due to cellular hypersensitivity (Granulomatous vasculitis)

- Giant cell arteritis
- Takayasu's arteritis
- Churg-Strauss disease (allergic granulomatosis)
- Wegener's granulomatosis
- Isolated CNS vasculitis

http://dx.doi.org/10.5772/55189

4.2. Classification based on caliber of blood vessel involved

i. Large vessel vasculitis:

- Giant cell arteritis
- Takayasu's arteritis

ii. Medium vessel vasculitis:

- Polyarteritis nodosa
- Kawasaki disease

iii. Small vessel vasculitis:

- Microscopic polyangiitis
- Leukocytoclastic vasculitis
- Wegener's granulomatosis
- Churg-Strauss disease

4.3. Classification based on cellular composition of the infiltrate

i. *Leukocytoclastic vasculitis* (LCV): Neutrophils are predominant. Cellular fragments and nuclear debris (leukocytoclasia) are found in the infiltrate.

- Polyarteritis nodosa
- Henoch-Schonlein purpura
- Vasculitis due to drugs, infections, and connective tissue diseases
- Erythema elevatum diutinum
- Granuloma faciale etc.

ii. Lymphocytic vasculitis:

- Lupus erythematosus
- Lymphoma
- Pityriasis lichenoides

iii. Eosinophilic vasculitis :

- Churg-Strauss vasculitis

iv. Granulomatous vasculitis :

- Wegener's granulomatosis and Churg-Strauss

v. Giant cell arteritis:

- Temporal arteritis

- Takayasu's arteritis

4.4. Clinical classification

i. Systemic necrotizing vasculitis :

- Polyarteritis nodosa
  - Classical
  - Microscopic polyangiitis
  - Allergic granulomatosis
  - Polyangiitis overlap
- Wegener's granulomatosis

ii. Giant cell vasculitis

- Temporal arteritis
- Takayasu's disease

iii. Predominantly Cutaneous small vessel vasculitis :

a. Idiopathic

b. Secondary:

- **Infection**: (Streptococcus, Staph, TB, Leprosy, Hep.B and C, HIV, Subacute bacterial endocarditis, EBV, parvovirus, Rickettsia)
- **Drugs**: Penicillin, sulpha, phenytoin, allopurinol, gold, thiazide, NSAIDs, Frusemide, quinidine, thiouracils, mefloquine
- **Connective tissue disease** (SLE, Sjogren's syndrome, RA, Scleroderma, Dermatomyositis)
- **Malignancy** (Lymphoma, leukemia, solid organ tumors)
- **Other diseases**: Cryoglobulinemia, complement deficiency, alpha1 antitrypsin deficiency Inflammatory bowel disease, Chronic active hepatitis, intestinal bypass surgery, primary biliary cirrhosis,Relapsing polychondritis

c. Clinical syndromes with leukocytoclastic vasculitis:

- Henoch-Schonlein purpura
- Urticarial vasculitis
- Serum sickness
- Erythema elevatum diutinum
- Granuloma faciale

- Hyperimmunoglobulinemia D
- Acute hemorrhagic edema of children
- Familial Mediterranean fever.

iv. Other vasculitic syndromes:

- Behcet's disease Buerger's disease
- Kawasaki's disease
- Isolated CNS vasculitis
- Cogan's syndrome

5. Immunodiagnostic approach

Primary systemic vasculitides were reclassified based on ANCA serology, the presence of immune deposits *in situ*, and the size of the vessels involved. WG, MPA and CSS were subsumed in the group of ANCA-associated vasculitides, which are characterized clinically by a WG, CSS or non-granulomatous MPA inflammation commonly involving the respiratory tract and ear–nose–throat (ENT) region and by a necrotizing pauci-immune (= no or minimal immune deposits) vasculitis typically affecting small- to medium-sized vessels.

ANCA are a heterogeneous group of autoantibodies that can be subdivided by indirect immunofluorescence tests (IFTs) and by enzyme-linked immunosorbent assays (ELISAs). IFTs can distinguish two major fluorescence patterns on ethanol-fixed human granulocytes: one of these patterns, classic cANCA, is highly specific for WG, while the other, perinuclear pANCA, is commonly seen in MPA (rarely in WG), but may be detected in a wide variety of other autoimmune conditions (e.g. systemic lupus erythematosus, rheumatoid arthritis, Felty's syndrome and chronic inflammatory bowel diseases with associated disorders).

The clinical utility of cANCA as a diagnostic marker for WG was recently confirmed in a large prospective European study undertaken with sera from vasculitis patients (sensitivity 60%, specificity 95%) [6]. However, when employed as a routine screening method for WG (defined according to ACR criteria) in patients with suspected vasculitis, the sensitivity of cANCA in a recent prospective single-centre study on 346 consecutive patients was only 28% (specificity for WG: 98%). The sensitivity rose to 83% if only biopsy-proven WG was considered [7]. A meta-analysis of 15 studies comprising 13 652 patients (including 736 cases of WG) yielded a pooled sensitivity of 66% and a specificity of 98% [8]. Taken together, these data show that the value of cANCA testing is limited by a rather low sensitivity; the greatest utility of cANCA testing may be in patients with suspected, but not yet proven, WG. This view is supported by a recent analysis of ANCA results in a large routine laboratory (Regional Immunology Laboratory, Belfast, UK). The overall positive predictive value for primary systemic vasculitides was 38% for all cANCA and only 20% for all pANCA. Specificity improved when only antinuclear antibody (ANA)-negative samples with a high ANCA titre were considered (cANCA 90%, pANCA 60%) [9]. In most, but not all cases, titres correlated with disease activity. Rising titres should alert the clinician to an increased risk of exacerbation, but are generally not regarded as an indication for intensifying therapy [10].

ELISAs are used to specify further the target antigens of ANCA, namely proteinase 3 (PR3; cANCA-positive samples have a 99% specificity for WG), myeloperoxidase (MPO; 80% specificity for MPA) [6], as well as less important target antigens such as cathepsin G, lacto-ferrin, lysozyme and human leucocyte elastase, which are not specific for any particular vasculitic disorder. Whether anti-bactericidal permeability increasing protein (BPI) ANCA offer further diagnostic perspectives in vasculitis is still unclear [11-13].

So, ANCA are not specific for ANCA-associated vasculitides and despite the high specificity of cANCA/PR3-ANCA for WG and of MPO-pANCA for MPA, an increasing number of 'false-positive' PR3-/MPO-ANCA have been described [10]. More recently, we and others have observed PR3-ANCA in subacute bacterial endocarditis, a condition sometimes associated with vasculitis [14]. Still, because ANCA test results are usually available before histological analyses are completed, ANCA serology remains the most important tool in the diagnostic repertoire for ANCA-associated vasculitides, especially in seriously ill patients suspected of having vasculitis. Under life-threatening conditions, therefore, therapy should be commenced based on clinical and serological findings! An overview of predominant immune phenomena in systemic vasculitides associated with the hypersensitivity reaction types (and the serological markers) is given in Table 2.

The incidence of ANCA in CSS is much lower than in WG and MPA, and their immunodiag-nostic significance is limited [6]. However, active CSS is characterized by increased eosinophils in conjunction with strongly elevated IgE and eosinophil cationic protein values [15].

Furthermore, endothelial cell damage in active AAV is indicated by markedly increased serum thrombomodulin (sTM) values [15]: in CSS, high levels of sTM correlate closely with the soluble interleukin-2 receptor, which has been shown to be a promising seromarker of disease activity in WG [16].

Because intermittent infections are a major differential diagnostic problem in seriously ill AAV patients (Table 3), a marker that distinguishes between the two conditions is urgently needed. Procalcitonin was recently shown to be normal in active autoimmune rheumatic disorders, but strongly elevated in concomitant bacterial infections and sepsis [17]. However, these findings have yet to be confirmed [18].

6. The mycotic process in endocarditis

Infective endocarditis (IE) is defined as an infection of the endocardial surface of the heart, which may include one or more heart valves, the mural endocardium, or a septal defect. Its intracardiac effects include severe valvular insufficiency, which may lead to intractable

	Henoch-Schönlein purpura	Cryoglobulin. vasculitis	MPA	WG	CSS
IgA immune deposits in vessels	+	–	–	–	–
IgG immune deposits in vessels	–	+	–	–	–
Cryoglobulins in blood and vessels	–	+	–	–	–
Hepatitis C viral genomes in blood[b] and vessels	–	HCV-RNA	–	–	–
ANCA in blood	–	–	MPO-ANCA	PR3-ANCA	(+)[a]
Missing Ig deposits ('pauci-immune')	–	–	+	+	+/–
Necrotizing granulomas	–	–	–	+[c]	+[c]
Asthma/eosinophilia (>10%)	–	–	–	–	+

[a]In about 30% of patients MPO-ANCA or PR3-ANCA were detected.

[b]Or in the cryoprecipitates.

[c]In particular in the respiratory tract.

Modified from [16].

Table 2. Differential diagnostic features of small vessel vasculitides

congestive heart failure and myocardial abscesses. IE also produces a wide variety of systemic signs and symptoms through several mechanisms, including both sterile and infected emboli and various immunological phenomena [19-21].

IE develops most commonly on the mitral valve, closely followed in descending order of frequency by the aortic valve, the combined mitral and aortic valve, the tricuspid valve, and, rarely, the pulmonic valve. Mechanical prosthetic and bioprosthetic valves exhibit equal rates of infection.

All cases of IE develop from a commonly shared process, as follows:

1. Bacteremia (nosocomial or spontaneous) that delivers the organisms to the surface of the valve

Wagner, 1991 [36]	GN, Osler nodes	Foc. segm. cresc. GN (IgM and C3 deposits)	*Streptococcus viridans*	nd	Recovery, ANCA neg.
Soto, 1994 [37]	Purpura, fever, weakness, haematuria, aneurysm	nd	*Streptococcus bovis*	Thickening of aortic valve	Mycotic intra-cran. cran. aneurysm. rupture
Subra, 1998 [38]	Nephrotic syndrome	Membranoproliferative GN	n.i.	Vegetations (mitral, aortic valves)	Improvement ANCA (+)
Subra, 1998 [38]	Fever, anaemia, purpura, GN	Foc. segm. cresc. GN (C1q and C3 deposits)	n.i.	Aortic vegetations	Improvement ANCA neg.
Choi, 2000 [39]	Fever, malaise, weight loss, splenomegaly	nd	*Streptococcus sanguis*	Mitral vegetations	Complete recovery ANCA neg.
Choi, 2000 [39]	Purpura, weight loss, malaise	nd	*S. viridans*	Mitral valve thickening	Complete recovery ANCA neg.

GN, glomerulonephritis; Foc. segm. cresc, focal segmental crescentic; nd, not done; s., Streptococcus; n.i., not isolated; cran., cranial; aneurysm., aneurysmatic; neg., negative; nd, not defined.

Reviewed and modified from [39].

Table 3. Summary of subacute bacterial endocarditis associated with PR3-ANCA

2. Adherence of the organisms
3. Eventual invasion of the valvular leaflets

The common denominator for adherence and invasion is nonbacterial thrombotic endocarditis, a sterile fibrin-platelet vegetation. The development of subacute IE depends on a bacterial inoculum sufficient to allow invasion of the preexistent thrombus. This critical mass is the result of bacterial clumping produced by agglutinating antibodies.

In acute IE, the thrombus may be produced by the invading organism (ie, *S aureus*) or by valvular trauma from intravenous catheters or pacing wires (ie, NIE/HCIE). *S aureus* can invade the endothelial cells (endotheliosis) and increase the expression of adhesion molecules and of procoagulant activity on the cellular surface. Nonbacterial thrombotic endocarditis may result from stress, renal failure, malnutrition, systemic lupus erythematosus, or neoplasia.

The Venturi effect also contributes to the development and location of nonbacterial thrombotic endocarditis. This principle explains why bacteria and the fibrin-platelet thrombus are deposited on the sides of the low-pressure sink that lies just beyond a narrowing or stenosis.

In patients with mitral insufficiency, bacteria and the fibrin-platelet thrombus are located on the atrial surface of the valve. In patients with aortic insufficiency, they are located on the ventricular side. In these examples, the atria and ventricles are the low-pressure sinks. In the case of a ventricular septal defect, the low-pressure sink is the right ventricle and the thrombus is found on the right side of the defect.

Nonbacterial thrombotic endocarditis may also form on the endocardium of the right ventricle, opposite the orifice that has been damaged by the jet of blood flowing through the defect (ie, the MacCallum patch).

1. Inflammatory diseases of unknown aetiology
    Systemic autoimmune diseases (e.g. vasculitides associated with systemic lupus erythematosus, Sjögren's syndrome, Behçet disease, and rheumatoid vasculitis)
    Local chronic inflammatory diseases (e.g. ulcerative colitis)
    Chronic granulomatous inflammation (Crohn's disease, sarcoidosis, etc.)
2. Infectious diseases
    Viruses (e.g. vasculitides associated with HIV, CMV, etc.)
    Bacteria (e.g. spirochaetales, mycobacteria, streptococci, tropheryma, whippeli, etc.)
    Parasites (e.g. *Ascaris* etc.)
    Fungi (e.g. *Aspergillus*)
3. Neoplasia
    Non-Hodgkin lymphoma
    Myeloproliferative diseases
    Solid tumours
    Atrial myxomas
4. Drug abuse (intoxication)
    Opioids (cocaine, morphine, etc.)
5. Drug-induced (casuistic)
    Antihypertensive (hydralazine)
    Antithyroid drugs (propylthiouracil, methimazole, carbamizole)
    Antibiotics (azithromycin, minocycline)
    Antifibrotic (penicillamine)
    Leukotriene receptor antagonist (zafirlukast, montelukast, pranlukast)

CMV, cytomegalovirus.

Table 4. Secondary vasculitides

The microorganisms that most commonly produce endocarditis (ie, *S aureus; Streptococcus viridans;* group A, C, and G streptococci; enterococci) resist the bactericidal action of complement and possess fibronectin receptors for the surface of the fibrin-platelet thrombus. Among the many other characteristics of IE-producing bacteria demonstrated in vitro and in vivo, some features include the following:

- Increased adherence to aortic valve leaflet disks by enterococci, *S viridans,* and *S aureus*
- Mucoid-producing strains of *S aureus*
- Dextran-producing strains of *S viridans*
- *S viridans* and enterococci that possess FimA surface adhesin

- Platelet aggregation by *S aureus* and *S viridans* and resistance of *S aureus* to platelet microbicidal proteins

Bacteremia (either spontaneous or due to an invasive procedure) infects the sterile fibrin-platelet vegetation described above. BSIs develop from various extracardiac types of infection, such as pneumonias or pyelonephritis, but most commonly from gingival disease. Of those with high-grade gingivitis, 10% have recurrent transient bacteremias (usually streptococcal species). Most cases of subacute disease are secondary to the bacteremias that develop from the activities of daily living (eg, brushing teeth, bowel movements).

Bacteremia can result from various invasive procedures, ranging from oral surgery to sclerotherapy of esophageal varices to genitourinary surgeries to various abdominal operations. The potential for invasive procedures to produce a bacteremia varies greatly. Procedures, rates, and organisms are as follows:

- Endoscopy - Rate of 0-20%; coagulase-negative staphylococci (CoNS), streptococci, diphtheroids
- Colonoscopy - Rate of 0-20%; *Escherichia coli, Bacteroides* species
- Barium enema - Rate of 0-20%; enterococci, aerobic and anaerobic gram-negative rods
- Dental extractions - Rate of 40-100%; *S viridans*
- Transurethral resection of the prostate - Rate of 20-40%; coliforms, enterococci, *S aureus*
- Transesophageal echocardiography - Rate of 0-20%; *S viridans,* anaerobic organisms, streptococci

Bacterial adherence to intravascular catheters depends on the response of the host to the presence of this foreign body, the properties of the organism itself, and the position of the catheter. Within a few days of insertion, a sleeve of fibrin and fibronectin is deposited on the catheter. *S aureus* adheres to the fibrin component.

S aureus also produces an infection of the endothelial cells (endotheliosis), which is important in producing the continuous bacteremia of *S aureus* BSIs. Endotheliosis may explain many cases of persistent methicillin-susceptible *S aureus* (MSSA) and methicillin-resistant S aureus (MRSA) catheter-related BSIs without an identifiable cause.

S aureus catheter-related BSIs occur even after an infected catheter is removed, apparently attributable to specific virulence factors of certain strains of *S aureus* that invade the adjacent endothelial cells. At some point, the staphylococci re-enter the bloodstream, resulting in bacteremia [22].

Four days after placement, the risk of infection markedly increases. Lines positioned in the internal jugular are more prone to infection than those placed in the subclavian vein. Colonization of the intracutaneous tract is the most likely source of short-term catheter-related BSIs. Among lines in place for more than 2 weeks, infection of the hub is the major source of bacteremia. In some cases, the infusion itself may be a reservoir of infection.

http://dx.doi.org/10.5772/55189

Colonization of heart valves by microorganisms is a complex process. Most transient bacteremias are short-lived, are without consequence, and are often not preventable. Bacteria rarely adhere to an endocardial nidus before the microorganisms are removed from the circulation by various host defenses.

Once microorganisms do establish themselves on the surface of the vegetation, the process of platelet aggregation and fibrin deposition accelerate at the site. As the bacteria multiply, they are covered by ever-thickening layers of platelets and thrombin, which protect them from neutrophils and other host defenses. Organisms deep in the vegetation hibernate because of the paucity of available nutrients and are therefore less susceptible to bactericidal antimicrobials that interfere with bacterial cell wall synthesis.

Complications of subacute endocarditis result from embolization, slowly progressive valvular destruction, and various immunological mechanisms. The pathological picture of subacute IE is marked by valvular vegetations in which bacteria colonies are present both on and below the surface.

The cellular reaction in SBE is primarily that of mononuclear cells and lymphocytes, with few polymorphonuclear cells. The surface of the valve beneath the vegetation shows few organisms. Proliferation of capillaries and fibroblasts is marked. Areas of healing are scattered among areas of destruction. Over time, the healing process falls behind, and valvular insufficiency develops secondary to perforation of the cusps and damage to the chordae tendineae. Compared with acute disease, little extension of the infectious process occurs beyond the valvular leaflets.

Levels of agglutinating and complement-fixing bactericidal antibodies and cryoglobulins are markedly increased in patients with subacute endocarditis. Many of the extracardiac manifestations of this form of the disease are due to circulating immune complexes. Among these include glomerulonephritis, peripheral manifestations (eg, Osler nodes, Roth spots, subungual hemorrhages), and, possibly, various musculoskeletal abnormalities. Janeway lesions usually arise from infected microemboli.

The microscopic appearance of acute bacterial endocarditis differs markedly from that of subacute disease. Vegetations that contain no fibroblasts develop rapidly, with no evidence of repair. Large amounts of both polymorphonuclear leukocytes and organisms are present in an ever-expanding area of necrosis. This process rapidly produces spontaneous rupture of the leaflets, of the papillary muscles, and of the chordae tendineae.

The complications of acute bacterial endocarditis result from intracardiac disease and metastatic infection produced by suppurative emboli. Because of their shortened course, immunological phenomena are not a part of acute IE.

W illiam Osler first used the term *mycotic aneurysm* in his 1885 Gulstonian Lecture series [23] to refer to an aneurysm resulting from an infectious process of the arterial wall, although a more accurate term might have been *endovascular infection* or *infective vasculitis*, because mycotic aneurysms are not due to a fungal organism.

Intracranial mycotic aneurysms (ICMAs) complicate about 2% to 3% of infective endocarditis (IE) cases, although as many as 15% to 29% of patients with IE have neurologic symptoms [24-26]. Of all intracerebral aneurysms, only 2% to 6% have an infectious etiology. Signs and symptoms of mycotic aneurysms may be misleading during the early stages, resulting in misdiagnosis and delays in treatment [27]. Early diagnosis of ICMA is the cornerstone of effective treatment.

Mycotic aneurysms can be divided into 4 types: [1] *embolic*, secondary to bacterial endocarditis (*embolomycotic aneurysms*); [2] *extravascular*, secondary to extension of contiguous infection from a septic focus neighboring an artery; [3] *cryptogenic* or primary bacteremic; and [4] direct contamination following arterial wall trauma, which may be postprocedural [28]. Aneurysms can occur in the cerebral circulation, usually at points of vessel bifurcation, or in the systemic circulation [29].

In IE-associated mycotic aneurysms, septic emboli are released from infected cardiac vegetations. These tiny septic emboli occlude the vasa vasorum or entire arterial lumen, which leads to damage to the muscular layer of the vessel. ICMA tend to occur in the more distal portions of the middle cerebral artery, near the surface of the brain, involving the secondary and tertiary branches. In contrast, berry aneurysms occur at proximal branch points in or near the circle of Willis [26]. The outcome depends upon the anatomical location of the embolus, the causative bacteria and associated virulence of the organism, underlying host defenses, and appropriate antibiotic therapy. Mycotic aneurysms can decrease, increase, remain the same in size, or even disappear during treatment for endocarditis [30].

Patients with bacterial intracranial aneurysms have variable neurological symptoms, and early symptoms of infection may be subtle. In ICMA, patients may have symptoms ranging from nonspecific, general complaints, including fever or headache, to neurological deficits or catastrophic intracranial hemorrhage. Laboratory results are typically suggestive of an underlying inflammatory process and may include leukocytosis, elevated erythrocyte sedimentation rate and/or C-reactive protein concentration, and anemia. Blood cultures are almost universally positive for microbial growth.

Computed tomographic angiography, magnetic resonance angiography (MRA), and catheter angiography are used to study the size, location, and morphology of intracranial aneurysms. Aneurysms 5 mm in diameter or larger can be detected by CTA and MRA. Smaller aneurysms are detected less reliably or detected in retrospect after comparison with cerebral angiography.[31-33]. Cerebral angiography is the gold standard and is often used in preoperative assessment and in determining prognosis[34]; however, it is not routinely recommended due to risk of complications associated with it. The size of the aneurysm during therapy can be safely and accurately monitored using CTA and MRA. In our patient, CTA was selected as the diagnostic tool.

Treatment of ICMA is controversial, in that the appropriate patients for surgical intervention, need for follow-up imaging, and most efficacious treatment are not well delineated in the medical literature. The appropriate treatment always involves medical and sometimes surgical therapies [35]. Moreover, there is no single uniformly accepted approach to the treatment of

ICMA in IE. The aim of therapy is to cure the underlying infection and avoid complications from the aneurysm. Some lesions will resolve with antibiotic therapy alone. The decision to pursue surgical management is complex and involves a number of factors, including the number, site, and anatomy of the aneurysm(s) and the comorbidities of the patient. Treatment options for unruptured aneurysms include observation or surgical approaches, such as craniotomy and clipping or endovascular coiling [36,37]. The surgical choice of treatment for ICMA is controversial, patient-specific, and is generally beyond the scope of this article. Four- to 6-week courses of pathogen-specific intravenous antibiotic are recommended. In addition, medical therapy should include control of hypertension and seizures. Therapy should be monitored with serial CTA or MRA, and surgical intervention is generally recommended for enlarging aneurysms in accessible locations. Ruptured aneurysms are treated emergently with surgery to prevent rebleeding if possible.

Staphylococcus aureus (~30%), *Salmonella* species (~15%), and less commonly viridans group streptococciaresomeofthecausitiveorganismsofmycoticaneurysmsinthepostantibioticera[38].

Recent reports suggest *Streptococcus pneumoniae,* including penicillin-resistant strains, are re-emerging as a cause of mycotic aneurysms [39]. Our patient was infected with *Streptococcus bovis,* a gram-positive cocci classified as group D streptococci. Endocarditis is the most significant clinical infection associated with *S bovis,* but bacteremia from enteric origins also occurs. *S bovis* accounts for 2% to 6% of streptococcal bloodstream isolates from hospitalized patients and for 2.4% to 25% of organisms associated with IE [40-44]. *S bovis* is a rare cause of ICMA, however. Interestingly, *S bovis* endocarditis or bacteremia is associated with concomitant undiagnosed gastrointestinal (GI) tumors in up to 56 % of patients [45]. GI diseases associated with *S bovis* endocarditis include colonic cancers, gastric ulcers, gastric cancer, duodenal ulcers, inflammatory bowel disease, colonic diverticula, angiodysplasia, and liver cirrhosis [40,46-48]. Thus, any patient with *S bovis* bacteremia should undergo screening for occult GI malignancy. Although our patient died before such screening could be completed, he did have a family history of gastric cancer and a personal history of colon cancer.

7. Bacterial causes of vasculitis

Bacterial seeding of vessels may lead to necrosis through direct bacterial action. Vessels may be seeded intraluminally at sites of endothelial injury or flow turbulence. Seeding of vasa vasora may cause destruction of vessels from the outside in. An injury of a large vessel by this mechanism is classically termed a "mycotic aneurysm."

Contiguous spread from an infected site to a vessel may occur. Vessels may also be seeded from within the lumen, as in subacute bacterial endocarditis in which septic emboli embed within the wall of smaller vessels, causing a "mycotic" process via a luminal route. Immune response to bacteria or to bacterial components may also lead to vasculitis, usually by immune-complex–mediated mechanisms[24].

In subacute bacterial endocarditis, direct spread via septic emboli and immune complex injury may occur.

Patients may present with evidence of elevated acutephase reactants, fever, malaise, myalgia, arthralgia, Osler's nodes, Janeway lesions, and septic infarcts [49,50].

Staphylococcus and streptococcus infections are common causes. Gram-negative organisms, other gram-positive cocci, fungi, and parasites may be causative as well, and their occurrence depends on the clinical setting [51-57].

Mycotic aneurysms resulting from septic emboli are common with staphylococcus, streptococcus, and *Salmonella* species [58-60]. Patients with subacute infections may develop cryoglobulins [61-63]. Bacteremia may present as leukocytoclastic vasculitis [64, 65]. Small-vessel vasculitis may be associated with post-streptococcal infection, distinct from endocarditis [66, 67].

The *Rickettsiae* are a group of obligate intracellular bacteria with tropism for vascular endothelium [68]. Infection results in widespread microvascular leak, local thrombosis, and ultimately multisystem failure if untreated. [69, 70].

Treponema pallidum and borrelia burgdorferi are also rare causes of infectious vasculitis [71].

In the lung, necrosis of vessels may occur from septic emboli or from contiguous spread in primary pneumonias. In the latter setting, *Pseudomonas aeruginosa* and *Legionella pneumophila* often cause direct necrosis via contiguous spread [72]. The presentation, however, is that of pneumonia.

Mycobacterial or fungal pulmonary infections may mimic Wegener's granulomatosis or Churg-Strauss vasculitis in eliciting a granulomatous reaction in vessels [73].

Spread of *Mycobacterium tuberculosis* to the aorta may be seen as a cause of tuberculous aortitis, coronary arteritis, and mycotic aneurysm [74-76]. *Aspergillus aeruginosa, Aspergillus fumigatus,* and *Mucor* may be characterized by direct vessel invasion and necrosis [59, 77, 78] *Coccidioides immitis* meningitis may be associated with vasculitis that can be confused with central nervous system

Angeitis [79, 80]. *Coccidioides immitis* may also present as an immune-complex–mediated disease with erythema nodosum, periarthritis predominantly of the ankles, and bihilar lymphadenopathy [81, 82]. This presentation is often confused with Löfgren's syndrome of sarcoidosis. While sarcoidosis as a cause of Löfgren's syndrome is more prevalent in eastern United States populations, *Coccidioides* immitis is a more likely cause of a Löfgren's-like presentation in the western United States.

Neisseria species may be associated with small-vessel vasculitis. In *Neisseria gonorrhea* infection, cutaneous papules vesiculate, then becomes necrotic [83]. In *N meningitides* infections, vasculitis may manifest in the skin and gastrointestinal tract with the endothelium showing necrosis and thrombosis [84-86]. In immunocompromised hosts, *Pseudomonas aeruginosa* and other gram-negative organisms can present as a large 1- to 5-cm macular erythema that develops central necrosis and peripheral edema and induration—a condition termed "ecthyma gangrenosum." Vessel thrombosis results from direct bacterial invasion of the vessels. Similar lesions may be seen in immunocompromised patients with disseminated *Pseudomonas,*

Nocardia, Aspergillus, Mucor, Curvularia, Pseudallescheria, Fusarium, Morganella, Metarrhizium, Xanthomonas, Klebsiella, E coli, and *Aeromonas* infections.[87-99].

Before AIDS, syphilis was the infectious agent known as the "great imposter," presenting as large- or medium size vessel disease (aortitis or coronary arteries) or as the small-vessel rash of secondary lues. Aortic aneurysms were insidious in clinical presentation. *Treponema pallidum* spirochetes were rarely detected in fibrosed and scarred vessels [100-102]. At least briefly, *Borrelia burgdorferi,* the causative agent of Lyme disease, was known as an "imposter." Vasculitic changes may be seen in the central nervous system, retina, and temporal arteries [103-116].

8. Viral causes of vasculitis

Our knowledge of viral pathogenesis has exploded in the last quarter of the twentieth century, accelerated in large part by epidemics of "emerging" viral diseases. Hepatitis C virus, discovered in 1989, has worldwide prevalence [25]. The10- to 20-year latent period before hepatic or rheumatic manifestations of disease explains the increasing number of cases of hepatitis C virus–mediated vasculitis currently being seen in the United States following the epidemic of new infections in the 1980s [26]. Prior to the discovery and characterization of hepatitis C virus in the late 1980s, the triad of arthritis, palpable purpura, and type II cryoglobulinemia was given the sobriquet "essential mixed cryoglobulinemia" and considered an idiopathic vasculitis.

Availability of diagnostic testing for hepatitis C virus demonstrated that almost all of these cases were associated with hepatitis C virus infection. Immune response to the virus elicits a response to the Fc portion of immunoglobulin with the majority of elicited antibody having the Wa idiotype [27,28].

Immune complexes of anti–Fc Wa idiotypic antibody and pre-existing antibody, and virus have the peculiar physical property of precipitating out of solution in the cold ("cryoglobulins"). Presumably, Wa idiotype recognizes a cross-reactive epitope found on hepatitis C virus and immunoglobulin. Extremities and skin are sufficiently cold so as to explain a predilection for small-vessel leukocytoclastic vasculitis of the skin; gravity enhances vascular injury in dependent distal vessels, giving rise to palpable purpura predominantly in the lower extremities. More severe cases may manifest visceral organ involvement including membranoproliferative glomerulonephritis and bowel involvement. Small- and mediumsized arteries may be involved as well, especially in the kidneys.

Hepatitis B virus (HBV) infection provides the classic example of virally mediated immune complex disease. A lymphocytic venulitis or neutrophilic vasculitis of small vessels with leukocytoclastic or fibrinoid changes presents typically as an "urticaria-arthritis syndrome."[29].

Immune complexes of hepatitis B virus surface antigen (HBsAg) and antibodies to hepatitis B virus surface antigen (HBsAb) circulate in the blood and are found deposited in vessels in association with complement [30, 31]. The long latency period of HBV allows time for an immune response to occur. Viral replication increases HBsAg load, and is temporally associated with jaundice [32]. The immune complexes eventually no longer form in antigen excess, and the serum sickness-like illness resolves. HBV has also been associated with large-vessel polyarteritis nodosa-like illness [33]. Onset is early in the course of chronic HBV hepatitis.

Immune complexes containing HBsAg, HBsAb, and complement are found in the vessel wall [34]. The determinants of small vessel versus larger vessel disease in the two syndromes of HBV infection are unknown.

Human immunodeficiency virus (HIV) patients may present with a variety of vasculitides. However, it is difficult to specifically attribute the various vasculitides seen to HIV because of frequent co-infections with other agents that may cause vasculitis in the absence of HIV infection.

Human T lymphotropic virus l infection may cause retinal, cutaneous, or central nervous system vasculitis [35-38].

The herpesviruses (cytomegalovirus, varicella-zoster, herpes simplex viruses 1 and 2, and herpes hominis) may be associated with retinal vasculitis in immunocompromised patients [39-45]. Varicella-zoster may also cause a diffuse central nervous system small arterial granulomatous vasculitis, or a small- and/or large-artery vasculopathy [46-48, 117]. Herpes simplex viruses 1 and 2 have been associated with cutaneous vasculitis and necrotizing arteritis of small and medium vessels [118-120]. Epstein-Barr virus has been suggested as a cause of both small- and large-vessel disease in a number of cases and short series [121-126]. However, the ability to demonstrate causality in many instances is made all the more difficult by the latency of herpesvirus infection.

Varicella zoster virus and CMV have been as well implicated in the etiopathogenesis of various vasculitides via numerous and overlapping mechanisms including direct microbial invasion of endothelial cells, immune complex mediated vessel wall damage and stimulation of autoreactive B and/or T cells through molecular mimicry and superantigens [71].

Vasculitis following varicella-herpes zoster infection occasionally develops in the form of a central neurological deficiency (locomotor deficiency with or without aphasia around one month after an ophthalmologic herpes zoster) or involving the retina or, more rarely, the skin or the kidneys. Vasculitis associated with cytomegaloviral infection,predominantly observed in immunodepressed patients, is diffuse and basically involving the digestive tube, notably the colon, the central nervous system and the skin [127].

Parvovirus B19 has been suggested as the causative agent of Wegener's granulomatosis and polyarteritis nodosa in a number of cases and short series [128-133]. However, the issue of latency and the failure to eliminate B19 from pooled blood products provides a cautionary note when considering causality [134-137]. Rare cases of vasculitis have similarly been reported following rubella virus, adenovirus, echovirus, coxsackievirus, parainfluenza virus, herpes simplex viruses, and hepatitis A virus infections [23, 138-148].

Ziegler et al demonstrated the presence of vasculitis in infected falcons by the West Nile virus. West Nile virus (WNV) is a zoonotic flavivirus that is transmitted by blood-suckling mosquitoes with birds serving as the primary vertebrate reservoir hosts (enzootic cycle). Some bird species like ravens, raptors and jays are highly susceptible and develop deadly encephalitis while others are infected subclinically only. Pathological findings in infected birds consistently included splenomegaly, non-suppurative myocarditis, meningoencephalitis and vasculitis. By immunohistochemistry WNV-antigens were demonstrated intralesionally. These results impressively illustrate the devastating and possibly deadly effects of WNV infection in falcons, independent of the genetic lineage and dose of the challenge virus used. Due to the relatively high virus load and long duration of viremia falcons may also be considered competent WNV amplifying hosts, and thus may play a role in the transmission cycle of this zoonotic virus.

Rare cases of vasculitis have similarly been reported following rubella virus, adenovirus, echovirus, coxsackievirus, parainfluenza virus, herpes simplex viruses, and hepatitis A virus infections [23, 138-148].

9. Parasitic causes of vasculitis

Toxocara canis presented in an adolescent as palpable purpura with additional features suggesting Henoch-Schönlein purpura [149]. *Cysticercus* has caused vasculitis and arachnoiditis as it infects the central nervous system [150] *Angiostrongylus* nematodes apparently caused a Wegener's granulomatosis-like pulmonary angiitis [151]. Loa loa, a filarial parasite, presented with cutaneous leukocytoclastic vasculitis

Author details

Jacques Choucair

Hotel Dieu de France hospital, Beirut, Lebanon

References

[1] Zeek, P. M. Periarteritis nodosa: a critical review. Am J Clin Pathol(1952). , 22, 777-90.

[2] Hunder, G. G. Vasculitis: diagnosis and therapy. Am J Med(1996). suppl. A):, 37-45.

[3] Jennette, J. C, Falk, R, Andrassy, K, et al. Nomenclature of systemic vasculitis. Proposal of an international conference. Arthritis Rheum(1994). , 37, 187-92.

[4] Coombs RRAGell PGH. The classification of allergic reactions underlying disease. In: Clinical aspects of immunology. Gell PGH, Coombs RRA, eds. Philadelphia: Davis, (1963).

[5] Hagen, E. C, Daha, M. R, Hermans, J, et al. Diagnostic value of standardized assays for anti-neutrophil cytoplasmic antibodies in idiopathic systemic vasculitis. Clin Nephrol(1998). , 53, 743-53.

[6] Rao, J. K, Allen, N. B, Feussner, J. R, & Weinberger, M. A prospective study of anti-neutrophil cytoplasmic antibody (cANCA) and clinical criteria in diagnosing Wegener's granulomatosis. Lancet(1995). , 346, 926-31.

[7] Rao, J. K, Weinberger, M, Oddone, E. Z, Allen, N. B, Lansman, P, & Feussner, J. R. The role of antineutrophil cytoplasmic antibody (cANCA) testing in the diagnosis of Wegener's granulomatosis. Ann Intern Med(1995). , 123, 925-32.

[8] Hagen, E. C, Daha, M. R, Hermans, J, et al. Diagnostic value of standardized assays for anti-neutrophil cytoplasmic antibodies in idiopathic systemic vasculitis. Clin Nephrol(1998). , 53, 743-53.

[9] Edgar JDMMcMillan SA, Bruce JN, Caulan SK. An audit of ANCA in routine clinical practice. Postgrad Med J(1995). , 71, 605-12.

[10] Csernok, W. L, & Immunodiagnostic, E. and pathophysiologic aspects of antineutrophil cytoplasmic antibodies in vasculitis. Curr Opin Rheumatol(1995). , 7, 11-9.

[11] Zhao, M. H, Jones, S. J, & Lockwood, C. M. Bactericidal/permeability increasing protein (BPI) is an important antigen for antineutrophil cytoplasmic autoantibodies (ANCA) in vasculitides. Clin Exp Immunol(1995). , 99, 49-56.

[12] Stoffel, M. P, Csernok, E, Herzberg, C, Johnston, T, Carroll, S. F, & Gross, W. L. Anti-neutrophil cytoplasmic antibodies (ANCA) directed against bactericidal/permeability increasing protein (BPI): A new seromarker for inflammatory bowel disease and associated disorders. Clin Exp Immunol(1996). , 104, 54-9.

[13] Schultz H, Csernok E, Johnston TW, Lockwood CM, Gross WL. Use of native and recombinant bactericidal/permeability increasing protein (BPI) as antigens for detection of BPI-ANCA. J Immunol Methods 1997;205:127-33.

[14] Lamprecht, P, Gadola, S, Schnabel, A, & Gross, W. L. ANCA, infectious endocarditis, glomerulonephritis and cryoglobulinemic vasculitis. Clin Nephrol(1998). letter).

[15] Schmitt, W. H, Csernok, E, Kobayashi, S, & Klinkenborg, A. Reinhold-Keller E, Gross WL. Churg-Strauss Syndrome: Serum markers of lymphocyte activation and endothelial damage. Arthritis Rheum(1997). , 41, 445-52.

[16] Schmitt, W. H, Heesen, C, Csernok, E, Rautmann, A, & Gross, W. L. Elevated serum levels of soluble interleukin-2 receptor (sIL-2R) in Wegener's granulomatosis (WG): Association with disease activity. Arthritis Rheum(1992). , 35, 1088-96.

[17] Stroemann, A, Künzel, K, Hiepe, S, Beier, W, Burmester, G. R, & Krause, A. Procalcitonin: Marker for bactericidal infections in patients with rheumatic diseases. Z Rheumatol(1996). suppl. 1):86.

[18] Moosig, F, & Csernok, E. Reinhold-Keller E, Schmitt WH, Gross WL. Elevated procalcitonin levels in active Wegener's granulomatosis. J Rheumatol(1998). , 25, 1531-3.

[19] Brusch, J. L. Infective endocarditis and its mimics in the critical care unit. In: Cunha BA, ed. *Infectious Diseases in Critical Care*. 2nd ed. New York, NY: Informa Healthcare; (2007). , 2007, 261-2.

[20] Karchmer, A. W. Infective endocarditis. In: *Braunwald's Heart Disease: A Textbook of Cardiovascular Medicine*. 7th ed. WB Saunders Co; (2005). , 2005, 1633-1658.

[21] Karchmer, A. W. Infective endocarditis. In: *Harrison's Principles of Internal Medicine*. 16th ed. McGraw-Hill; (2005). , 2005, 731-40.

[22] Xiong, Y. Q, Fowler, V. G, Yeaman, M. R, Perdreau-remington, F, Kreiswirth, B. N, & Bayer, A. S. Phenotypic and genotypic characteristics of persistent methicillin-resistant Staphylococcus aureus bacteremia in vitro and in an experimental endocarditis model. *J Infect Dis*. Jan 15 (2009). , 199(2), 201-8.

[23] Osler, W. Malignant endocarditis (Gulstonian Lecture I). *Lancet*. (1885). , 1, 415-418.

[24] Chan, F. Y, Crawford, E. S, Coselli, J. S, & Safi, H. J. Williams TW Jr. In situ prosthetic graft replacement for mycotic aneurysm of the aorta. *Ann Thorac Surg*. (1989). , 47(2), 193-203.

[25] Bohmfalk, G. L, Story, J. L, & Wissinger, J. P. Brown WE Jr. Bacterial intracranial aneurysm. *J Neurosurg*. (1978). , 48(3), 369-382.

[26] Jones HR JrSiekert RG. Neurological manifestations of infective endocarditis. Review of clinical and therapeutic challenges. *Brain*. (1989). Pt 5):1295-1213.

[27] Leo, P. J, Pearl, J, & Tsang, W. Mycotic aneurysm: a diagnostic challenge. *Am J Emerg Med*. (1996). , 14(1), 70-73.

[28] Cloft, H. J, Kallmes, D. F, Jensen, M. E, Lanzino, G, & Dion, J. E. Endovascular treatment of ruptured, peripheral cerebral aneurysms: parent artery occlusion with short guglielmi detachable coils. *AJNR Am J Neuroradiol*. (1999). , 20(2), 308-310.

[29] Shaikholeslami, R, Tomlinson, C. W, Teoh, K. H, Molot, M. J, & Duke, R. J. Mycotic aneurysm complicating staphylococcal endocarditis. *Can J Cardiol*. (1999). , 15(2), 217-222.

[30] Ziment, I. Nervous system complications in bacterial endocarditis. *Am J Med*. (1969). , 47(4), 593-607.

[31] Walsh, D. W, Ho, V. B, & Haggerty, M. F. Mycotic aneurysm of the aorta: MRI and MRA features. *J Magn Reson Imaging*. (1997). , 7(2), 312-315.

[32] Huston, J. rd, Nichols DA, Luetmer PH, et al. Blinded prospective evaluation of sensitivity of MR angiography to known intracranial aneurysms: importance of aneurysm size. *AJNR Am J Neuroradiol.* (1994). , 15(9), 1607-1614.

[33] Schwartz, R. B, Tice, H. M, Hooten, S. M, Hsu, L, & Stieg, P. E. Evaluation of cerebral aneurysms with helical CT: correlation with conventional angiography and MR angiography. *Radiology.* (1994). , 192(3), 717-722.

[34] Benjamin, M. E. Cohn EJ Jr, Purtill WA, Hanna DJ, Lilly MP, Flinn WR. Arterial reconstruction with deep leg veins for the treatment of mycotic aneurysms. *J Vasc Surg.* (1999). , 30(6), 1004-1015.

[35] Johnston, S. C, Wilson, C. B, Halbach, V. V, et al. Endovascular and surgical treatment of unruptured cerebral aneurysms: comparison of risks. *Ann Neurol.* (2000). , 48(1), 11-19.

[36] Bederson, J. B, Awad, I. A, Wiebers, D. O, et al. Recommendations for the management of patients with unruptured intracranial aneurysms: a statement for healthcare professionals from the Stroke Council of the American Heart Association. *Stroke.* (2000). , 31(11), 2742-2750.

[37] Johnston, S. C, Zhao, S, Dudley, R. A, Berman, M. F, & Gress, D. R. Treatment of unruptured cerebral aneurysms in California. *Stroke.* (2001). , 32(3), 597-605.

[38] Brown, S. L, Busuttil, R. W, Baker, J. D, Machleder, H. I, Moore, W. S, & Barker, W. F. Bacteriologic and surgical determinants of survival in patients with mycotic aneurysms. *J Vasc Surg.* (1984). , 1(4), 541-547.

[39] Brouwer, R. E, Van Bockel, J. H, & Van Dissel, J. T. *Streptococcus pneumoniae,* an emerging pathogen in mycotic aneurysms? *Neth J Med.* (1998). , 52(1), 16-21.

[40] Ballet, M, Gevigney, G, Gare, J. P, Delahaye, F, Etienne, J, & Delahaye, J. P. Infective endocarditis due to *Streptococcus bovis*. A report of 53 cases. *Eur Heart J.* (1995). , 16(12), 1975-1980.

[41] Murray, H. W, & Roberts, R. B. *Streptococcus bovis* bacteremia and underlying gastrointestinal disease. *Arch Intern Med.* (1978). , 138(7), 1097-1099.

[42] Selton-suty, C, Hoen, B, Delahaye, F, et al. Comparison of infective endocarditis in patients with and without previously recognized heart disease. *Am J Cardiol.* (1996). , 77(12), 1134-1137.

[43] Cabell, C. H, Jollis, J. G, Peterson, G. E, et al. Changing patient characteristics and the effect on mortality in endocarditis. *Arch Intern Med.* (2002). , 162(1), 90-94.

[44] Roberts, R. B. Streptococcal endocarditis: the viridans and beta hemolytic streptococci. In: Kaye D, ed. *Infective Endocarditis.* 2nd ed. New York: Raven Press; (1992).

[45] Hoen, B, Briancon, S, Delahaye, F, et al. Tumors of the colon increase the risk of developing *Streptococcus bovis* endocarditis: case-control study. *Clin Infect Dis.* (1994). , 19(2), 361-362.

[46] Zarkin, B. A, Lillemoe, K. D, Cameron, J. L, Effron, P. N, Magnuson, T. H, & Pitt, H. A. The triad of *Streptococcus bovis* bacteremia, colonic pathology, and liver disease. *Ann Surg.* (1990). , 211(6), 786-791.

[47] Kupferwasser, I, Darius, H, Muller, A. M, et al. Clinical and morphological characteristics in *Streptococcus bovis* endocarditis: a comparison with other causative microorganisms in 177 cases. *Heart.* (1998). , 80(3), 276-280.

[48] Friedrich, I. A, Wormser, G. P, & Gottfried, E. B. The association of remote *Streptococcus bovis* bacteremia with colonic neoplasia. *Am J Gastroenterol.* (1982). , 77(2), 82-84.

[49] Kodo, K, Hida, M, Omori, S, Mori, T, Tokumura, M, Kuramochi, S, et al. Vasculitis associated with septicemia: case report and review of the literature. Pediatr Nephrol (2001). , 16, 1089-1092.

[50] Conti, T, & Barnet, B. The diagnostic challenge of infective endocarditis: cutaneous vasculitis leading to the diagnosis of infective endocarditis. J Am Board Fam Pract (2001). , 14, 451-456.

[51] Mylonakis E CSBInfective endocarditis in adults. N Engl J Med (2001). Steitz A, Orth T, Feddersen A, Fischer T, Marker-Hermann E, Husmann M. A case of endocarditis with vasculitis due to *Actinobacillus actinomycetemcomitans:* a 16S rDNA signature for distinction from related organisms. Clin Infect Dis 1998; 27:224-225., 345(18), 1318-1330.

[52] Steitz, A, Orth, T, Feddersen, A, Fischer, T, Marker-hermann, E, & Husmann, M. A case of endocarditis with vasculitis due to *Actinobacillus actinomycetemcomitans:* a 16S rDNA signature for distinction from related organisms. Clin Infect Dis (1998). , 27, 224-225.

[53] Cohen, C. A, Almeder, L. M, Israni, A, & Maslow, J. N. *Clostridium septicum* endocarditis complicated by aortic-ring abscess and aortitis. Clin Infect Dis (1998). , 26, 495-496.

[54] Elzouki, A. Y, Akthar, M, & Mirza, K. Brucella endocarditis associated with glomerulonephritis and renal vasculitis. Pediatr Nephrol (1996). , 10, 748-751.

[55] Bani-sadr, F, Hamidou, M, Richard, P, Tiab, M, Lalande, S, & Grolleau, J. Y. Cutaneous vasculitis and acute renal failure disclosing endocarditis caused by *Actinobacillus actinomycetemcomitans*). Presse Med (1993).

[56] Gladstone, J. L, Friedman, S. A, Cerruti, M. M, & Jomain, S. L. Treatment of *Candida* endocarditis and arteritis. J Thorac Cardiovasc Surg (1976). , 71, 835-838.

[57] Martinez, A. J, Sotelo-avila, C, Alcala, H, & Willaert, E. Granulomatous encephalitis, intracranial arteritis, and mycotic aneurysm due to a free-living ameba. Acta Neuropathol (Berl) (1980). , 49, 7-12.

[58] Vyas, S. K, Law, N. W, & Loehry, C. A. Mycotic aneurysm of left subclavian artery. Br Heart J (1993). , 69, 455-456.

[59] Jenckes GA IIIAspergillus aortitis. J Thorac Cardiovasc Surg (1990). , 99, 375-376.

[60] Julke, M, & Leu, H. J. Extra-aortic aneurysms. Analysis of 163 aneurysms in 142 patients). Schweiz Med Wochenschr (1985). , 115, 10-13.

[61] La Civita LFadda P, Olivieri I, Ferri C. Cryoglobulinaemic vasculitis as presenting manifestation of infective endocarditis. Ann Rheum Dis (2002). , 61, 89-90.

[62] Yerly, P, Chuard, C, Pugin, P, & Regamey, C. Cryoglobulins and endocarditis, a case report.) Rev Med Suisse Romande (2001). , 121, 573-576.

[63] Agarwal, A, Clements, J, Sedmak, D. D, & Imler, D. Nahman NS Jr, Orsinelli DA, et al. Subacute bacterial endocarditis masquerading as type III essential mixed cryoglobulinemia. J Am Soc Nephrol (1997). , 8, 1971-1976.

[64] Lum, P. N, Woo, P. C, Wong, S. S, & Yuen, K. Leukocytoclastic vasculitis complicating *Klebsiella pneumoniae* bacteremia. Diagn Microbiol Infect Dis (2000). , 37, 275-277.

[65] Garcia-porrua, C, & Gonzalez-gay, M. A. Bacterial infection presenting as cutaneous vasculitis in adults. Clin Exp Rheumatol (1999). , 17, 471-473.

[66] Houston, T. P. Small-vessel vasculitis following simultaneous influenza and pneumococcal vaccination. N Y State J Med (1983). , 83, 1182-1183.

[67] David, J, Ansell, B. M, & Woo, P. Polyarteritis nodosa associated with streptococcus. Arch Dis Child (1993). , 69, 685-688.

[68] Walker, D. H, Cain, B. G, & Olmstead, P. M. Laboratory diagnosis of Rocky Mountain spotted fever by immunofluorescent demonstration of Rickettsia in cutaneous lesions. Am J Clin Pathol (1978). , 69, 619-623.

[69] George, F, Brouqui, P, Boffa, M. C, Mutin, M, Drancourt, M, Brisson, C, et al. Demonstration of *Rickettsia conorii*-induced endothelial injury in vivo by measuring circulating endothelial cells, thrombomodulin, and von Willebrand factor in patients with Mediterranean spotted fever. Blood (1993). , 82, 2109-2116.

[70] Davi, G, Giammarresi, C, Vigneri, S, Ganci, A, & Ferri, C. Di Francesco L, et al. Demonstration of *Rickettsia conorii*-induced coagulative and platelet activation in vivo in patients with Mediterranean spotted fever. Thromb Haemost (1995). , 74, 631-634.

[71] Clin Dev Immunol(2004). Sep-Dec;11(3-4):227-31

[72] Reich, J. M. Pulmonary gangrene and the air crescent sign. Thorax (1993). , 48, 70-74.

[73] Henocq, E, Hutinel, B, Jacob, J, & Olivier, C. Immunopathologic aspects of recurrent phlebitis and nodular vascularitis. Therapeutic applications). Phlebologie (1976). , 29, 125-132.

[74] Strnad, B. T, Mcgraw, J. K, Heatwole, E. V, & Clark, P. Tuberculous aneurysm of the aorta presenting with uncontrolled hypertension. J Vasc Interv Radiol (2001). , 12, 521-523.

[75] Allins, A. D, Wagner, W. H, Cossman, D. V, Gold, R. N, & Hiatt, J. R. Tuberculous infection of the descending thoracic and abdominal aorta: case report and literature review. Ann Vasc Surg (1999). , 13, 439-444.

[76] Tuder, R. M, Renya, G. S, & Bensch, K. Mycobacterial coronary arteritis in a heart transplant recipient. Hum Pathol (1986). , 17, 1072-1074.

[77] Nenoff, P, Kellermann, S, Horn, L. C, Keiner, S, Bootz, F, & Schneider, S. al. Case report. Mycotic arteritis due to *Aspergillus fumigatus* in a diabetic with retrobulbar aspergillosis and mycotic meningitis. Mycoses (2001). , 44, 407-414.

[78] Oaks, T. E, Pae, W. E, Pennock, J. L, Myers, J. L, & Pierce, W. S. Aortic rupture caused by fungal aortitis: successful management after heart transplantation. J Heart Transplant (1988). , 7, 162-164.

[79] De Carvalho, C. A, Allen, J. N, Zafranis, A, & Yates, A. J. Coccidioidal meningitis complicated by cerebral arteritis and infarction. Hum Pathol (1980). , 11, 293-296.

[80] Kobayashi, R. M, Coel, M, Niwayama, G, & Trauner, D. Cerebral vasculitis in coccidioidal meningitis. Ann Neurol (1977). , 1, 281-284.

[81] Whitaker, D. C, & Lynch, P. J. Erythema nodosum and coccidioidomycosis. Ariz Med (1979). , 36, 887-889.

[82] Body, B. A. Cutaneous manifestations of systemic mycoses. Dermatol Clin (1996). , 14, 125-135.

[83] Mastrolonardo, M, Loconsole, F, Conte, A, & Rantuccio, F. Cutaneous vasculitis as the sole manifestation of disseminated gonococcal infection: case report. Genitourin Med (1994). , 70, 130-131.

[84] Garcia-patos, V, Barnadas, M. A, Domingo, P, Esquius, J, & De Moragas, J. M. Cutaneous vasculitis during bacteremia caused by meningococcus serogroup B). Rev Clin Esp (1992). , 190, 311-313.

[85] Dearaujomartins-romeo, D, Garcia-porrua, C, & Gonzalez-gay, M. A. Cutaneous vasculitis is not always benign. Rev Rhum Engl Ed (1999).

[86] Seaton, R. A, Nathwani, D, Dick, J, & Smith, D. Acute meningococcaemia complicated by late onset gastrointestinal vasculitis. J Infect (2000). , 41, 190-191.

[87] Versapuech, J, Leaute-labreze, C, Thedenat, B, Taieb, A, & Ragnaud, J. M. Ecthyma gangrenosum caused by *Pseudomonas aeruginosa* without septicemia in a neutropenic patient). Rev Med Interne (2001)., 22, 877-880.

[88] Bonduel, M, Santos, P, Turienzo, C. F, Chantada, G, & Paganini, H. Atypical skin lesions caused by *Curvularia* sp. and *Pseudallescheria boydii* in two patients after allogeneic bone marrow transplantation. Bone Marrow Transplant (2001)., 27, 1311-1313.

[89] Mull, C. C, Scarfone, R. J, & Conway, D. Ecthyma gangrenosum as a manifestation of *Pseudomonas* sepsis in a previously healthy child. Ann Emerg Med (2000). , 36, 383-387.

[90] Wu, B. Y, Peng, C. T, Tsai, C. H, & Chiu, H. H. Community-acquired *Pseudomonas aeruginosa* bacteremia and sepsis in previously healthy infants. Acta Paediatr Taiwan (1999)., 40, 233-236.

[91] Fergie, J. E, Huang, D. B, Purcell, K, & Milligan, T. Successful treatment of *Fusarium solanae* ecthyma gangrenosum in a child with acute lymphoblastic leukemia in relapse. Pediatr Infect Dis J (2000)., 19, 579-581.

[92] Del Pozo JGarcia-Silva J, Almagro M, Martinez W, Nicolas R, Fonseca E. Ecthyma gangrenosum-like eruption associated with *Morganella morganii* infection. Br J Dermatol (1998)., 139, 520-521.

[93] Burgner, D, Eagles, G, Burgess, M, Procopis, P, Rogers, M, Muir, D, et al. Disseminated invasive infection due to *Metarrhizium anisopliae* in an immunocompromised child. J Clin Microbiol (1998)., 36, 1146-1150.

[94] Repiso, T, Garcia-patos, V, Martin, N, Creus, M, Bastida, P, & Castells, A. Disseminated fusariosis. Pediatr Dermatol (1996)., 13, 118-121.

[95] Martino, P, Gastaldi, R, Raccah, R, & Girmenia, C. Clinical patterns of *Fusarium* infections in immunocompromised patients. J Infect Dis (1994). Suppl 1):7-15.

[96] Jang, T. N, Wang, F. D, Wang, L. S, Liu, C. Y, & Liu, I. M. *Xanthomonas maltophilia* bacteremia: an analysis of 32 cases. J Formos Med Assoc (1992)., 91, 1170-1176.

[97] Stotka, J. L, & Rupp, M. E. *Klebsiella pneumoniae* urinary tract infection complicated by endophthalmitis, perinephric abscess, and ecthyma gangrenosum. South Med J (1991)., 84, 790-793.

[98] Edelstein, H, & Cutting, H. O. *Escherichia coli* as cause of ecthyma gangrenosum. Postgrad Med (1986)., 79, 44-45.

[99] Harris, R. L, Fainstein, V, Elting, L, Hopfer, R. L, & Bodey, G. P. Bacteremia caused by *Aeromonas* species in hospitalized cancer patients. Rev Infect Dis (1985). , 7, 314-320.

[100] Cheng, T. O. Syphilitic aortitis is dying but not dead. Catheter Cardiovasc Interv (2001)., 52, 240-241.

[101] Aizawa, H, Hasegawa, A, Arai, M, Naganuma, F, Hatori, M, Kanda, T, et al. Bilateral coronary ostial stenosis and aortic regurgitation due to syphilitic aortitis. Intern Med (1998)., 37, 56-59.

[102] Samson, L, Chalaoui, J, & Paradis, B. Case of the day. General. Syphilitic aortitis, with saccular aneurysm of the descending aorta and fusiform aneurysm of the ascending aorta. Radiographics (1990)., 10, 508-510.

[103] Oksi, J, Kalimo, H, Marttila, R. J, Marjamaki, M, Sonninen, P, Nikoskelainen, J, et al. Intracranial aneurysms in three patients with disseminated Lyme borreliosis: cause or chance association? J Neurol Neurosurg Psychiatry (1998)., 64, 636-642.

[104] Keil, R, Baron, R, Kaiser, R, & Deuschl, G. Vasculitis course of neuroborreliosis with thalamic infarct). Nervenarzt (1997)., 68, 339-341.

[105] Oksi, J, Kalimo, H, Marttila, R. J, Marjamaki, M, Sonninen, P, Nikoskelainen, J, et al. Inflammatory brain changes in Lyme borreliosis. A report on three patients and review of literature. Brain (1996)., 119, 2143-2154.

[106] Leys, A. M, Schonherr, U, Lang, G. E, Naumann, G. O, Goubau, P, Honore, A, et al. Retinal vasculitis in Lyme borreliosis. Bull Soc Belge Ophtalmol (1995)., 259, 205-214.

[107] Giang, D. W. Central nervous system vasculitis secondary to infections, toxins, and neoplasms. Semin Neurol (1994)., 14, 313-319.

[108] Smith, J. L, Winward, K. E, Nicholson, D. F, & Albert, D. W. Retinal vasculitis in Lyme borreliosis. J Clin Neuroophthalmol (1991)., 11, 7-15.

[109] Lang, G. E, Schonherr, U, & Naumann, G. O. Retinal vasculitis with proliferative retinopathy in a patient with evidence of *Borrelia burgdorferi* infection. Am J Ophthalmol (1991)., 111, 243-244.

[110] Pizzarello, L. D. MacDonald AB, Semlear R, DiLeo F, Berger B. Temporal arteritis associated with *Borrelia* infection. A case report. J Clin Neuroophthalmol (1989)., 9, 3-6.

[111] Lock, G, Berger, G, & Grobe, H. Neuroborreliosis: progressive encephalomyelitis with cerebral vasculitis). Monatsschr Kinderheilkd (1989)., 137, 101-104.

[112] Veenendaal-hilbers, J. A, Perquin, W. V, Hoogland, P. H, & Doornbos, L. Basal meningovasculitis and occlusion of the basilar artery in two cases of *Borrelia burgdorferi* infection. Neurology (1988)., 38, 1317-1319.

[113] Meier, C, & Grehl, H. Vasculitic neuropathy in the Garin-Bujadoux- Bannwarth syndrome. A contribution to the understanding of the pathology and pathogenesis of the neurological complications in Lyme borreliosis). Dtsch Med Wochenschr (1988)., 113, 135-138.

[114] Uldry, P. A, Regli, F, & Bogousslavsky, J. Cerebral angiopathy and recurrent strokes following *Borrelia burgdorferi* infection. J Neurol Neurosurg Psychiatry (1987). , 50, 1703-1704.

[115] MacDonald ABGiant cell arteritis and *Borrelia* infection. J Clin Neuroophthalmol (1987)., 7, 180-181.

[116] Camponovo, F, & Meier, C. Neuropathy of vasculitic origin in a case of Garin-Boujadoux-Bannwarth syndrome with positive *Borrelia* antibody response. J Neurol (1986)., 233, 69-72.

[117] Caruso, J. M, Tung, G. A, & Brown, W. D. Central nervous system and renal vasculitis associated with primary varicella infection in a child. Pediatrics (2001). E9.

[118] Koo, E. H, & Massey, E. W. Granulomatous angiitis of the central nervous system: protean manifestations and response to treatment. J Neurol Neurosurg Psychiatry (1988)., 51, 1126-1133.

[119] Schmitt, J. A, Dietzmann, K, Muller, U, & Krause, P. Granulomatous vasculitis-an uncommon manifestation of herpes simplex infection of the central nervous system). Zentralbl Pathol (1992)., 138, 298-302.

[120] Shiozi, Y, Takeshima, M, Itoshima, T, Nose, S, & Hamaya, K. Granulomatous angiitis of the central nervous system complicated by the syndrome of inappropriate antidiuretic hormone). No To Shinkei (1995)., 47, 595-599.

[121] Ban, S, Goto, Y, Kamada, K, Takahama, M, Watanabe, H, Iwahori, T, et al. Systemic granulomatous arteritis associated with Epstein-Barr virus infection. Virchows Arch (1999)., 434, 249-254.

[122] Lande, M. B, Mowry, J. A, & Houghton, D. C. White CR Jr, Borzy MS. Immune complex disease associated with Epstein-Barr virus infectious mononucleosis. Pediatr Nephrol (1998)., 12, 651-653.

[123] Murakami, K, Ohsawa, M, Hu, S. X, Kanno, H, Aozasa, K, & Nose, M. Large-vessel arteritis associated with chronic active Epstein-Barr virus infection. Arthritis Rheum (1998)., 41, 369-373.

[124] Nakagawa, A, Ito, M, Iwaki, T, Yatabe, Y, Asai, J, & Hayashi, K. Chronic active Epstein-Barr virus infection with giant coronary aneurysms. Am J Clin Pathol (1996)., 105, 733-736.

[125] Muso, E, Fujiwara, H, Yoshida, H, Hosokawa, R, Yashiro, M, Hongo, Y, et al. Epstein-Barr virus genome-positive tubulointerstitial nephritis associated with Kawasaki disease-like coronary aneurysms. Clin Nephrol (1993)., 40, 7-15.

[126] Kikuta, H, Sakiyama, Y, Matsumoto, S, Hamada, I, Yazaki, M, Iwaki, T, et al. Detection of Epstein-Barr virus DNA in cardiac and aortic tissues from chronic, active Epstein-Barr virus infection associated with Kawasaki disease-like coronary artery aneurysms. J Pediatr (1993)., 123, 90-92.

[127] Cohen, P, & Guillevin, L. Presse Med. (2004). Nov 6;33(19 Pt 2):1371-84.

[128] Naides, S. J. Rheumatic manifestations of parvovirus B19 infection. Rheum Dis Clin North Am (1998). , 24, 375-401.

[129] Aygoren-pursun, E, & Scharrer, I. A multicenter pharmacosurveillance study for the evaluation of the efficacy and safety of recombinant factor VIII in the treatment of patients with hemophilia A. German Kogenate Study Group. Thromb Haemost (1997). , 78, 1352-1356.

[130] Corman, L. C, & Dolson, D. J. Polyarteritis nodosa and parvovirus B19 infection. Lancet (1992).

[131] Delannoy, D, Balquet, M. H, & Savinel, P. Vasculitis with mixed cryoglobulin in a case of human parvovirus B19 infection. Presse Med (1993).

[132] Finkel, T. H, Torok, T. J, Ferguson, P. J, Durigon, E. L, Zaki, S. R, et al. Chronic parvovirus B19 infection and systemic necrotizing vasculitis: opportunistic infection or aetiological agent? Lancet (1994). , 343, 1255-1258.

[133] Martinelli, C, Azzi, A, Buffini, G, Comin, C. E, & Leoncini, F. Cutaneous vasculitis due to human parvovirus B19 in an HIV-infected patient: report of a case. AIDS (1997). , 11, 1891-1893.

[134] Erdman, D. D, Anderson, B. C, Torok, T. J, Finkel, T. H, & Anderson, L. J. Possible transmission of parvovirus B19 from intravenous immune globulin. J Med Virol (1997). , 53, 233-236.

[135] Prowse, C, Ludlam, C. A, & Yap, P. L. Human parvovirus B19 and blood products. Vox Sang (1997). , 72, 1-10.

[136] Yee, T. T, Cohen, B. J, Pasi, K. J, & Lee, C. A. Transmission of symptomatic parvovirus B19 infection by clotting factor concentrate. Br J Haematol (1996). , 93, 457-459.

[137] Flunker, G, Peters, A, Wiersbitzky, S, Modrow, S, & Seidel, W. Persistent parvovirus B19 infections in immunocompromised children. Med Microbiol Immunol (1998). , 186, 189-194.

[138] Inman, R. D, Hodge, M, Johnston, M. E, Wright, J, & Heathcote, J. Arthritis, vasculitis, and cryoglobulinemia associated with relapsing hepatitis A virus infection. Ann Intern Med (1986). , 105, 700-703.

[139] Press, J, Maslovitz, S, & Avinoach, I. Cutaneous necrotizing vasculitis associated with hepatitis A virus infection. J Rheumatol (1997). , 24, 965-967.

[140] Costa, M. M, Lisboa, M, Romeu, J. C, Caldeira, J, & De Q, V. Henoch-Schönlein purpura associated with coxsackie-virus B1 infection. Clin Rheumatol (1995). , 14, 488-490.

[141] Okano, M, Thiele, G. M, Sakiyama, Y, Matsumoto, S, & Purtilo, D. T. Adenovirus infection in patients with Kawasaki disease. J Med Virol (1990). , 32, 53-57.

[142] Embil, J. A, Mcfarlane, E. S, Murphy, D. M, Krause, V. W, & Stewart, H. B. Adenovirus type 2 isolated from a patient with fatal Kawasaki disease. Can Med Assoc J (1985).

[143] Chia, J. K, & Bold, E. J. Life-threatening leukocytoclastic vasculitis with pulmonary involvement due to echovirus 7. Clin Infect Dis (1998)., 27(5), 1326-1327.

[144] Riikonen, R. S. Retinal vasculitis caused by rubella. Neuropediatrics (1995). , 26, 174-176.

[145] Duhaut, P, Bosshard, S, Calvet, A, Pinede, L, Demolombe-rague, S, Dumontet, C, et al. Giant cell arteritis, polymyalgia rheumatica, and viral hypotheses: a multicenter, prospective case-control study. Groupe de Recherche sur l'Arterite a Cellules Geantes. J Rheumatol (1999)., 26, 361-369.

[146] Forster, W, Bialasiewicz, A. A, Busse, H, & Coxsackievirus, B. associated panuveitis. Br J Ophthalmol (1993)., 77, 182-183.

[147] Corbeel, L, Gewillig, M, & Baeten, E. Casteels-Van Daele M, Eggermont E. Carotid and coronary artery involvement in infantile periarteritis nodosa possibly induced by Coxsackie B4 infection. Favourable course under corticosteroid treatment. Eur J Pediatr (1987)., 146, 441-442.

[148] Roden, V. J, Cantor, H. E, Connor, O, Schmidt, D. M, & Cherry, R. R. JD. Acute hemiplegia of childhood associated with Coxsackie A9 viral infection. J Pediatr (1975). , 86, 56-58.

[149] Hamidou, M. A, Gueglio, B, Cassagneau, E, Trewick, D, & Grolleau, J. Y. Henoch-Schönlein purpura associated with *Toxocara canis* infection. J Rheumatol (1999). , 26, 443-445.

[150] Revuelta, R, Juambelz, P, Balderrama, J, & Teixeira, F. Contralateral trigeminal neuralgia: a new clinical manifestation of neurocysticercosis: case report. Neurosurgery (1995)., 37, 138-139.

[151] Pirisi, M, Gutierrez, Y, Minini, C, Dolcet, F, Beltrami, C. A, Pizzolito, S, et al. Fatal human pulmonary infection caused by an *Angiostrongylus*-like nematode. Clin Infect Dis (1995)., 20, 59-65.

Chapter 7

Vasculitis and Vasculopathy in Rheumatic Diseases

Mislav Radić and Josipa Radić

Additional information is available at the end of the chapter

http://dx.doi.org/10.5772/55056

1. Introduction

Vessels and the vascular endothelium are involved in the pathogenesis of inflammatory rheumatic diseases a family of related disorders that include rheumatoid arthritis (RA), systemic lupus erythematosus (SLE) and systemic sclerosis (SSc). In these conditions vascular involvement is very important. This chapter aims to give an overview of the prevalence of the different forms of vasculopathy/vasculitis that can be encountered in the RA, SLE and SSc patients, describe their pathogenesis, and address their impact on disease severity and outcome. All of these rheumatic diseases involve some level of underlying vasculitis.

SSc is a connective tissue disease characterized by fibrosis and vasculopathy involving multiple organ systems. Many clinical complications of SSc are due to dysfunction of vascular beds throughout the body. Involvement of the microvasculature leads to cutaneous and mucosal telangiectasias, digital ulcers, and tissue ischemia. If medium-sized blood vessels are involved, manifestations include gangrene, digital loss, renal crisis, and pulmonary arterial hypertension. While occlusive vasculopathy is a well-recognized feature of SSc, less is known about the occurrence and the consequences of frank vascular inflammation. Albeit rare, typical vasculitis with inflammatory infiltrates damaging blood vessels has been reported in patients with systemic sclerosis. The distinction between SSc vasculopathy and SSc-associated vasculitis can be difficult to make based on clinical presentation alone, but knowledge of the underlying pathogenesis and histopathology can be very helpful. In the current pathogenic model of SSc, a vascular injury of unknown cause leads to endothelial apoptosis and initiates the process of SSc vasculopathy. Continuous endothelial dysfunction likely contributes to activation of adventitial fibroblasts with resultant intimal proliferation, eventual luminal narrowing, and tissue hypoxia. Histopathology of SSc vasculopathy reflects the underlying pathogenesis, with myofibroblast proliferation and matrix deposit in the subendothelial layer leading to obliterative thickening of vessel walls. Inflammatory infiltrates are absent, and the internal elastic lamina remains intact. In contrast to vasculopathy, concurrent vasculitis in SSc shows histopathologic evidence of inflammation, with presence of mononuclear infiltrates and destruction of the vascular wall. However, vasculitis is known to occur even in the setting of a disease predisposing towards vasculopathy, and histology is required to distinguish the two pathogenic processes.

SLE is a connective tissue autoimmune disease, where vasculopathy is one of the typical symptoms. It is reported in 10-40% of patients. It occurs more often in women (80%) than in men and may precede the development of a full-blown SLE. The differentiation of the type of vascular complications is very difficult, sometimes impossible, and requires an in-depth immune, histopathologic and imaging diagnostic approaches, and extensive clinical experience. It may play a key role in the choice of treatment strategy and prediction of the patient prognosis. Therefore, the awareness of the etiology, pathophysiology, the clinical and histopathogical setting, and SLE associated vascular complications is of great clinical significance. Vascular lesions in SLE are commonly known as the lupus vasculopathy; a typical lupus vasculitis with inflammatory and vascular wall necrosis and a thrombus in the lumen of affected artery occurs less often. SLE-associated vasculitis may present different clinical courses. The broad spectrum of symptoms includes mild forms affecting only cutaneous vessels, and also severe, catastrophic forms, with organ complications development, and vasculitis within the internal organs. Lupus vasculopathy is usually seen in cutaneous vessels, in renal glomeruli, coronary and brain vessels, the brain, lung alveoli and less often in the gastrointestinal tract. It has to be stressed that cutaneous lupus vasculopathy in systemic lupus erythematosus occurs most often, and is reported in 94% of patients with lupus vasculitis.

Systemic rheumatoid vasculitis is a multisystem autoimmune inflammatory condition of small and medium-sized vessels that typically affects a subset of patients with longstanding seropositive RA and alters the course and prognosis of the disease. Mortality rates are high, with significant morbidity. Systemic rheumatoid vasculitis refers to patients with rheumatoid arthritis, a chronic disease with painful inflammation of the joints, who also develop inflammatory disease in small and medium-sized blood vessels. The reason why systemic rheumatoid vasculitis develops in some RA patients and not others is not clear. Genetic factors may be involved. Viral infections and drug reactions have been suggested as causes of systemic rheumatoid vasculitis. The blood vessels most often involved are arteries that bring blood to the skin, nerves, and internal organs. Veins can also be involved. When systemic rheumatoid vasculitis involves the small arteries and veins that nourish the skin of the fingertips and skin around the nails, small pits in the fingertips or small sores causing pain and redness around the nails can occur. Involvement of somewhat larger arteries and veins of the skin can cause a painful red rash that often involves the legs. If the skin is very inflamed, ulcers can occur and infection becomes a complicating risk. Systemic rheumatoid vasculitis that injures the nerves can cause loss of sensation, numbness and tingling, or potentially weakness or loss of function of the hands and/or feet. The rare systemic rheumatoid vasculitis of larger arteries can cause complete absence of blood flow to tissue sites supplied by the affected vessel (termed occlusion, resulting in infarction), which can cause gangrene of fingers or toes, stomach pain, cough, chest pain, heart attack, and/or a stroke if the brain is involved. This form of systemic rheumatoid vasculitis can also be accompanied by general symptoms such as fever, loss of appetite, weight loss, and loss of energy. Higher titers of rheumatoid factors, antibodies to cyclic citrullinated peptides (anti CCP), and circulating immune complexes with lower C4 levels are detected in the sera of patients with RA and vasculitis, compared with patients with RA only. Deposition of rheumatoid factor-containing immune complexes likely contributes to vessel inflammation and damage through binding to cell surface Fc receptors, activation of the complement cascade, and release of proinflammatory cytokines.

2. Systemic sclerosis (SSc)

2.1. SSc vasculopathy

SSc is a connective tissue disease characterized by fibrosis and vasculopathy involving multiple organ systems. Classification into diffuse or limited cutaneous forms depends on the extent of skin thickening, with the former affecting areas proximal to the elbows or knees, and the latter limited to the face and distal extremities [1]. Systemic sclerosis (scleroderma) has two very different subsets: limited scleroderma and diffuse scleroderma. These can be identified by differences in clinical findings and by the temporal relationship to vasospasm. Limited scleroderma is so named because skin involvement is limited to the hands and face. Limited SSc is characterized by calcinosis, Raynaud's phenomenon, esophageal dysmotility, sclerodactyly, and telangiectasia (CREST syndrome). The most common cause of death in limited scleroderma is pulmonary hypertension or pulmonary fibrosis. Because Raynaud's phenomenon is a near universal prodrome, there are long-standing suggestions that the initial event in limited SSc may affect the vasculature [2]. Even in localized SSc, which has fewer systemic features, Raynaud's progresses to peripheral ischemia with digital ulceration and loss of fingers [3]. Although the vasospasm associated with Raynaud's phenomenon may be prodromal, it is not itself a sufficient cause of the disease because symptoms of vasospasm can precede diagnosis of limited SSc by many years, and the incidence of SSc in the population of people with Raynaud's phenomenon is very low [4]. Diffuse SSc appears with a much wider extent of skin involvement. Patients with diffuse SSc are prone to kidney crisis and pulmonary fibrosis. These patients develop Raynaud's phenomenon within 1 year of onset of symptoms but they tend to not have it as a prodrome. Both limited and diffuse SSc patients have ischemic changes in their digits (80%–95% have Raynaud's phenomenon), some with ulcers, gangrene, and loss of fingers [3]. Many clinical complications of SSc are due to dysfunction of vascular beds throughout the body. Involvement of the microvasculature leads to cutaneous and mucosal telangiectasias, digital ulcers, and tissue ischemia. If medium-sized blood vessels are involved, manifestations include gangrene, digital loss, renal crisis, and pulmonary arterial hypertension [5]. While occlusive vasculopathy is a well-recognized feature of SSc, less is known about the occurrence and the consequences of frank vascular inflammation. The distinction between SSc vasculopathy and vasculitis can be difficult to make based on clinical presentation alone, but knowledge of the underlying pathogenesis and histopathology can be very helpful. In the current pathogenic model of SSc, a vascular injury of unknown cause leads to endothelial apoptosis and initiates the process of SSc vasculopathy. Autoantibodies, reperfusion injury, infection, and defects in vascular repair have all been implicated as possible triggers [6]. Increased levels of endothelial cells in the circulation have been cited as evidence that the intactness of the vascular lining is jeopardized [6, 7]. Subsequent endothelial dysfunction results in the imbalance of vasoactive factors: decreased levels of vasodilators such as endothelial nitric oxide synthase and prostacyclin syntheses, as well as increased levels of the vasoconstrictor endothelin-1 and vascular endothelial growth factor [8, 9]. Continuous endothelial dysfunction likely contributes to activation of adventitial fibroblasts with resultant intimal proliferation, eventual luminal narrowing, and tissue hypoxia [7, 10]. Intimal hyperplasia, or more correctly the formation of a neointima, is a common response to arterial injury, and it is a characteristic feature of the arteries in SSc. The best evidence for intimal hyperplasia in SSc is found in a remarkable autopsy series reported by D'Angelo et al. [11] that is summarized in Table 1.

System	Pathology
Pulmonary	interstitial fibrosis and arterial thickening fibrotic pleuritis
Coronary	myocardial fibrosis arteriolar concentric intimal thickening pericarditis fibrous and adhesive
Gastrointestinal	esophageal atrophy and fibrosis lesions of reflux small intestine atrophy and fibrosis large intestine atrophy and fibrosis
Renal	artery hyperplasia and bone marrow thickening, fibrinoid necrosis
Skeletal muscle	atrophy round cell myositis
Arterioles	noninflammatory intimal proliferation in two or more organ systems inflammatory polyarteritis

Table 1. Summary of vascular pathology findings in SSc

Characteristic vascular changes in scleroderma also occur at the capillary level. The change most studied in the clinical literature is at the level of the nail beds. Changes in the nailfold capillaries are one of the first signs in SSc [12]. Because these changes have only been described by nail bed microscopy, little is known about the mechanism of this change. However, the morphology seen in the scleroderma nail beds closely resembles changes seen when vascular endothelial growth factor (VEGF) is overexpressed locally [13], and nailfold changes appear to be associated with very high levels of circulating VEGF [14]. These abnormalities have led to speculation that endothelial death is a primary and ongoing process in SSc. Although there is evidence from in vitro studies that SSc serum may contain antiangiogenic or other agents that are toxic to endothelium, apoptotic change or even increased endothelial turnover has not been demonstrated in vivo [15, 16]. Endothelin-1 (ET-1) is a prototypical endothelial cell-derived product, and endothelial damage leads to increased production of ET-1. Since ET-1 is a vasoconstrictive agent, loss of normal vessel compliance and vasorelaxation may be induced by increased levels of ET-1. In addition, ET-1 promotes fibroblast synthesis of collagen [17]. ET-1 upregulates expression of adhesion molecules, which promote the homing of pathogenic leukocytes to the skin. Further, ET-1 can also induce myofibroblast differentiation in fibroblasts [18]. ET-1 can induce connective tissue growth factor (CTGF), and may mediate the induction of collagen synthesis by activation of CTGF [19]. Circulating ET-1 levels have been observed in patients with diffuse SSc with widespread fibrosis and those with limited SSc and hypertensive disease [20], suggesting that soluble ET-1 levels may be a marker of fibrosis and vascular damage. Thus, ET is suggested to significantly contribute to fibrogenesis, linking between vasculopathy, and fibrosis, and the blockade of ET signalling may lead to the reduction of fibrosis. *In vitro*, SSc fibroblasts synthesized increased amounts of ET-1, and further, bosentan reduced the contractile ability of the SSc fibroblasts [18]. Therefore, a blocking ET-1 might be expected as a benefit in reducing pulmonary fibrosis. Recently, bosentan is demonstrated to reduce the number of newly formation of digital ulcers associated with SSc [21]. Additionally, bosentan may reduce the sclerosis of the skin in a pilot study [22].

Nitric oxide (NO) is a strong vasodilator and inhibits the biochemical effect of ET-1. However, ET-1 induces inducible NO syntheses (iNOS) expression in endothelial cells [23], and iNOS expression is detected in the endothelial cells in the lesion skin of SSc [24]. So far, several reports have shown impaired NO production in SSc [24, 25], which may contribute to the vascular pathogenesis of the arteriolar intimal proliferation in SSc. Thus, an imbalance between vasoconstriction and vasodilatation can lead to ischemia-reperfusion injury, endothelial damage and subsequent increased collagen gene expression *via* hypoxia. Hypoxia induces ECM proteins in cultured fibroblasts, and vascular endothelial growth factor (VEGF) overexpression may be caused in response to chronic hypoxia condition [26].

Histopathology of SSc vasculopathy reflects the underlying pathogenesis, with myofibroblast proliferation and matrix deposit in the subendothelial layer leading to obliterate thickening of vessel walls. Inflammatory infiltrates are absent, and the internal elastic lamina remains intact [27].

In contrast to vasculopathy, concurrent vasculitis in SSc shows histopathologic evidence of inflammation, with presence of mononuclear infiltrates and destruction of the vascular wall. Notably, both vasculopathic and vasculitic changes were seen in five of nine (55%) digital amputation specimens from SSc patients, emphasizing that small vessel vasculitis and stenosing vasculopathy may coexist[27]. Further support has come from autopsy studies of SSc patients, where 24% of 58 cases showed noninflammatory intimal proliferation in two or more organs, but 9% had features of inflammatory polyarteritis [11]. Thus, vasculitis is known to occur even in the setting of a disease predisposing towards vasculopathy, and histology is required to distinguish the two pathogenic processes.

2.2. Large-vessel vasculitis associated with SSc

Giant cell arteritis is a common vasculitis of the elderly involving large- and medium-sized arteries, typically the temporal, ophthalmic, vertebral, and axillary arteries as well as the aorta. The American College of Rheumatology (ACR) criteria include at least three of the following: (1) onset at age 50, (2) new headache, (3) claudication of the jaw or tongue, (4) temporal artery tenderness to palpation or decreased pulsation, (5) ESR 50 mm/h, and (6) temporal artery biopsy showing vasculitis with mononuclear inflammatory infiltrate or granulomatous inflammation with presence of giant cells [28]. While giant cell arteritis is relatively common among the vasculitides, it has only been reported in three cases of concurrent SSc, all of which were women in their sixth decade with limited skin involvement [29-31].

Takayasu arteritis is a relatively rare large vessel vasculitis (incidence 0.4–2/million/year) affecting mostly young women of Asian origin although the incidence among the middleaged with atherosclerosis has been rising [32, 33]. The aorta and its main branches are typically involved. ACR diagnostic criteria include at least three of the following: (1) onset before age 40, (2) claudication of an extremity, (3) decreased brachial artery pulse, (4) 10 mmHg in systolic blood pressure between the arms, (5) bruit over the subclavian arteries or aorta, and (6) stenosis/occlusion of the aorta, its major branches, or large arteries in proximal upper or lower extremities [34]. Similar to giant cell arteritis, the histopathology in Takayasu arteritis shows mononuclear infiltrates in the vessel wall, intimal thickening, and destruction of elastic laminas, giant cell formation, and expansion of the adventitial layer. Elastic lamina destruction can lead to aneurysm formation while transmural inflammation drives intimal proliferation, adventitial scarring, and vascular lumen narrowing. Four cases of Takayasu arteritis in the setting of SSc have been reported. As the overwhelming majority of patients with Takaysu arteritis are female, all four of these cases were women, with ages ranging from 29 to 68 [35-38]. Three of the patients had diffuse skin involvement of SSc.

2.3. Medium- and small-vessel vasculitis associated with SSc

Polyarteritis nodosa (PAN) is a necrotizing vasculitis affecting medium-sized vessels, with a constellation of clinical findings that reflect multiorgan involvement. It can be associated with hepatitis B viral infection. PAN can be distinguished from the small-vessel vasculitides such as microscopic polyangiitis by the absence of antineutrophil cytoplasmic antibodies. The ACR diagnostic criteria for PAN include at least three of the following: (1) weight loss 4 kg, (2) livedo reticularis, (3) testicular pain or tenderness, (4) myalgias, weakness, or leg tenderness, (5) mono- or polyneuropathy, (6) hypertension, (7) elevated blood creatinine or urea, (8) serum hepatitis B antigen or antibody, (9) aneurysms or occlusions of visceral arteries, or (10) granulocytes on biopsy of small- or medium-sized arteries [39]. A recent retrospective study of 348 patients with PAN found general symptoms in 93.1%, neurologic involvement in 79%, and skin involvement in about 50% [40]. Five-year relapse-free survival was 59.4% for nonhepatitis-B-associated PAN and 67% for HBV-associated PAN. Only one case of PAN has been described in a 28-year-old woman with diffuse SSc, characterized by Raynaud's phenomenon and skin sclerosis over the hands, arms, and chest [41].

http://dx.doi.org/10.5772/55056

Primary angiitis of the central nervous system (PACNS) is a rare poorly characterized entity affecting small- and medium-sized vessels of the central nervous system (CNS) but not organs or vessels outside the CNS. In general, PACNS is distinguished from secondary CNS vasculitis with the exclusion of infections, malignancy, systemic vasculitis or connective tissue disease, or drug-induced vasculitis. Clinical presentations of PACNS include confusion, new onset headache, seizures, stroke or cerebral hemorrhage, and myelopathy [42]. The duration from symptom onset to diagnosis can range from 3 days to 3 years [43]. Multiple laboratory data abnormalities can occur but none is specific for the diagnosis, with ESR described to be normal in a number of cases. Characteristic changes on cerebral angiography include multifocal segmental stenosis, dilatation, or occlusion of small- and medium-sized leptomeningial and intracranial vessels as well as formation of collateral vessels. Further supportive evidence can be obtained from leptomeningeal or parenchymal biopsies, which are specific but not sensitive for vasculitis given the focal segmental nature of the disease; therefore, a negative biopsy does not rule out the diagnosis. Histology can show either granulomas in small vessel walls, lymphocytic infiltrates, or necrotizing vasculitis [43]. The rarity and heterogeneity complicate classification, diagnosis, and management. Calabrese and Mallek have proposed the following diagnostic criteria for PACNS: (1) recent onset of headache, confusion, or multifocal neurologic deficits, (2) cerebral angiographic changes suggestive of vasculitis, (3) exclusion of systemic disease or infection, and (4) leptomeningeal or parenchymal biopsy to confirm vasculitis and to exclude infection, malignancy, and noninflammatory vascular occlusive disease [44]. However, only one case of PACNS has been described in SSc [41].

2.4. Mixed cryoglobulinemia and cryofibrinogenemiaassociated with SSc

Mixed cryoglobulinemia is the presence of polyclonal immunoglobulins that precipitate in the serum with cold exposure, often secondary to a connective tissue disease such as systemic lupus erythematosus or Sjogren's syndrome. The presence of cryoglobulins (CGs) may be asymptomatic or may lead to manifestations of the cryoglobulinemic syndrome, including purpura, arthralgia, myalgia, glomerulonephritis, and peripheral neuropathy [45]. The diagnosis of the latter entails a combination of clinical presentation, laboratory testing showing the presence of circulating cryoglobulins, and histopathologic appearance such as leukocytoclastic vasculitis (most common). Similarly, cryofibrinogenemia is the presence of cold-induced precipitants in the plasma but not in the serum. Connective tissue diseases, malignancy, and infection have been known to be associated with this condition, which can be asymptomatic or can manifest as painful ulcers, purpura, or perniosis, reflecting possible underlying cold-induced thromboses, increased blood viscosity, or vascular reactivity. The diagnosis of clinically significant cryofibrinogenemia requires not only circulating cryofibrinogen (CF) but also clinical features and histopathologic evidence of small-vessel thrombosis and perivascular infiltrate [46]. For both mixed cryoglobulinemia and cryofibrinogenemia, treating the underlying disease (whether infection, connective tissue disease, or malignancy) can sometimes improve symptoms. Plasmapheresis and immunosuppression with glucocorticoids and/or cytotoxic therapy have also been used in severe disease although with unclear efficacy.

Connective tissue diseases have been associated with the presence of both CG and CF, perhaps more so than CF alone [47]. In the few studies and reports involving SSc, these cold-induced precipitants do not appear to trigger symptoms. In one study, one out of 19 patients with both CG and CF carried the diagnosis of SSc [47]. In another study, 10 out of 20 SSc patients had the presence of polyclonal IgG and IgM cryoglobulins in the serum, but none exhibited clinical signs of cryoglobulinemic syndrome [48]. In one report of long-standing SSc with the presence of cryoglobulins (both IgG and IgM), the patient presented with paresthesias, transient aphasia, vision changes, and delirium. Cerebral angiogram was normal, and electroencephalogram revealed generalized slowing of action potentials, and computed tomography of the extremities revealed calcinosis. While peripheral neuropathy can be a manifestation of mixed cryoglobulinemia, central nervous system involvement would be highly unusual; therefore it, is unclear whether the presence of cryoglobulins in this case is an incidental finding. Another man with long-standing SSc presented with sudden onset gangrene in the fingers and toes after cold exposure and was found to have very elevated cryofibrinogen [49].

2.5. Behcet's disease associated with SSc

Behcet's disease is characterized by recurrent oral aphthous ulcers and other systemic manifestations believed to be due to systemic vasculitis, including genital aphthous ulcers, ocular disease, skin involvement, gastrointestinal ulcers, neurologic disease, and arthritis. It is more common along the ancient Silk Road, with 0.11% prevalence in Turkey and 2.6% per 100,000 in Southern China [50]. Diagnosis is made based on clinical features including presence of recurrent oral aphthae plus two of the following without other systemic disease: (1) recurrent genital aphthae, (2) eye lesions including uveitis or retinal vasculitis, (3) skin lesions including erythema nodosum, pseudovasculitis, papulopustular lesions, or acneiform nodules, or (4) positive pathergy test [51]. Treatment for mucocutaneous and joint disease includes colchicine (mixed results), glucocorticoids, and other immunosuppressives such as azathioprine. More serious disease with internal organ involvement has been treated with cyclophosphamide and high-dose steroids. Overviewing the literature, only two cases of Behcet's disease with concurrent SSc have been reported [52, 53].

2.6. Relapsing polychondritis associated with SSc

Relapsing polychondritis (RPC) is an inflammatory disease of unknown etiology involving cartilagenous tissues in multiple organs, typically the ears, nose, eyes, respiratory tract, and joints. Vascular and neurologic complications have also been reported. Association with systemic vasculitis, connective tissue disease, or myelodysplastic syndrome occurs in up to one-third of the cases. The original diagnostic criteria by McAdam required three of six clinical manifestations: (1) bilateral auricular chondritis, (2) nonerosive seronegative polyarthritis, (3) nasal chondritis, (4) respiratory tract chondritis, (5) ocular inflammation, or (6) cochlear and/or vestibular dysfunction [54]. The criteria were later modified to include the presence of three or more of the above, one clinical manifestation with corroborating histology, or chondritis at more than two sites responsive to steroids or diamino-diphenyl sulfone [55]. Only one case of RPC has been reported in association with SSc [56]

2.7. ANCA-associated vasculitis (AAV) in SSc patients

The spectrum of necrotizing small-vessel vasculitis known as ANCA-associated vasculitis (AAV) includes Wegener's granulomatosis (WG), microscopic polyangiitis (MPA), and Churg-Strauss syndrome (CSS). While formally classified as small-vessel vasculitis, AAV can involve medium-sized vessels. Cytoplasmic antineutrophil cytoplasmic antibodies (c-ANCAs) directed against proteinase 3 (PR3) are more commonly found in WGs whereas perinuclear ANCAs (p-ANCA) targeting myeloperoxidase (MPO) are more frequently seen in MPA and CSS. Variable organ involvement makes diagnosis a challenge, with alveolar hemorrhage and crescentic glomerulonephritis frequently occurring in WG and MPA, while polyneuropathy can be seen in ANCA-associated CSS [57]. Disease stage can range from localized without end-organ damage to severe generalized with organ failure. Of all the small vessel vasculitides, AAV is the most frequently reported in association with SSc, raising the question whether an overlap syndrome exists that combines features from both diseases. A study by Rho et al. found 31 reports containing 63 cases of AAV in SSc up to 1994 [58].

While lumen-occlusive vasculopathy is a prominent feature of SSc, frank vasculitis may also occur. Coexistent SSc and vasculitis have been reported for vessels of all sizes, either before or after SSc diagnosis, and in either SSc subtype (limited or diffuse).

3. Systemic lupus erythematosus (SLE)

3.1. Vascular involvement in SLE

SLE is a connective tissue autoimmune disease, where vasculopathy is one of the most typical symptoms [59]. Vascular involvement is frequent in SLE patients and represents the most frequent cause of death in established disease. In this context, vasculopathy can be directly aetiologically implicated in the pathogenesis of the disease, presenting as an acute/subacute manifestation of lupus (e.g., antiphospholipid syndrome (APS), lupus vasculitis). Besides overt vessel obstruction, vascular disease in lupus, especially when affecting medium- and small-sized vessels, may contain both vasculopathic and vasculitic pathophysiologic parameters.

Livedoid vasculopathy, a condition which can be observed in patients with systemic lupus erythematosus/antiphospholipid syndrome or specific forms of systemic vasculitis (mainly polyarteritis nodosa and cryoglobulinemia), is associated with chronic ulcerations of the lower extremities and characterized by uneven perfusion [60]. The pathogenesis of livedoid vasculopathy has not been fully elucidated, or rather, cannot be solely attributed to a particular mechanism, as both hypercoagulable states, as well as autoimmune diseases, appear to associate with and contribute to its development [61].

The typical histological findings show dermal blood vessel occlusion [62]. The histopathological findings of intravascular fibrin, segmental hyalinization, and endothelial proliferation clearly support the thrombotic parameter of its pathogenesis [63]. The presence of immunoreactants in the vessel wall and circulating immune complexes (such as rheumatoid factor) are in favor of its immunological component; the absence however of fibrinoid necrosis and inflammatory infiltration of the vessel wall differentiates livedoid vasculopathy from true vasculitides.

It is reported in 10–40% of patients. It occurs more often in women (80%) than in men and may precede the development of a full-blown SLE [64]. Vascular lesions in SLE are commonly known as the lupus vasculopathy; a typical lupus vasculitis with inflammatory and vascular wall necrosis and a thrombus in the lumen of affected artery occurs less often [65-67]. However, the rate of thrombotic events is higher in patients with disease of recent onset, when compared to patients with other autoimmune diseases and remains so throughout the course of the disease [68]; in the LUMINA study, which included multiethnic SLE patients of recent diagnosis, age, damage accrual at enrolment, and antiphospholipid antibodies, as well as the use of higher dosages of glucocorticoids were associated with a shorter time interval to thrombotic events [69]. Appel et al. [66] provided an SLE vasculopathy classification including: non complicated vascular deposits of immune complexes, noninflammatory necrotic vasculopathy, thrombotic microangiopathy and true lupus vasculitis. Of all lupus vasculitis, cases more than 60% is leucocytoclastic inflammation, 30% is vasculitis with cryoglobulinemia, and systemic vasculitis resembling polyarteritis nodosa constitutes about 6% of SLE vasculitides patients [66, 70-72]. Other clinical syndromes of vasculopathy in patients from the discussed group include thrombocytopenia with thrombotic purpura, venous thrombosis, antiphospholipid syndrome and urticaria vasculitis, reported in 5% of SLE patients [66]. The SLE associated vasculitis may present different clinical courses. The broad spectrum of symptoms includes mild forms affecting only cutaneous vessels, and also severe, catastrophic forms, with organ complications development, and vasculitis within the internal organs [73, 74]. Lupus vasculitis is usually seen in cutaneous vessels, in renal glomeruli, coronary and brain vessels, the brain, lung alveoli and less often in the gastrointestinal tract [59]. It has to be stressed that cutaneous lupus vasculopathy in SLE occurs most often, and is reported in 94% of patients with lupus vasculitis [75, 76]. Mild forms are characterized by purpura, urticaria lesions or bullous lesions of extremities, and livedo reticularis on the trunk.

It has been demonstrated that internal organ vessels are affected in 18% of SLE vasculitis patients. Renal vasculitis takes the shape of focal segmental glomerulitis with development of fibrinoid necrosis [59]. Lung vasculitis takes the form of necrotic alveolar capillaritis predisposing to pulmonary hemorrhage [59]. Brain vasculitis occurs only in about 10% of SLE patients, and associated clinical symptoms are very variable; from a mild cognitive dysfunction to severe psychosis and convulsions, local ischemia and strokes [59, 77]. The peripheral nervous system may also be affected by lupus vasculopathy leading to multifocal inflammatory mononeuropathies [59]. Mesothelium vasculitis may also occur and lead to gastrointestinal hemorrhage or perforation [59]

3.2. Antiphospholipid syndrome

The clinical APS, an autoimmune syndrome usually developing in the context of SLE, is a condition defined as a predisposition for arterial and/or venous thromboses and/or recurrent miscarriages or other obstetric emergencies (e.g., premature birth, preeclampsia) in association with hematologic abnormalities and specific antibodies targeted against phospholipid-binding plasma proteins [78]. It has been suggested that endothelial damage of whatever origin exposes endothelial cell phospholipids, which enables the adhesion of antibodies directed against phospholipids (aPL) [75]. The pathogenetic action mechanisms of aPL antibodies are variable. When binding with membrane phospholipids aPL antibodies may inhibit reactions catalyzed by them in the coagulation cascade, for example through inhibition of C and S protein activation [79]. These antibodies may also activate endothelial cells thrombin formation [79]. The binding of aPL antibodies with platelet membrane phospholipids binding protein predisposes to platelet activation and adhesion, with consequent thrombus formation. These antibodies probably also participate in the complement system activation [79]. As a result, the aPL antibodies demonstrate proadhesive, proinflammatory and prothrombotic effects on endothelial cells [79].Thrombosis within the context of APS may occur even in histologically normal vessels. However, in the majority of aPL-positive patients, seropositivity *per se* does not suffice for the development of clinical events. Thrombotic events seem to occur more readily in SLE patients with coexistent atherosclerosis [80]. Recently, the presence of micro-angiopathy, defined as capillary microhemorhages, and diagnosed with the aid of capillaro-scopy, has been proposed as an augmentary screening tool for aPL-seropositive patients who are prone to develop clinical thrombotic manifestations [81].

3.3. Lupus vasculitis

Distinction of inflammatory lupus vasculitis from APS, which may present with similar clinical manifestations, is of major significance in terms of clinical management. Inflammatory vascular disease is triggered by the in situ formation, or the deposition, of immune complexes within the vessel wall.

Vasculitis may manifest in as high as 56% of SLE patients throughout their life, in contrast to antiphospholipid syndrome which has a prevalence of 15%. Patients with vasculitis are mainly male and tend to be of younger age [82]. Antibodies against endothelial cells have been identified as a major endothelial cell cytotoxic effector and have been implicated in the pathogenesis of several connective tissue diseases, predominantly vasculitides [83]. More than 80% of systemic lupus erythematosus patients are positive for antiendothelial cell antibodies (AECAs) [84]. Other forms of SLE-related vasculitis include drug-induced vasculitis [85] and infection-induced vasculitis [86] either through direct compromise of the vascular wall by pathogens, or through antigen-induced autoimmune and inflammatory processes. Some drugs may play a role in the induction of inflammatory vascular lesions in SLE. The drug molecule may act as a hapten, which as a result of autoantigen binding alters the antigen properties. Several SLE inducing drugs are listed below: penicillins, allopurinol, thiazides, pyrazolones, retinoids, streptokinase, cytokines, monoclonal antibodies, chinolons, hydan-toin, carbamazepine and other anticonvulsants [59, 87]. Vasculitis may be a result of direct attack of microorganisms on the blood vessel wall or may be caused by infected thrombotic mass [74]. Hepatitis C virus may take part in vasculitis development, with the cryoglobulin presence [88]]. There is an unexplained relationship between blood cryoglobulins and hepatitis C [74]. The following mechanisms leading to viral and bacterial vasculitis in SLE have been suggested: [1] the viruses directly attack the vascular wall inducing an inflammatory process,

[2] some of them, as cytomegalovirus, may permeate and activate endothelial cells leading to vasculitis and [3] bacterial *Staphylococcus* antigens, as for example neutral phosphatase, may bind with basement membranes and adhere specifically to IgG, which in turn induces an immune response and an inflammatory process.

4. Rheumatoid arthritis (RA)

RA is a chronic inflammatory systemic disorder which primarily involves the joint synovial membrane. The purpose of this chapter section is to describe the occurrence and pathophysiology of vasculitis and vasculopathy in RA.

4.1. Rheumatoid vasculitis

Rheumatoid vasculitis typically affects small and medium-size blood vessels. It is associated with high rates of premature mortality with up to 40% of patients dying by 5 years as well as significant morbidity due to both organ damage from vasculitis and consequences of the treatment [89, 90]. Diagnostic criteria for systemic rheumatoid vasculitis were proposed in 1984 by Scott et al. [91], although the classification of RA-associated vasculitis remains poorly codified. It shares many characteristics with a classic polyarteritis nodosa and may affect peripheral nerves, causing mononeuritis multiplex, skin, gastrointestinal tract, and other organs, but it is not usually associated with the development of microaneurysms [92]. High levels of circulating immune complexes have been observed in patients with rheumatoid vasculitis [93], and in particular high serum levels of rheumatoid factor are often detected at the time of onset of vasculitis [94]. Deposition of immune complexes most likely contributes to small vessel inflammation and organ damage. Anti CCP levels also tend to be higher in patients with RA who have systemic vasculitis than in those who do not. Rheumatoid vasculitis has been reported in a substantial number of patients with RA [95]. It is more common in men and patients with longstanding disease [91]. The annual incidence of rheumatoid vasculitis in men to be 15.8 per million and in women, 9.4 per million [95]. Nevertheless, the 30-year incidence of vasculitis in patients with RA was estimated to be 3.6% [96].

Predictors of vasculitis in RA patients include clinical and generic factors (Table 2) [97-103]. Smoking, which is also a risk factor for development of RA in the general population [104], is associated with an increased risk of vasculitis among patients with RA [99, 100]. Rheumatoid nodules early during the disease predict the occurrence of systemic rheumatoid vasculitis [97, 98]. However, genetic predisposition toward developed RA, as HLA-DRB1-shared epitope genotypes is strongly associated with extraarticular disease manifestations such as rheumatoid vasculitis [101, 102]. In particular, double dose of RA-associated HLADRB1*04 alleles is associated with an increased risk of vasculitis [105]. Rheumatoid vasculitis is associated with an increased mortality as compared with that in patients with RA in general [89]. In particular, a poor survival has been observed after diagnosis of vasculitis-related neuropathy [106]. In such patients, a low serum level of complement factor C4 is a negative prognostic marker [90].

The increased mortality may be due to a high risk of cardiovascular comorbidity [107, 108] and severe infections [109].

Marker	Pathophysiological explanation
Rheumatoid nodules	sign of microvascular extraarticular inflammation
Smoking	vascular damage, immunomodulation
HLA-DRB1*04/04 double gene dose	selection and activation of T cells
HLA-C*3 allele	activation of cytotoxic CD28null T cells
KIR2DS2 allele	activation of cytotoxic CD28null T cells

KIR, killer immunoglobulin-like receptors

Table 2. Predictors for vasculitis in RA patients

According to the data from the literature very little is known of what events trigger the development of vasculits in RA patients at a particular time point. This probably includes a number of different infectious agents and other immune exposures. For example, rare cases of rheumatoid vasculitis following influenza vaccination have been described [110].

4.2. Clinical manifestations of rheumatoid vasculits

Rheumatoid vasculitis often affects more than single organ. Patients may develop nailfold infarcts and leg ulcers. These patients may go on to have more widespread vascular disease but usually do not [111]. Cutaneous manifestations of rheumatoid vasculitis may present as digital digital infarcts, livedo, palpable purpura, bulla, ulcerations, painful nodules, or gangrene. Histologically, rheumatoid vasculitis involves blood vessels of the small arteries, and all layers of the vessel wall are infiltrated by neutrophils, lymphocytes, and plasma cells. Cutaneous manifestation of rheumatoid vasculitis is classified into three grades: severe, moderate, and mild. The severe type presents with digital gangrene, nail fold infarcts, large cutaneous ulcers; the moderate type presents with palpable purpura; and the mild type presents with nailfold telangiectasias with thromboses, minute digital ulcerations, petechiae, and livedo reticularis. Minor bleeding from the nail folds, finger pulp, and the edge of the nails results from digital infarcts (isolated nailfold vasculitis) [112]. RA patients who develop leg ulcers and digital ulcers should be more closely monitored, especially patients who have high titers of rheumatoid factor, positive anti CCPs, cryoglobulins, and low complements, as more ominous manifestations of RA are more likely to occur in these patients [113]. The diagnosis of leg ulcers in patients with RA is often associated with trivial trauma. There is often an underlying vasculitis, which promotes the lesion.

Systemic vasculitis in RA usually occurs in patients who have longstanding disease, generally of more than 10-year duration. Even so, it may occur at any time during the disease course, and, irrespective of when it occurs, it is associated with a poor prognosis. From a clinical standpoint, patients have more severe RA with destructive joint disease and other features of extraarticular disease [98]. Patients with Felty's syndrome are particularly prone to develop rheumatoid vasculitis. The appearance of rheumatoid vasculitis may be associated with a rise in acute-phase markers, including the sedimentation rate and C-reactive protein, together with longstanding thrombocytosis and anemia of chronic disease [98]. RA-associated vasculitis may involve any blood vessel bed in the body, including cerebral, mesenteric, and coronary arteries [114]. More severe features of rheumatoid vasculitis are frank infarctions of the digits and mononeuritis multiplex [113, 115]. Unfortunately, patients with systemic rheumatoid vasculitis may develop mononeuritis multiplex [116]. Mononeuritis in RA often begins with numbness and then progresses to tingling and muscle weakness. Initially, the mononeuritis is asymmetric but may become symmetrical. Other early manifestations of rheumatoid vasculitis include pericarditis and scleritis. Rheumatoid vasculitis is also strongly associated with the presence of rheumatoid nodules, and most RA patients with vasculitis have nodulosis [98]. Rheumatoid vasculitis may also affect the coronary arteries. In the kidney, renal artery involvement, as occurs in polyarteritis nodosa with vasculitis, may cause renal failure, although the disorder should be distinct from polyarteritis nodosa [117, 118].

Rheumatoid vasculitis is an unusual complication of RA, which has profound impact on disease severity and life expectancy of patients who develop this extraarticular disease manifestation.

4.3. Angiogenesis in RA

RA is the rheumatic disease in which the role of angiogenesis has been studied most extensively; it is characterized by excessive angiogenesis [119]. Proangiogenic mediators associated with RA include the following: growth factors such as VEGF; cytokines such as TNF-α (which has many effects in addition to angiogenesis); chemokines such as IL-8; and other mediators, including ET-1. VEGF, an endothelial selective mitogen that is secreted predominantly by macrophages, is an important cytokine in both angiogenesis and vasculogenesis [120]. In RA, VEGF expression is induced by hypoxia. Hypoxic environment of the inflamed RA joint activates the VEGF gene via binding of hypoxia inducible factor. This in turn augments IL-1 or transforming growth factor (TGF)-β induced synovial fibroblast VEGF [121], which contributes significantly to angiogenesis in the synovium and progression of RA. Evidence of the importance of TNF-α as a proangiogenic mediator in RA is illustrated by the effect of giving anti-TNF-a to patients with RA. Administration of anti-TNF-α drugs to patients with RA leads to vascular deactivation, including decreased angiogenesis and endothelial cell markers [122]. Chemokines are also very important in angiogenesis in RA. Recent studies have shown that the chemokine IL-8/CXC chemokine ligand (CXCL)8 plays a role in the pathogenesis of RA synovitis. This molecule is angiogenic and appears to be responsible for much of the macrophage-derived angiogenic activity seen in RA [123]. In addition to its well recognized effects as a potent endogenous vasoconstrictor and smooth muscle mitogen, ET-1 also appears to have proangiogenic effects in some rheumatic diseases. In patients with RA, levels of ET-1 in synovial fluid, serum and plasma are elevated in comparison with those in normal individuals [124-127]. Although this clearly does not demonstrate a causal role for ET-1 in the pathophysiology of RA, it may suggest some degree of involvement.

http://dx.doi.org/10.5772/55056

4.4. Vasculopathy in RA

Atherogenesis is a precocious feature in RA, as extraarticular manifestation of the syndrome, and might be defined as rheumatoid vasculopathy. RA has been associated with precocious and accelerated atherosclerosis [128-134] and with increased CV morbidity and mortality [135]. Notably, atherosclerosis has been proposed as extraarticular manifestation of the disease [130]. Several disease-related mechanisms may be involved in the development of premature vascular damage in RA, including increased synthesis of proinflammatory mediators (such as cytokines, chemokines, adhesion molecules), autoantibodies against endothelial cell components, perturbations in T-cell subsets, genetic polymorphisms, hyperhomocysteinemia, oxidative stress, and abnormal vascular repair, as well as iatrogenic factors [136, 137]. Hyperhomocysteinemia, which is a common finding in patients with RA, is a further contributor to the impaired endothelial function, potentiates the oxidation of lipoproteins, and has prothrombotic effects [138]. Inflammation severity was found to be associated with functional and structural arterial wall changes in patients with recent RA onset, and early control of inflammation is associated with improved arterial function that may reduce atherosclerosis progression [139].

5. Conclusion

Vascular damage in humans develops on various grounds. It may be inflammatory or noninflammatory. The damages may be induced by environmental factors (toxic agents, medications, microorganisms), through cancer as a paraneoplastic syndrome, or may be directly associated with an active immune process. Distinguishing between noninflammatory vasculopathy and vasculitis can pose a significant diagnostic challenge in the absence of histological examination. Vasculitis should not be confused with *vasculopathy*, which simply means something is wrong with the blood vessels, although it's usually not vasculitis. When a blood vessel becomes inflamed and narrowed, blood supply to that area can become partially or completely blocked. Complete blockage is called *occlusion*; it causes the vessel wall to swell and makes things stick to the wall -- so a clot forms. When vasculitis interferes with circulation in any part of the body, it causes local tenderness and pain. If the blood vessels are close to the skin, characteristic *rashes* occur. Depending on where the blockage occurs, almost any organ in the body can be affected. However, vasculopathy can also block blood vessels, but it does not cause the fever, pain, and local tenderness associated with vasculitis.

As this chapter illustrates, vascular involvement is an important part in the RA, SLE and SSc pathogenesis. Vasculitis in RA is generally associated with longstanding disease, has an important impact on s patient's well being and markedly influences patient life expectancy. Predictors of vasculitis in RA patients include clinical and genetic factors. Vaculitis in RA generally affects small and medium-seized vessels. It shares many characteristics with a classic polyarteritis nodosa and may affect peripheral nerves, causing mononeuritis multiplex, skin, gastrointestinal tract and other organs. It is not usually associated with the development of microaneurysms. Atherogenesis is a precocious feature in RA, as extraarticular manifestation of the syndrome, and might be defined as rheumatoid vasculopathy. Several disease-related mechanisms may be involved in the development of premature vascular damage in RA. Increased synthesis of proinflammatory mediators, autoantibodies against endothelial cell components, perturbations in T-cell subsets, genetic polymorphisms, hyperhomocysteinemia, oxidative stress and abnormal vascular repair are associated with atherosclerosis in RA.

Vascular involvement in SLE may be of inflammatory or thrombotic origin. Both mechanisms involve the immune system. The activation and consequent endothelial lesions play a very important role in the disease pathogenesis. The common hypothesis for vasculopathy in SLE concerns the endothelial deposition of circulating immune complexes. There are many various autoantibodies in SLE as circulating immune complexes which directly or indirectly affect endothelial cells, causing chronic vessel wall damage. Furthermore, vasculitis in SLE is proatherogenic condition and is characterized by leucocytes activation and production of cytokine and other inflammatory mediators.

Although SSc is considered a fibrosing disease, vascular involvement plays a major role in pathogenesis and organ dysfunction. SSc vascular disease involves vasculopathy with luminal occlusion, thrombosis and vasospasm. The vascular pathology in SSc is not necessarily an inflammatory process and would be better be characterised as a vasculopathy in the absence of vasculitis. In the current pathogenic model of SSc, a vascular injury of unknown cause leads to endothelial apoptosis and initiates the process of SSc vasculopathy. Histopathology of SSc vasculopathy reflects the underlying pathogenesis, with myofibroblast proliferation and matrix deposit in the subendothelial layer leading to obliterative thickening of vessel walls. Inflammatory infiltrates are absent, and the internal elastic lamina remains intact. In contrast to vasculopathy, concurrent vasculitis in SSc shows histopathological evidence of inflammation with presence of mononuclear infiltrates and destruction of the vascular wall.

Author details

Mislav Radić[1] and Josipa Radić[2]

1 Division of Rheumatology and Clinical Immunology, University Hospital Centre Split, University of Split School of Medicine, Split, Croatia

2 Division of Nephrology, University Hospital Centre Split, University of Split School of Medicine, Split, Croatia

References

[1] Medsger, T. A. Jr. Natural history of systemic sclerosis and the assessment of disease activity, severity, functional status, and psychologic well-being. Rheumatic diseases clinics of North America. (2003). , 29(2), 255-73.

[2] LeRoy ECSystemic sclerosis. A vascular perspective. Rheumatic diseases clinics of North America. (1996)., 22(4), 675-94.

[3] Maricq, H. R. Capillary abnormalities, Raynaud's phenomenon, and systemic sclerosis in patients with localized scleroderma. Archives of dermatology. (1992)., 128(5), 630-2.

[4] Carpentier, P. H, Satger, B, Poensin, D, & Maricq, H. R. Incidence and natural history of Raynaud phenomenon: A long-term follow-up (14 years) of a random sample from the general population. Journal of vascular surgery : official publication, the Society for Vascular Surgery [and] International Society for Cardiovascular Surgery, North American Chapter. (2006)., 44(5), 1023-8.

[5] Ebert, E. C. Gastric and enteric involvement in progressive systemic sclerosis. Journal of clinical gastroenterology. (2008)., 42(1), 5-12.

[6] Kahaleh, B. Vascular disease in scleroderma: mechanisms of vascular injury. Rheumatic diseases clinics of North America. (2008)., 34(1), 57-71.

[7] Fleming, J. N, Nash, R. A, & Mahoney, W. M. Jr., Schwartz SM. Is scleroderma a vasculopathy? Current rheumatology reports. (2009)., 11(2), 103-10.

[8] Muller-ladner, U, Distler, O, Ibba-manneschi, L, Neumann, E, & Gay, S. Mechanisms of vascular damage in systemic sclerosis. Autoimmunity. (2009)., 42(7), 587-95.

[9] Mulligan-kehoe, M. J, & Simons, M. Vascular disease in scleroderma: angiogenesis and vascular repair. Rheumatic diseases clinics of North America. (2008)., 34(1), 73-9.

[10] Wigley, F. M. Vascular disease in scleroderma. Clinical reviews in allergy & immunology. (2009).

[11] Dangelo, W. A, Fries, J. F, Masi, A. T, & Shulman, L. E. Pathologic Observations in Systemic Sclerosis (Scleroderma)- a Study of 58 Autopsy Cases and 58 Matched Controls. American Journal of Medicine. (1969)., 46(3), 428-9.

[12] Nagy, Z, & Czirjak, L. Nailfold digital capillaroscopy in 447 patients with connective tissue disease and Raynaud's disease. Journal of the European Academy of Dermatology and Venereology : JEADV. (2004)., 18(1), 62-8.

[13] Birkenhager, R, Schneppe, B, Rockl, W, Wilting, J, Weich, H. A, & Mccarthy, J. E. Synthesis and physiological activity of heterodimers comprising different splice forms of vascular endothelial growth factor and placenta growth factor. The Biochemical journal. (1996). Pt 3):703-7.

[14] Distler, O, Distler, J. H, Scheid, A, Acker, T, Hirth, A, Rethage, J, et al. Uncontrolled expression of vascular endothelial growth factor and its receptors leads to insufficient skin angiogenesis in patients with systemic sclerosis. Circulation research. (2004)., 95(1), 109-16.

[15] Mulligan-kehoe, M. J, Drinane, M. C, Mollmark, J, Casciola-rosen, L, Hummers, L. K, Hall, A, et al. Antiangiogenic plasma activity in patients with systemic sclerosis. Arthritis Rheum. (2007). , 56(10), 3448-58.

[16] Jun, J. B, Kuechle, M, Harlan, J. M, & Elkon, K. B. Fibroblast and endothelial apoptosis in systemic sclerosis. Current opinion in rheumatology. (2003). Epub 2003/10/22., 15(6), 756-60.

[17] Horstmeyer, A, Licht, C, Scherr, G, Eckes, B, & Krieg, T. Signalling and regulation of collagen I synthesis by ET-1 and TGF-beta1. The FEBS journal. (2005). , 272(24), 6297-309.

[18] Shi-wen, X, Denton, C. P, Dashwood, M. R, Holmes, A. M, Bou-gharios, G, Pearson, J. D, et al. Fibroblast matrix gene expression and connective tissue remodeling: role of endothelin-1. The Journal of investigative dermatology. (2001). , 116(3), 417-25.

[19] Shephard, P, Hinz, B, Smola-hess, S, Meister, J. J, Krieg, T, & Smola, H. Dissecting the roles of endothelin, TGF-beta and GM-CSF on myofibroblast differentiation by keratinocytes. Thrombosis and haemostasis. (2004). , 92(2), 262-74.

[20] Vancheeswaran, R, Magoulas, T, Efrat, G, Wheeler-jones, C, Olsen, I, Penny, R, et al. Circulating endothelin-1 levels in systemic sclerosis subsets--a marker of fibrosis or vascular dysfunction? The Journal of rheumatology. (1994). , 21(10), 1838-44.

[21] Korn, J. H, Mayes, M, Cerinic, M. M, Rainisio, M, Pope, J, Hachulla, E, et al. Digital ulcers in systemic sclerosis- Prevention by treatment with bosentan, an oral endothelin receptor antagonist. Arthritis Rheum-Us. (2004). , 50(12), 3985-93.

[22] Kuhn, A, Haust, M, Ruland, V, Weber, R, Verde, P, Felder, G, et al. Effect of bosentan on skin fibrosis in patients with systemic sclerosis: a prospective, open-label, non-comparative trial. Rheumatology. (2010). , 49(7), 1336-45.

[23] Hirata, Y, Emori, T, Eguchi, S, Kanno, K, Imai, T, Ohta, K, et al. Endothelin Receptor Subtype-B Mediates Synthesis of Nitric-Oxide by Cultured Bovine Endothelial-Cells. J Clin Invest. (1993). , 91(4), 1367-73.

[24] Yamamoto, T, Katayama, I, & Nishioka, K. Nitric oxide production and inducible nitric oxide synthase expression in systemic sclerosis. Journal of Rheumatology. (1998). , 25(2), 314-7.

[25] Takagi, K, Kawaguchi, Y, Hara, M, Sugiura, T, Harigai, M, & Kamatani, N. Serum nitric oxide (NO) levels in systemic sclerosis patients: correlation between NO levels and clinical features. Clin Exp Immunol. (2003). , 134(3), 538-44.

[26] Beyer, C, Schett, G, Gay, S, & Distler, O. Distler JHW. Hypoxia Hypoxia in the pathogenesis of systemic sclerosis. Arthritis research & therapy. (2009).

[27] Herrick, A. L, Oogarah, P. K, Freemont, A. J, Marcuson, R, & Haeney, M. Jayson MIV. Vasculitis in Patients with Systemic-Sclerosis and Severe Digital Ischemia Requiring Amputation. Ann Rheum Dis. (1994)., 53(5), 323-6.

[28] Hunder, G. G, Bloch, D. A, Michel, B. A, Stevens, M. B, Arend, W. P, Calabrese, L. H, et al. The American-College-of-Rheumatology 1990 Criteria for the Classification of Giant-Cell Arteritis. Arthritis Rheum-Us. (1990)., 33(8), 1122-8.

[29] Perezjimenez, F, Lopezrubio, F, Canadillas, F, Jimenezalonso, J, & Jimenezpereperez, J. Giant-Cell Arteritis Associated with Progressive Systemic-Sclerosis. Arthritis Rheum-Us. (1982)., 25(6), 717-8.

[30] Hupp, S. L. Giant-Cell Arteritis Associated with Progressive Systemic-Sclerosis. J Clin Neuro-Ophthal. (1989)., 9(2), 126-30.

[31] Sari-kouzel, H, Herrick, A. L, Freemont, A. J, Marcuson, R. W, & Jayson, M. I. Giant cell arteritis in a patient with limited cutaneous systemic sclerosis. Rheumatology. (1999)., 38(5), 479-80.

[32] Reinhold-keller, E, Herlyn, K, Wagner-bastmeyer, R, & Gross, W. L. Stable incidence of primary systemic vasculitides over five years: Results from the German vasculitis register. Arthrit Rheum-Arthr. (2005)., 53(1), 93-9.

[33] Seyahi, E, Ugurlu, S, Cumali, R, Balci, H, Seyahi, N, Yurdakul, S, et al. Atherosclerosis in Takayasu arteritis. Ann Rheum Dis. (2006)., 65(9), 1202-7.

[34] Arend, W. P, Michel, B. A, Bloch, D. A, Hunder, G. G, Calabrese, L. H, Edworthy, S. M, et al. The American-College-of-Rheumatology 1990 Criteria for the Classification of Takayasu Arteritis. Arthritis Rheum-Us. (1990)., 33(8), 1129-34.

[35] Passiu, G, Vacca, A, Sanna, G, Cauli, A, Laudadio, M, Garau, P, et al. Takayasu's arteritis overlapping with systemic sclerosis. Clinical and experimental rheumatology. (1999)., 17(3), 363-5.

[36] Yago, T, Ota, S, & Nishinarita, M. A case of systemic sclerosis complicated by Takayasu's arteritis]. Ryumachi [Rheumatism]. (2002)., 42(3), 605-9.

[37] Kocabay, G, Tiryaki, B, Ekmekci, A, & Inanc, M. Takayasu arteritis associated with systemic sclerosis. Modern rheumatology / the Japan Rheumatism Association. (2006)., 16(2), 120-1.

[38] Kim, T. J, Uhm, W. S, Song, S. Y, & Jun, J. B. Unilateral weak radial pulse in a patient with systemic sclerosis: Takayasu's arteritis or thoracic outlet syndrome? Rheumatology international. (2007). Epub 2006/12/23., 27(8), 789-90.

[39] Lightfoot, R. W. Jr., Michel BA, Bloch DA, Hunder GG, Zvaifler NJ, McShane DJ, et al. The American College of Rheumatology 1990 criteria for the classification of polyarteritis nodosa. Arthritis Rheum. (1990)., 33(8), 1088-93.

[40] Pagnoux, C, Seror, R, Henegar, C, Mahr, A, & Cohen, P. Le Guern V, et al. Clinical features and outcomes in 348 patients with polyarteritis nodosa: a systematic retro-

spective study of patients diagnosed between 1963 and 2005 and entered into the French Vasculitis Study Group Database. Arthritis Rheum. (2010). , 62(2), 616-26.

[41] Kang, M. S, Park, J. H, & Lee, C. W. A case of overlap between systemic sclerosis and cutaneous polyarteritis nodosa. Clin Exp Dermatol. (2008). , 33(6), 781-3.

[42] Calabrese, L. H, Duna, G. F, & Lie, J. T. Vasculitis in the central nervous system. Arthritis Rheum-Us. (1997). , 40(7), 1189-201.

[43] Lie, J. T. Primary (granulomatous) angiitis of the central nervous system: a clinicopathologic analysis of 15 new cases and a review of the literature. Human pathology. (1992). , 23(2), 164-71.

[44] Calabrese, L. H, & Mallek, J. A. Primary angiitis of the central nervous system. Report of 8 new cases, review of the literature, and proposal for diagnostic criteria. Medicine. (1988). , 67(1), 20-39.

[45] Brouet, J. C, Clauvel, J. P, Danon, F, Klein, M, & Seligmann, M. Biologic and clinical significance of cryoglobulins. A report of 86 cases. The American journal of medicine. (1974). , 57(5), 775-88.

[46] Jantunen, E, Soppi, E, Neittaanmaki, H, & Lahtinen, R. Essential cryofibrinogenaemia, leukocytoclastic vasculitis and chronic purpura. Journal of internal medicine. (1993). , 234(3), 331-3.

[47] Blain, H, Cacoub, P, Musset, L, Costedoat-chalumeau, N, Silberstein, C, Chosidow, O, et al. Cryofibrinogenaemia: a study of 49 patients. Clin Exp Immunol. (2000). , 120(2), 253-60.

[48] Husson, J. M, Druet, P, Contet, A, Fiessinger, J. N, & Camilleri, J. P. Systemic sclerosis and cryoglobulinemia. Clinical immunology and immunopathology. (1976). , 6(1), 77-82.

[49] Barrett, M. C, Prendiville, J. S, Pardy, B. J, & Cream, J. J. Cryofibrinogenaemia and acute gangrene in systemic sclerosis. Postgraduate medical journal. (1986). , 62(732), 935-6.

[50] Yurdakul, S, Hamuryudan, V, & Yazici, H. Behcet syndrome. Current opinion in rheumatology. (2004). , 16(1), 38-42.

[51] Criteria for diagnosis of Behcet's diseaseInternational Study Group for Behcet's Disease. Lancet. (1990). , 335(8697), 1078-80.

[52] Choy, E, Kingsley, G, & Panayi, G. Systemic sclerosis occurring in a patient with Adamantiades-Behcet's disease. Br J Rheumatol. (1993). , 32(2), 160-1.

[53] Yokota, K, Hirano, M, Akiba, H, Adachi, D, Takeishi, M, Akiyama, Y, et al. A case of Behcet's disease with esophageal ulcers complicated with systemic sclerosis, chronic hepatitis C, and pancytopenia]. Nihon Rinsho Men'eki Gakkai kaishi = Japanese journal of clinical immunology. (2004). , 27(3), 164-70.

[54] Mcadam, L. P, Hanlan, O, Bluestone, M. A, & Pearson, R. CM. Relapsing polychondritis: prospective study of 23 patients and a review of the literature. Medicine. (1976). , 55(3), 193-215.

[55] Damiani, J. M, & Levine, H. L. Relapsing polychondritis--report of ten cases. The Laryngoscope. (1979). Pt 1):929-46.

[56] Sugisaki, K, Takeda, I, Kanno, T, & Kasukawa, R. A case report of relapsing polychondritis with an auricular ulcer complicated by systemic sclerosis]. Ryumachi [Rheumatism]. (2002). , 42(3), 610-7.

[57] Holle, J. U, & Gross, W. L. ANCA-associated vasculitides: pathogenetic aspects and current evidence-based therapy. Journal of autoimmunity. (2009).

[58] Rho, Y. H, Choi, S. J, Lee, Y. H, Ji, J. D, & Song, G. G. Scleroderma associated with ANCA-associated vasculitis. Rheumatology international. (2006). , 26(5), 465-8.

[59] Cruz, D. D. Vasculitis in systemic lupus erythematosus. Lupus. (1998). , 7(4), 270-4.

[60] Criado, P. R, Rivitti, E. A, Sotto, M. N, Valente, N. Y, Aoki, V, Carvalho, J. F, et al. Livedoid vasculopathy: an intringuing cutaneous disease. Anais brasileiros de dermatologia. (2011). , 86(5), 961-77.

[61] Sopena, B, Perez-rodriguez, M. T, Rivera, A, Ortiz-rey, J. A, Lamas, J, & Freire-dapena, M. C. Livedoid vasculopathy and recurrent thrombosis in a patient with lupus: seronegative antiphospholipid syndrome? Lupus. (2010). , 19(11), 1340-3.

[62] Shimizu, A, Tamura, A, Yamanaka, M, Amano, H, Nagai, Y, & Ishikawa, O. Case of livedoid vasculopathy with extensive dermal capillary thrombi. The Journal of dermatology. (2010). , 37(1), 94-7.

[63] Khenifer, S, Thomas, L, Balme, B, & Dalle, S. Livedoid vasculopathy: thrombotic or inflammatory disease? Clin Exp Dermatol. (2010). , 35(7), 693-8.

[64] Sen, D, & Isenberg, D. A. Antineutrophil cytoplasmic autoantibodies in systemic lupus erythematosus. Lupus. (2003). , 12(9), 651-8.

[65] Sung, J. M, Hsu, S. C, Chen, F. F, & Huang, J. J. Systemic lupus erythematosus presented as non-inflammatory necrotizing vasculopathy-induced ischemic glomerulopathy and small vessels-related ischemic cardiomyopathy. Lupus. (2002). , 11(7), 458-62.

[66] Appel, G. B, Pirani, C. L, & Dagati, V. Renal Vascular Complications of Systemic Lupus-Erythematosus. Journal of the American Society of Nephrology. (1994). , 4(8), 1499-515.

[67] Jayne, D. The clinical features and pathology of vasculitis associated with anti-myeloperoxidase autoantibodies. Japanese journal of infectious diseases. (2004). S, 16-7.

[68] Romero-diaz, J, Vargas-vorackova, F, Kimura-hayama, E, Cortazar-benitez, L. F, Gijon-mitre, R, Criales, S, et al. Systemic lupus erythematosus risk factors for coronary artery calcifications. Rheumatology (Oxford). (2012). , 51(1), 110-9.

[69] Burgos, P. I, & Mcgwin, G. Jr., Reveille JD, Vila LM, Alarcon GS. Factors predictive of thrombotic events in LUMINA, a multi-ethnic cohort of SLE patients (LXXII). Rheumatology (Oxford). (2010). , 49(9), 1720-5.

[70] Carlson, J, & Chen, K. R. Cutaneous vasculitis update: Neutrophilic muscular vessel and eosinophilic, granulomatous, and lymphocytic vasculitis syndromes. Am J Dermatopath. (2007). , 29(1), 32-43.

[71] Carlson, J. A, & Chen, K. R. Cutaneous vasculitis update: Small vessel neutrophilic vasculitis syndromes. Am J Dermatopath. (2006). , 28(6), 486-506.

[72] Sunderkotter, C, Bonsmann, G, Sindrilaru, A, & Luger, T. Management of leukocytoclastic vasculitis. J Dermatol Treat. (2005). , 16(4), 193-206.

[73] Carlson, J. A, Cavaliere, L. F, & Grant-kels, J. M. Cutaneous vasculitis: diagnosis and management. Clin Dermatol. (2006). , 24(5), 414-29.

[74] Kallenberg CGMHeeringa P. Pathogenesis of vasculitis. Lupus. (1998). , 7(4), 280-4.

[75] Calamia, K. T, & Balabanova, M. Vasculitis in systemic lupus erythematosis. Clin Dermatol. (2004). , 22(2), 148-56.

[76] Zecevic, R. D, Vojvodic, D, Ristic, B, Pavlovic, M. D, Stefanovic, D, & Karadaglic, D. Skin lesions--an indicator of disease activity in systemic lupus erythematosus? Lupus. (2001). , 10(5), 364-7.

[77] Meroni, P. L, Tincani, A, Sepp, N, Raschi, E, Testoni, C, Corsini, E, et al. Endothelium and the brain in CNS lupus. Lupus. (2003). , 12(12), 919-28.

[78] Rodriguez-garcia, J. L, Bertolaccini, M. L, Cuadrado, M. J, Sanna, G, Ateka-barrutia, O, & Khamashta, M. A. Clinical manifestations of antiphospholipid syndrome (APS) with and without antiphospholipid antibodies (the so-called'seronegative APS'). Ann Rheum Dis. (2012). , 71(2), 242-4.

[79] Tenedios, F, Erkan, D, & Lockshin, M. D. Cardiac involvement in the antiphospholipid syndrome. Lupus. (2005). , 14(9), 691-6.

[80] Frostegard, J. Systemic lupus erythematosus and cardiovascular disease. Lupus. (2008). , 17(5), 364-7.

[81] Pyrpasopoulou, A, Triantafyllou, A, Anyfanti, P, Douma, S, & Aslanidis, S. Capillaroscopy as a screening test for clinical antiphospholipid syndrome. Eur J Intern Med. (2011). EE9., 158.

[82] Cieslik, P, Hrycek, A, & Klucinski, P. Vasculopathy and vasculitis in systemic lupus erythematosus. Polskie Archiwum Medycyny Wewnetrznej. (2008).

[83] Guilpain, P, & Mouthon, L. Antiendothelial cells autoantibodies in vasculitis-associated systemic diseases. Clinical reviews in allergy & immunology. (2008).

[84] Praprotnik, S, Blank, M, Meroni, P. L, Rozman, B, Eldor, A, & Shoenfeld, Y. Classification of anti-endothelial cell antibodies into antibodies against microvascular and macrovascular endothelial cells- The pathogenic and diagnostic implications. Arthritis Rheum-Us. (2001). , 44(7), 1484-94.

[85] Dobre, M, Wish, J, & Negrea, L. Hydralazine-Induced ANCA-Positive Pauci-immune Glomerulonephritis: A Case Report and Literature Review. Renal Failure. (2009). , 31(8), 745-8.

[86] Avcin, T, Canova, M, Guilpain, P, & Guillevin, L. Kallenberg CGM, Tincani A, et al. Infections, connective tissue diseases and vasculitis. Clinical and experimental rheumatology. (2008). SS26., 18.

[87] Radic, M. Martinovic Kaliterna D, Radic J. Drug-induced vasculitis: a clinical and pathological review. The Netherlands journal of medicine. (2012). , 70(1), 12-7.

[88] Ramos-casals, M, & Font, J. Mycophenolate mofetil in patients with hepatitis C virus infection. Lupus. (2005). SS72., 64.

[89] Erhardt, C. C, Mumford, P. A, Venables, P. J, & Maini, R. N. Factors predicting a poor life prognosis in rheumatoid arthritis: an eight year prospective study. Annals of the rheumatic diseases. (1989). , 48(1), 7-13.

[90] Puechal, X, Said, G, Hilliquin, P, Coste, J, Job-deslandre, C, Lacroix, C, et al. Peripheral neuropathy with necrotizing vasculitis in rheumatoid arthritis. A clinicopathologic and prognostic study of thirty-two patients. Arthritis and rheumatism. (1995). , 38(11), 1618-29.

[91] Scott, D. G, Bacon, P. A, & Tribe, C. R. Systemic rheumatoid vasculitis: a clinical and laboratory study of 50 cases. Medicine. (1981). , 60(4), 288-97.

[92] Pagnoux, C, Mahr, A, Cohen, P, & Guillevin, L. Presentation and outcome of gastrointestinal involvement in systemic necrotizing vasculitides: analysis of 62 patients with polyarteritis nodosa, microscopic polyangiitis, Wegener granulomatosis, Churg-Strauss syndrome, or rheumatoid arthritis-associated vasculitis. Medicine. (2005). , 84(2), 115-28.

[93] Scott DGIBacon PA, Allen C, Elson CJ, Wallington T. Igg Rheumatoid-Factor, Complement and Immune-Complexes in Rheumatoid Synovitis and Vasculitis- Comparative and Serial Studies during Cyto-Toxic Therapy. Clin Exp Immunol. (1981). , 43(1), 54-63.

[94] Turesson, C, Jacobsson, L. T, Sturfelt, G, Matteson, E. L, Mathsson, L, & Ronnelid, J. Rheumatoid factor and antibodies to cyclic citrullinated peptides are associated with severe extra-articular manifestations in rheumatoid arthritis. Annals of the rheumatic diseases. (2007). , 66(1), 59-64.

[95] Watts, R. A, Carruthers, D. M, Symmons, D. P, & Scott, D. G. The incidence of rheumatoid vasculitis in the Norwich Health Authority. British journal of rheumatology. (1994)., 33(9), 832-3.

[96] Turesson, C, Fallon, O, Crowson, W. M, Gabriel, C. S, Matteson, S. E, & Extra-articular, E. L. disease manifestations in rheumatoid arthritis: incidence trends and risk factors over 46 years. Annals of the rheumatic diseases. (2003)., 62(8), 722-7.

[97] Voskuyl, A. E, Zwinderman, A. H, Westedt, M. L, Vandenbroucke, J. P, Breedveld, F. C, & Hazes, J. M. Factors associated with the development of vasculitis in rheumatoid arthritis: results of a case-control study. Annals of the rheumatic diseases. (1996)., 55(3), 190-2.

[98] Turesson, C, Mcclelland, R. L, Christianson, T, & Matteson, E. Clustering of extraarticular manifestations in patients with rheumatoid arthritis. The Journal of rheumatology. (2008)., 35(1), 179-80.

[99] Struthers, G. R, Scott, D. L, Delamere, J. P, Sheppeard, H, & Kitt, M. Smoking and rheumatoid vasculitis. Rheumatology international. (1981)., 1(3), 145-6.

[100] Turesson, C, Schaid, D. J, Weyand, C. M, Jacobsson, L. T, Goronzy, J. J, Petersson, I. F, et al. Association of HLA-C3 and smoking with vasculitis in patients with rheumatoid arthritis. Arthritis and rheumatism. (2006)., 54(9), 2776-83.

[101] Weyand, C. M, Xie, C, & Goronzy, J. J. Homozygosity for the HLA-DRB1 allele selects for extraarticular manifestations in rheumatoid arthritis. The Journal of clinical investigation. (1992)., 89(6), 2033-9.

[102] Turesson, C, Schaid, D. J, Weyand, C. M, Jacobsson, L. T, Goronzy, J. J, Petersson, I. F, et al. The impact of HLA-DRB1 genes on extra-articular disease manifestations in rheumatoid arthritis. Arthritis research & therapy. (2005). R, 1386-93.

[103] Yen, J. H, Moore, B. E, Nakajima, T, Scholl, D, Schaid, D. J, Weyand, C. M, et al. Major histocompatibility complex class I-recognizing receptors are disease risk genes in rheumatoid arthritis. J Exp Med. (2001)., 193(10), 1159-67.

[104] Silman, A. J, & Newman, J. MacGregor AJ. Cigarette smoking increases the risk of rheumatoid arthritis- Results from a nationwide study of disease-discordant twins. Arthritis and rheumatism. (1996)., 39(5), 732-5.

[105] Gorman, J. D, David-vaudey, E, Pai, M, Lum, R. F, & Criswell, L. A. Particular HLA-DRB1 shared epitope genotypes are strongly associated with rheumatoid vasculitis. Arthritis and rheumatism. (2004)., 50(11), 3476-84.

[106] Turesson, C, Fallon, O, Crowson, W. M, Gabriel, C. S, & Matteson, S. E. EL. Occurrence of extraarticular disease manifestations is associated with excess mortality in a community based cohort of patients with rheumatoid arthritis. Journal of Rheumatology. (2002)., 29(1), 62-7.

[107] Maradit-kremers, H, Nicola, P. J, Crowson, C. S, Ballman, K. V, & Gabriel, S. E. Cardiovascular death in rheumatoid arthritis: a population-based study. Arthritis and rheumatism. (2005). , 52(3), 722-32.

[108] Turesson, C, Mcclelland, R. L, Christianson, T. J, & Matteson, E. L. Severe extra-articular disease manifestations are associated with an increased risk of first ever cardiovascular events in patients with rheumatoid arthritis. Annals of the rheumatic diseases. (2007). , 66(1), 70-5.

[109] Doran, M. F, Crowson, C. S, Pond, G. R, Fallon, O, & Gabriel, W. M. SE. Predictors of infection in rheumatoid arthritis. Arthritis and rheumatism. (2002). , 46(9), 2294-300.

[110] Iyngkaran, P, Limaye, V, Hill, C, Henderson, D, Pile, K. D, & Rischmueller, M. Rheumatoid vasculitis following influenza vaccination. Rheumatology (Oxford). (2003). , 42(7), 907-9.

[111] Watts, R. A, Carruthers, D. M, & Scott, D. G. Isolated nail fold vasculitis in rheumatoid arthritis. Annals of the rheumatic diseases. (1995). , 54(11), 927-9.

[112] Jorizzo, J. L, & Daniels, J. C. Dermatologic conditions reported in patients with rheumatoid arthritis. Journal of the American Academy of Dermatology. (1983). , 8(4), 439-57.

[113] Geirsson, A. J, Sturfelt, G, & Truedsson, L. Clinical and serological features of severe vasculitis in rheumatoid arthritis: prognostic implications. Annals of the rheumatic diseases. (1987). , 46(10), 727-33.

[114] Achkar, A. A, Stanson, A. W, Johnson, M, Srivatsa, S. S, Dale, L. C, & Weyand, C. M. Rheumatoid Vasculitis Manifesting as Intraabdominal Hemorrhage. Mayo Clin Proc. (1995). , 70(6), 565-9.

[115] Bywaters EGLPeripheral Vascular Obstruction in Rheumatoid Arthritis and Its Relationship to Other Vascular Lesions. Annals of the rheumatic diseases. (1957). , 16(1), 84-103.

[116] Said, G, & Lacroix, C. Primary and secondary vasculitic neuropathy. J Neurol. (2005). , 252(6), 633-41.

[117] Boers, M, & Croonen, A. M. Dijkmans BAC, Breedveld FC, Eulderink F, Cats A, et al. Renal Findings in Rheumatoid-Arthritis- Clinical Aspects of 132 Necropsies. Annals of the rheumatic diseases. (1987). , 46(9), 658-63.

[118] Ball, J. Rheumatoid Arthritis and Polyarteritis Nodosa. Annals of the rheumatic diseases. (1954). , 13(4), 277-90.

[119] Koch, A. E. The role of angiogenesis in rheumatoid arthritis: recent developments. Annals of the rheumatic diseases. (2000). , 59, 65-71.

[120] Koch, A. E, Harlow, L. A, Haines, G. K, Amento, E. P, Unemori, E. N, Wong, W. L, et al. Vascular Endothelial Growth-Factor- a Cytokine Modulating Endothelial Function in Rheumatoid-Arthritis. J Immunol. (1994). , 152(8), 4149-56.

[121] Cho, M. L, Cho, C. S, Min, S. Y, Kim, S. H, Lee, S. S, Kim, W. U, et al. Cyclosporine inhibition of vascular endothelial growth factor production in rheumatoid synovial fibroblasts. Arthritis and rheumatism. (2002). , 46(5), 1202-9.

[122] Paleolog, E. M, Young, S, Stark, A. C, Mccloskey, R. V, Feldmann, M, & Maini, R. N. Modulation of angiogenic vascular endothelial growth factor by tumor necrosis factor alpha and interleukin-1 in rheumatoid arthritis. Arthritis and rheumatism. (1998). , 41(7), 1258-65.

[123] Koch, A. E, Polverini, P. J, Kunkel, S. L, Harlow, L. A, Dipietro, L. A, Elner, V. M, et al. Interleukin-8 as a Macrophage-Derived Mediator of Angiogenesis. Science. (1992). , 258(5089), 1798-801.

[124] Haq, A, Ramahi, K, Al-dalaan, A, & Al-sedairy, S. T. Serum and synovial fluid concentrations of endothelin-1 in patients with rheumatoid arthritis. J Med. (1999).

[125] Miyasaka, N, Hirata, Y, Ando, K, Sato, K, Morita, H, Shichiri, M, et al. Increased Production of Endothelin-1 in Patients with Inflammatory Arthritides. Arthritis and rheumatism. (1992). , 35(4), 397-400.

[126] Pache, M, Kaiser, H. J, Haufschild, T, Lubeck, P, & Flammer, J. Increased endothelin-1 plasma levels in giant cell arteritis: A report on four patients. Am J Ophthalmol. (2002). , 133(1), 160-2.

[127] Nahir, A. M, Hoffman, A, Lorber, M, & Keiser, H. R. Presence of Immunoreactive Endothelin in Synovial-Fluid- Analysis of 22 Cases. Journal of Rheumatology. (1991). , 18(5), 678-80.

[128] Jonsson, S. W, Backman, C, Johnson, O, Karp, K, Lundstrom, E, Sundqvist, K. G, et al. Increased prevalence of atherosclerosis in patients with medium term rheumatoid arthritis. Journal of Rheumatology. (2001). , 28(12), 2597-602.

[129] Kumeda, Y, Inaba, M, Goto, H, Nagata, M, Henmi, Y, Furumitsu, Y, et al. Increased thickness of the arterial intima-media detected by ultrasonography in patients with rheumatoid arthritis. Arthritis and rheumatism. (2002). , 46(6), 1489-97.

[130] Van Doornum, S, Mccoll, G, & Wicks, I. P. Accelerated atherosclerosis- An extraarticular feature of rheumatoid arthritis? Arthritis and rheumatism. (2002). , 46(4), 862-73.

[131] Gonzalez-gay, M. A, Gonzalez-juanatey, C, & Martin, J. Rheumatoid arthritis: A disease associated with accelerated atherogenesis. Semin Arthritis Rheu. (2005). , 35(1), 8-17.

[132] Szekanecz, Z, & Kerekes, G. Der H, Sandor Z, Szabo Z, Vegvari A, et al. Accelerated atherosclerosis in rheumatoid arthritis. Ann Ny Acad Sci. (2007). , 1108, 349-58.

[133] Gerli, R, Sherer, Y, Bocci, E. B, Vaudo, G, Moscatelli, S, & Shoenfeld, Y. Precocious atherosclerosis in rheumatoid arthritis- Role of traditional and disease-related cardiovascular risk factors. Ann Ny Acad Sci. (2007). , 1108, 372-81.

[134] Szekanecz, Z, & Koch, A. E. Vascular involvement in rheumatic diseases:'vascular rheumatology'. Arthritis research & therapy. (2008).

[135] Sokka, T, Abelson, B, & Pincus, T. Mortality in rheumatoid arthritis: (2008). update. Clin Exp Rheumatol. 2008;26(5):SS61., 35.

[136] Sattar, N, Mccarey, D. W, Capell, H, & Mcinnes, I. B. Explaining how "high-grade" systemic inflammation accelerates vascular risk in rheumatoid arthritis. Circulation. (2003). , 108(24), 2957-63.

[137] Kaplan, M. J. Management of cardiovascular disease risk in chronic inflammatory disorders. Nat Rev Rheumatol. (2009). , 5(4), 208-17.

[138] Roubenoff, R, Dellaripa, P, Nadeau, M. R, Abad, L. W, Muldoon, B. A, Selhub, J, et al. Abnormal homocysteine metabolism in rheumatoid arthritis. Arthritis and rheumatism. (1997). , 40(4), 718-22.

[139] Hannawi, S, Marwick, T. H, & Thomas, R. Inflammation predicts accelerated brachial arterial wall changes in patients with recent-onset rheumatoid arthritis. Arthritis research & therapy. (2009).

Chapter 8

Treatment of ANCA-Associated Vasculitis in Adults

Aurore Fifi-Mah and Cheryl Barnabe

Additional information is available at the end of the chapter

http://dx.doi.org/10.5772/54290

1. Introduction

Vasculitis is the general term used to describe diseases associated with inflammation of the blood vessels. This inflammation results in end-organ ischemia and damage with life-threatening consequences. Treatment is tailored to the type of vasculitis the patient has, prognostic features and disease severity. Two main treatment phases are recognized: induction of remission, and maintenance of remission. In this chapter we will focus on the treatment of ANCA-associated vasculitis (AAV), namely: Granulomatosis with polyangiitis (GPA), formerly Wegener's Granulomatosis; Eosinophilic granulomatosis with polyangiitis (EGPA), formerly Churg-Strauss Syndrome, and Microscopic Polyangiitis (MPA). Patients with Polyarteritis nodosa (PAN) were included in the initial therapeutic trials of these diseases, therefore some of the studies results have been applied to that population as well.

We introduce first the historical use of glucocorticoids, which are uniformly incorporated in the treatment protocols of therapeutic trials. Cyclophosphamide is recommended for the induction of remission in AAV, and in particular for generalized and severe disease. CYCLOPS, a trial of oral versus intravenous cyclophosphamide, demonstrated that intravenous dosing was as effective in inducing remission with a reduced cumulative dose, and with fewer episodes of leucopenia, but in long-term follow-up relapse was more common in the intravenous treatment group. NORAM compared the use of methotrexate compared to oral cyclophosphamide for induction of remission in patients with limited GPA, and concluded that methotrexate was nearly as effective as cyclosphosphamide in achieving remission, but in long-term follow-up more corticosteroids and further immunosuppressive agents were required. More recently, rituximab use for the induction of remission was studied in the RAVE and RITUXVAS clinical trials. Rituximab was proven to be effective as cyclophosphamide, but without a reduction in the rate of infection as had been expected. Plasma exchange in combination with oral cyclophosphamide for patients with severe renal involvement significantly decreases the risk of end-stage renal disease compared to intravenous steroids and oral cyclophosphamide, but without a significant difference in patient survival.

Maintenance of remission is typically with oral cyclophosphamide, azathioprine or methotrexate, with demonstrated efficacy in the CYCAZAREM and WEGENT studies. Leflunomide is also effective, and mycophenolate mofetil is less effective than azathioprine but is an alternative agent should the others not be tolerated. Etanercept therapy does not have a role in maintenance therapy given its inefficacy and toxicity in patients exposed to cyclophosphamide. Other anti-TNF agents, rituximab, Intravenous Immunoglobulin (IVIg), 15-Deoxyspergualin, antithymocyte globulin and alemtuzumab (CAMPATH-1H) have shown some benefit for refractory or relapsing disease and require further evaluation.

We conclude the chapter by discussing the use of trimethoprim-sulfamethoxazole (T/S) use in localized disease, as well as a specific focus on the treatment evidence in EGPA with and without poor prognostic factors.

2. ANCA-associated vasculitis (AAV)

AAV refers to primary forms of vasculitis targeting the small and medium sized arteries. These were initially differentiated on the basis of clinical features in the 1990 American College of Rheumatology (ACR) classification [1-4]. Further refinements to the classification criteria and new nomenclature have evolved from the initial classification criteria. In 1994, the Chapel Hill Consensus Conference group incorporated vessel size and pathological features to define the different primary vasculitides. They also introduced the use of antibodies to discriminate between vasculitis of the small vessels [5]. Anti-neutrophil cytoplasmic antibodies (ANCA) were initially described in 1985 in patients with segmental necrotizing and crescentic glomerulonephritis [6] but were later identified in patients with GPA, EGPA and MPA, and are associated with these conditions with high sensitivity and specificity [7].

There are two major types of ANCA recognized by indirect immunofluorescence (IIF). The perinuclear pattern, or P-ANCA, is characterized by immunofluorescence seen at the periphery of the nucleus of alcohol-fixed neutrophils. The cytoplasmic pattern, or C-ANCA, is characterized by diffuse staining of the cytoplasm. C-ANCA has a specificity for proteinase 3 (PR3), most frequently associated with GPA. P-ANCA has a specificity for myeloperoxidase (MPO), and is most commonly seen in MPA and EGPA.

Although the etiopathogenesis of AAV is not yet well understood, immune system dysregulation and abnormal inflammatory responses ensue. Therapies which alter immune system signaling and response are used to halt perpetuation of the inflammatory response to prevent end-organ damage and suppress disease activity.

3. Outcomes without treatment and determining prognosis

Because these diseases have a high mortality rate (82% of mortality in GPA at one year without treatment) [8] and relapse frequently (38% of patients with AAV will experience

http://dx.doi.org/10.5772/54290

a relapse within 5 years despite treatment) [9] treatment protocols have reflected the need to obtain rapid control of disease activity and maintain long-term immunosuppression while reducing drug toxicity. This is the basis for an induction phase of treatment to achieve remission followed by a maintenance phase to reduce the risk of relapse. Guillevin et al. developed the Five Factor Score [10] to identify factors associated with poor prognosis at the time of diagnosis. They initially analysed 342 patients with MPA, EGPA and PAN, and the five factors associated with increased mortality were: renal failure with creatinine greater than 140 μmol/L, proteinuria greater than 1 gram/day, cardiac involvement, central nervous system involvement, or severe gastro-intestinal involvement. In patients with none of these features, the 5 year survival rate was 88.1%. With 1 of these features, the 5 year survival rate declined to 74.1%, and with 2 or more of these features the survival rate was only 54.1%. The analysis of a larger group of 1108 patients with GPA, MPA, EGPA and PAN in 2009 [11] resulted in the identification of new prognosis factors associated with an increase in 5-year mortality rate. These include age > 65 years, cardiac involvement, gastro-intestinal involvement, and renal failure with creatinine >150 μmol/L. The presence of ear, nose and throat symptoms in patients with GPA and EGPA is associated with a lower relative risk of death.

4. Categorization of disease severity to guide initial treatment agent

As reflected in the European League Against Rheumatism (EULAR) treatment guidelines [12] the initial immunosuppressive agent choice is dictated by the extent and severity of the disease. The European Vasculitis Study (EUVAS) disease categorisation [13] separates disease severity into localized disease, early systemic disease, generalized, severe and refractory disease.

Category	Definition
Localised	Upper and/or lower respiratory tract disease without any other systemic involvement or constitutional symptoms
Early Systemic	Any, without organ-threatening or life-threatening disease
Generalised	Renal or other organ threatening disease, serum creatinine <500 μmol/liter (5.6 mg/dl)
Severe	Renal or other vital organ failure, serum creatinine "/>500 μmol/litre (5.6 mg/dl)
Refractory	Progressive disease unresponsive to glucocorticoids and cyclophosphamide

Table 1. Categorization of disease severity to guide initial treatment in anti-neutrophilic cytoplasmic antibodies (ANCA)-associated vasculitis [13]

We will now review in detail the evidence for the agents recommended in these treatment guidelines, as well as new evidence arising since their development.

5. Induction of remission

5.1. Glucocorticoids

Efficacy: Glucocorticoids are the first line treatment to rapidly control inflammation and prevent further organ damage in patients with active AAV. There is no trial evidence to support the use, dose or route of steroids traditionally used in AAV but certainly experience has solidified their clinical use. In all the randomized trials glucocorticoids were used in combination with immunosuppressants and is it not possible to know their effect alone. A report in 1957 of 17 patients with PAN revealed that the use of glucocorticoids alone lead to 80% survival at 12 months compared to 64% in an untreated group [14]. However the superiority of cortisone was not maintained at 3 years [14, 15].

In randomized controlled studies of remission induction, prednisone is started at 1 mg/kg then tapered to a low dose (e.g. 5 mg at 18 months in CYCLOPS) [16] or completely stopped at 12 months (NORAM) [17] or even 6 months (WGET [18], RAVE [19]). The complete weaning of steroids is not necessarily desirable as shown by a meta-analysis done by Walsh et al [20]. Continuation of low dose prednisone (5-7.5 mg/day) was associated with a lower relapse rate of 14% (95%CI 10-19%) compared to a relapse rate of 43% (95%CI 33-52%) in those with complete glucocorticoid discontinuation.

The European Vasculitis Study group (EUVAS) guidelines for the treatment of AAV [12] indicate that high dose prednisolone or prednisone at 1 mg/kg be used for the first month, then tapered to no less than 15 mg at 3 months and 10 mg or lower during the maintenance phase of treatment. In instances where rapid control of disease is necessary, parenteral methylprednisolone (1 g daily for 3 days) should be used in addition to oral glucocorticoids.

A clinical trial currently in progress named 'plasma exchange and glucocorticoid dosing in the treatment of ANCA-associated vasculitis' (PEXIVAS) (ClinicalTrials.gov Identifier: NCT00987389) will address the question of dose and tapering schedule of glucocorticoids. The trial design will compare the standard dosing of glucocorticoids (similar to the recommendations of EUVAS) compared to a reduced dose regimen. All patients will receive between 1 and 3 g of intravenous methylprednisolone over 1 to 3 days, then daily oral glucocorticoid, which may consist of prednisone or prednisolone and administered through a weight-based protocol. Based on body weight, all participants will receive either 50, 60 or 75 mg/day of oral glucocorticoid for 7 days. Participants in the standard-dose group will continue at 50, 60 or 75 mg/day for 7 additional days and taper to between 12.5 and 20 mg/day at 3 months and 5 mg/day at 6 months. Participants in the low-dose group will continue at 25, 30 or 40 mg/day for 7 days and taper to between 6 and 10 mg/day by 3 months and 5 mg/day by 6 months.
All patients will receive 5 mg/day from 6 months to 12 months after randomisation.

Safety: Multiple adverse consequences of steroid therapy are recognized, including weight gain and fat redistribution, fluid retention and hypertension, irritability and difficulty sleeping, cataracts and glaucoma, elevated blood sugars and skin thinning. It is critical to minimize steroid exposure while suppressing disease activity. It is common practice to prescribe therapy to reduce the risk of glucocorticoid-induced osteoporosis. Vitamin D supplementation and

http://dx.doi.org/10.5772/54290

Calcium intake should fall in line with local treatment recommendations, and bisphosphonates are typically necessary for patients as they will be exposed to prolonged steroid use. Additional considerations are prophylaxis against opportunistic infections such as *Pneumocystis jiroveci* with Trimethoprim/Sulfamethoxazole (T/S), and stress-dose steroids for critical illness.

5.2. Induction of remission in generalized and severe AAV

5.2.1. *Cyclophosphamide*

Efficacy: Cyclophosphamide is typically reserved for patients with severe or generalized AAV, or if a poor prognostic factor is present. In 1973, Fauci and Wolff published their experience of treating 18 patients with GPA and systemic involvement with oral cyclophosphamide [21]. Twelve patients achieved remission, and 6 were able to discontinue immunosuppression after several months. They later reported on a larger cohort of 85 patients with GPA treated with a protocol of oral cyclophosphamide of 2 mg/kg/day and high dose prednisone of 1 mg/kg /day [22]. They were followed prospectively over 21 years with 93% achieving complete remission and a mean survival of 48 months although 29% relapsed. This work also highlighted the toxicity of this drug, such as gonadal failure, cystitis in 34% of patients, and 1 patient developing lymphoma.

In an effort to reduce the toxicity associated with the prolonged used of cyclophosphamide, Hoffman et al [23] designed a protocol of intravenous pulses, similar to the National Institute of Health (NIH) study of treatment of severe lupus nephritis [24]. Fourteen patients with GPA, 12 with relapsing disease previously treated with daily oral cyclophosphamide, received monthly pulses of 1g/m^2 of cyclophosphamide for 6 months along with high dose oral glucocorticoids. If remission was achieved the pulses were reduced in frequency to every 2 months for 6 months then every 3 months for a total of 1.5 years. Glucocorticoids were tapered and stopped over this time period. Unfortunately, although 93% improved initially, only 21% had sustained remission. Thirty six percent (4 patients) had experienced toxicity, mostly attributable to infections, but confounded by the concomitant use of high doses of prednisone.

A subsequent 18 month European open-label randomized controlled multicenter clinical trial, CYCLOPS [16], of pulse versus daily oral cyclophosphamide in 149 newly diagnosed patients with AAV (including GPA, MPA and renal limited vasculitis) with renal involvement and a creatinine between 150 and 500 umol/L was performed. Patients in the intravenous pulse group received cyclophosphamide 15 mg/kg every 2 weeks for the first 3 pulses then continued either intravenous pulse (15 mg/kg) or oral pulse (5 mg/kg for 3 consecutive days), every 3 weeks afterwards until remission and then for another 3 months. The oral cyclophosphamide group received 2 mg/kg daily until remission then 1.5 mg/kg for another 3 months. Remission maintenance was with azathioprine at a dose of 2 mg/kg for 18 months. The cyclophosphamide doses were adjusted for renal function and age, as well as leukocyte count, with a maximum dose of 1.2 g in the pulse group and 200 mg in the daily oral group. Both groups were also treated with oral glucocorticoids during induction, with initially 1 mg/kg (maximum 80 mg) used, but with progressive tapering to 12.5 mg at 3 months and 5 mg at 18 months.

The administration route of cyclophosphamide did not affect the remission rate, with 88% of subjects randomized to pulse therapy and 88% of subjects randomized to daily oral therapy in remission at 9 months. Both groups had a median time to remission of 3 months (range of 0.5 to 8 months in the pulse group and 1 to 7.5 months in the daily oral group). The cumulative dose in the oral group was higher than the pulse group (median 15.9 g vs. 8.2 g) with a lower rate of leukopenia in the pulse group.

The long-term follow-up of these studies was recently reported [25]. Retrospective chart information was available for 134 out of 148 patients, and 1 patient was subsequently excluded as their diagnosis was changed to EGPA. The median follow-up was 4.3 years. An increased relapse rate was observed in the pulse group compared to the daily oral group. Fifteen (20.8%) of the daily oral group and 30 (39.5%) of the pulse group had at least one relapse. However there was no difference in survival, renal function nor adverse events between groups. The presence of PR3-ANCA was independently associated with an increase risk of relapse (hazard ratio 2.47 (95%CI 1.32-4.59, p=0.004).

A meta-analysis [26] of randomized trials [27-29] comparing daily oral versus intravenous pulse of cyclophosphamide concluded that pulse therapy was significantly less likely to fail in remission induction (odds ratio (OR) 0.29 (95% CI 0.12-0.73) and had a significantly lower risk of infection (OR: 0.45 (95% CI 0.23-0.89)) and leucopenia (OR 0.36 (95% CI 0.17-0.78)). There was a non-significant increase in the relapse odds in the pulse cyclophosphamide group (OR 1.79 (95%CI 0.85-3.75).

Safety: Although cyclophosphamide has been the mainstay of treatment for generalized and severe forms of AAV, there are several limitations to its use. First, there are significant adverse events associated with this drug even at the lower cumulative dose achieved through pulse therapy. Infertility is a concern in individuals of childbearing age, and bladder toxicity and malignancy are associated with increased morbidity and mortality [30-32]. The development of leukopenia significantly increases the risk of bacterial infection, and renders the patient susceptible to opportunistic infections. Table 2 provides dose adjustment recommendations based on the patient's age, renal function and leukocyte nadir to reduce the risk of toxicity.

5.2.2. Rituximab

Efficacy: The use of Rituximab, an anti-CD20 monoclonal antibody depleting B lymphocytes, has been reported in several case series and case reports to be effective in patients with generalized, severe and refractory disease [33]. This was subsequently confirmed by 2 randomized controlled trials published in 2010, "Rituximab in ANCA-associated Vasculitis" (RAVE) [19] and "Randomised Trial of Rituximab Versus Cyclophosphamide for Generalized ANCA-Associated Vasculitis" (RITUXVAS) [34]. In these two studies rituximab was non-inferior and/or equivalent to cyclophosphamide in inducing remission in AAV. Rituximab was superior to cyclophosphamide in relapsing patients.

RAVE [19] was a North American multicentre, randomized, double blind, controlled therapeutic trial where 197 patients with new or relapsing ANCA positive GPA and MPA without severe renal disease (creatinine less than 354 umol/L) or severe alveolar hemorrhage (not

	Age	Creatinine	Leukocyte nadir (10-14 days)	Leukocyte count
IV cyclosphamide: 15 mg/kg Max dose: 1.2 g	>60: reduce dose by 2.5 mg/kg per pulse >70: reduce dose by 5 mg/kg per pulse	300 to 500 µmol/L (3.4 to 5.7 mg/dL) reduce pulse by 2.5 mg/kg	2 to 3 x10^9/L reduce dose of subsequent pulse by 20% 1 to 2 x10^9/L reduce dose of subsequent pulse by 40%	
Daily Oral cyclophosphamide 2 mg/kg Max dose: 200 mg	>60 reduce dose by 25% >70 reduce dose by 50%			< 4x10^9/L stop drug until >4 reduce dose by 25% <1x10^9/L restart at 50 mg then increase weekly as tolerated

Table 2. Adjusted cyclophosphamide dose according to age, renal function and leukocyte count [16]

requiring a ventilator). The study was designed as a non-inferiority trial comparing intravenous rituximab (375 mg/m^2 of body surface weekly for 4 weeks) to daily oral cyclophosphamide (2mg/kg). Both groups received methylprednisolone 1 g for one to three pulses, followed by prednisone 1 mg/kg. The primary end point was defined as a Birmingham Vasculitis Activity Score for Wegener's Granulomatosis (BVAS/WG) [35] of 0 and the complete discontinuation of prednisone at 6 months. Once remission was achieved by 3 to 6 months, maintenance therapy was initiated in the cyclophosphamide group with azathioprine (2 mg/kg), however the Rituximab group did not receive maintenance therapy. There was no difference in the primary outcome at 6 months between the 2 groups. Sixty-three of the 99 patients in the rituximab group (64%) reached the primary end point, as compared with 52 of 98 in the control group (53%), and met the criterion for non-inferiority (P<0.001). However, among patients with relapsing disease at baseline, rituximab was more efficacious than cyclophosphamide, with 34 of 51 patients in the rituximab group (67%) reaching the primary end point, as compared with only 21 of 50 in the control group (42%) (p=0.01). In an oral presentation at the American College of Rheumatology Annual Meeting in November 2011, the extended follow-up to 18 months was reported. One single course of rituximab without maintenance therapy was as effective as 18 months of induction and maintenance therapy with cyclophosphamide followed by azathioprine. Complete remission was achieved and sustained at 6, 12, and 18 months in 64%, 47%, and 39% of subjects in the rituximab arm, comparable at 53%, 39%, and 33% of subjects in the cyclophosphamide/azathioprine arm, respectively. Disease flares in the two treatment arms did not differ in number or severity, and no unexpected safety issues were detected. Patients at highest risk for flare had GPA, were PR3 positive, were without major renal disease, and had relapsing disease at baseline. Disease flares in the rituximab treated subjects occurred only after the return of detectable levels of B cells.

RITUXVAS [34] was a European multicenter, open label, randomized trial of rituximab compared to intravenous cyclophosphamide in 44 patients with newly diagnosed ANCA-associated vasculitis with renal involvement [34]. Subjects in the rituximab group received both rituximab (375 mg/m^2 per week for 4 consecutive weeks) and intravenous cyclophosphamide (15 mg/kg) with the first and third rituximab infusions. They did not receive any maintenance therapy. If they had progressive disease within the first 6 months, a third dose of intravenous cyclophosphamide was permitted. Subjects in the control group received intravenous cyclophosphamide (15 mg/kg), every 2 weeks for the first three doses then every 3 weeks for 3 to 6 months until remission, followed by azathioprine for maintenance. Both treatment arms received 1 g of intravenous methylprednisolone and then oral prednisone at 1 mg/kg per day initially, with a reduction to 5 mg per day at the end of 6 months. The primary outcome was sustained remission and rates of serious adverse events at 12 months. Thirty-three subjects were enrolled in the rituximab group and 11 in the control group. Sustained remission was observed in 25 of 33 patients in the rituximab group (76%) and 9 of 11 patients in the control group (82%) (p=0.68). Six of the 33 subjects in the rituximab group (18%) and 2 of the 11 patients in the control group (18%) died. Among the survivors, sustained remission rates at 12 months were equal, and observed in 93% of the rituximab group and 90% of the control group (p=0.80). The median time to remission was 90 days (interquartile range, 79 to 112) in the rituximab group and 94 days (interquartile range, 91 to 100) in the control group (p=0.87). At 12 months of follow-up, 4 of 27 subjects in the rituximab group (15%) and 1 of 10 subjects in the control group (10%) suffered a relapse (p=0.70). This study also demonstrated efficacy in serious renal disease. Among the 9 subjects who were on dialysis at study entry, 6 of the 8 subjects randomized to the rituximab group attained sustained remission, and 5 no longer required dialysis.

Safety: Unfortunately, rituximab use was not associated with a lower rate of serious adverse events in either study, although there were more episodes of leukopenia in subjects randomized to cyclophosphamide. In the RAVE study, there were no significant differences between the treatment groups in the numbers of total adverse events, serious adverse events, or non –disease related adverse events. During the first 6 months of the trial, solid malignant tumors were diagnosed in 1 patient in each group; 2 patients in the control group and 1 in the rituximab group died. Six malignant conditions developed in 5 additional patients after 6 months. Four of those patients had been assigned initially to rituximab and one had been assigned to cyclophosphamide. Among patients with exposure to rituximab during the trial, malignant conditions developed in 6 of 124 (5%), as compared with 1 of 73 patients without exposure to rituximab (1%, p=0.26). In RITUXVAS, severe adverse events were similar between groups (rituximab group 42% and 36% in the standard care group). Infection rates were similar (rituximab group incidence rate 0.66/patient year vs 0.60/patient year in the standard care group). Dialysis patients were particular prone to adverse events, with 3 of the 9 dying, and 7 of 9 with at least one serious adverse event.

5.2.3. Plasma exchange

The rationale for the physical removal of ANCA by plasma exchange is based on the demonstration of the pathogenic role of ANCA in animal models of AAV [36, 37]. Corticosteroids and cyclophosphamide are used concomitantly to suppress inflammation and autoantibody production.

A study of patients with severe renal involvement of GPA and MPA causing rapidly progressive glomerulonephritis was designed to compare intravenous (IV) methylprednisolone and plasma exchange [38]. One hundred and thirty-seven patients with creatinine >500 umol/l were enrolled in this open label, randomized trial and 69% were on dialysis for less than 2 weeks at study entry. Both groups received oral cyclophosphamide (2.5 mg/kg/day reduced to 1.5 mg/kg/day at 3 months and stopped at 6 months), followed by azathioprine (2 mg/kg/day). Oral prednisolone was tapered from 1 mg/kg/day at entry to 0.25 mg/kg/day by week 10,15 mg/day at 3 months and10mg/day from 5 to12 months. The IV methylprednisolone group (n=67) received 1000 mg/day for three consecutive days, and the subjects in the plasma exchange group (n=70) underwent a total of seven plasma exchanges within 14 days of study entry, with a plasma exchange volume of 60 ml/kg on each occasion and volume replacement with 5% albumin mandated in the protocol. The primary outcome measure was renal recovery at 3 months, defined by patient survival, dialysis independence, and serum creatinine <500 umol/l (5.8 mg/dl).

There was a significant decrease in the risk of end-stage renal disease in the plasma exchange group compared to IV methylprednisolone but there was no significant difference in patient survival at 12 months. By 3 months, renal recovery had occurred in 33 (49%) of 67 of the IV methylprednisolone group and 48 (69%) of 70 of the plasma exchange group (95%CI for the difference 18 to 35%; $p = 0.02$). This effect was sustained to 12 months from entry with only two from each group progressing to end stage renal disease after initial recovery, with a risk reduction of 24% (95%CI 6.1 to 41) at 12 months. At 12 months, 43% of subjects in the IV methylprednisolone group and 59% of subjects in the plasma exchange group remained alive and independent of dialysis ($p = 0.008$). The hazard ratio for end stage renal disease over 12 months for plasma exchange versus IV methylprednisolone was 0.47 (95%CI 0.24 to 0.91; $p = 0.03$). Subject survival at 3 and 12 months respectively was 84% and 76% in the IV methylprednisolone group and 84% and 73% in the plasma exchange group (log rank test $p = 0.68$). Mortality was 25.5% at 12 months, and the major causes of death were infection (n = 19), pulmonary hemorrhage (n = 6), and cardiovascular disease (n = 4). Most deaths occurred during the first 3 months, when corticosteroid dosages were highest and vasculitis was most active. After 3 months, there was a higher mortality in those who had failed to recover renal function.

5.3. Induction of remission in early systemic disease

5.3.1. Methotrexate

The treatment of AAV with cyclophosphamide is associated with significant toxicity and morbidity as previously discussed. Alternative immunosuppression to reduce this risk have been studied. The "Non-Renal Wegener's Granulomatosis Treated Alternatively with Methotrexate" (NORAM) [17] trial was designed to test the hypothesis than methotrexate could replace cyclophosphamide for remission induction. NORAM was a non-inferiority, unblinded, prospective, randomized, controlled trial in early systemic GPA and MPA, without organ-threatening or life-threatening disease and a creatinine of less than 150 umol/

L. More than 90% of patients had GPA. In total, 49 subjects were treated with methotrexate (15 mg/week orally escalating to a maximum of 20–25 mg/week by 12 weeks), which was then maintained until month 10 and then tapered and discontinued by month 12. A total of 46 subjects received oral cyclophosphamide (2 mg/kg/day (maximum 150 mg/day) until remission), for a minimum of 3 and a maximum of 6 months. Dose alterations were made for subjects >60 years of age, and the drug was withdrawn if the total white blood cell count fell below 4 x10^9/liter. At remission, cyclophosphamide was reduced to 1.5 mg/kg/day until month 10, when it was tapered and discontinued by month 12. Both treatment groups received oral prednisolone 1 mg/kg/day, tapered to 15 mg/day at 12 weeks and 7.5 mg/day by 6 months, and discontinued by 12 months. The primary end point was induction of remission within 6 months. Between month 12 to 18, patients received no immunosuppressant agents.

At 6 months, 90% of subjects randomized to methotrexate and 94% of subjects randomized to cyclophosphamide achieved remission (p=0.041). The median time to remission was 3 months (range 1–9) in the methotrexate group and 2 months (range 1–5) in the cyclophosphamide group (p=0.19 log rank test). Of the subjects who achieved remission during the treatment period, 70% of the subjects randomized to methotrexate and 47% of subjects randomized to cyclophosphamide had a relapse, with the time to relapse being significantly longer in the cyclophosphamide group (median 15 months, range 4-17) compared to the methotrexate group (median 13 months, range 2-17) (P =0.023 log rank test). Leukopenia was more common in the cyclophosphamide group and liver dysfunction was more common in the methotrexate group.

The long term follow-up of patients treated in the NORAM study was recently reported [39]. Data was obtained on all 95 original subjects with a median duration of follow-up of 6 years. Subjects in the methotrexate group required a longer duration of corticosteroid therapy during the trial period of 18 months (median 15 months, interquartile range (IQR) 12-18) compared to 12 months (IQR 12-15) in the cyclophosphamide group, p=0.005). During subsequent follow-up, the median duration of corticosteroid therapy during months 19-60 was 3.0 years in the methotrexate group and only 1.5 years in the cyclophosphamide group (p=0.004). After the trial period of 18 months, patients' treatment was left at the discretion of their physicians. Physicians were asked to provide information regarding drugs used to manage disease flare such as cyclophosphamide, methotrexate, azathioprine and mycophenolate mofetil. Exposure to cyclophosphamide and these other agents was also longer in the methotrexate group (p=0.037; and p=0.031, respectively).

Overall, the cumulative relapse-free survival from the time of first remission was 69% after 1 year, 32% after 3 years, and 24% after 5 years of follow-up, demonstrating a trend to being higher in the cyclophosphamide group (p=0.056, logrank test). The cumulative overall survival did not differ between treatment arms (p=0.88, log-rank test) and was 98% after 1 year, 93% after 3 years, and 89% after 5 years. The number of serious infections did not differ between treatment groups. The authors have concluded that methotrexate therapy was associated with less effective long-term disease control as compared to cyclophosphamide.

6. Maintenance of remission

The relapse rate of AAV is high, as demonstrated by the different induction trials, and occur frequently during a drug withdrawal period [32, 39]. Therefore it is important to maintain long-term immunosuppression, while limiting drug toxicity. When a standardized treatment of induction of remission followed by maintenance therapy is applied, the relapse rate in GPA can be reduced from 76.8% (in cohorts treated before 1993) to 50% (in cohorts treated after 1999) over 5 years follow-up [40]. Several studies have provided different drug alternatives for maintenance of remission.

6.1. Azathioprine

An 18 month prospective open label study (CYCAZAREM) compared the use of oral cyclophosphamide to azathioprine in the maintenance phase, with 155 subjects with GPA, MPA and renal limited vasculitis recruited from 39 hospitals in 11 European countries [41]. All subjects had received the same remission-induction therapy, consisting of daily oral cyclophosphamide (2 mg/kg) and prednisolone (initially 1 mg/kg/day, with the dose tapered to 0.25 mg/kg/day by 12 weeks). Renal vasculitis was the most common form of organ involvement, occurring in 94 percent of the patients in the study. Patients attaining remission by 3 months, and those attaining remission between 3 and 6 months, were randomly assigned to treatment with azathioprine (2 mg/kg/day) or to continue cyclophosphamide therapy at a lower dose (1.5 mg/kg/day). Both treatment groups continued to receive prednisolone 10 mg daily. At 12 months after study entry, both groups received azathioprine at a dose of 1.5 mg/kg/day and prednisolone 7.5 mg daily. The primary end point was relapse, either major (threatened function of the kidney, lung, brain, eye, motor nerve or gut) or minor (affecting at least three other items in the Birmingham Vasculitis Activity Score (BVAS)) [42].

Of the initial 155 subjects, clinical remission was achieved in 93% overall, with 77% reaching this target by 3 months and 16% between 3 and 6 months. These patients were randomly assigned to cyclophosphamide (73 patients) or azathioprine (71 patients). Azathioprine was demonstrated to be equivalent to cyclophosphamide for maintenance therapy. Sixteen percent in the azathioprine group had relapses, compared to 14% in the cyclophosphamide group ($p=0.65$). Five patients in each group had a major relapse. The most frequent adverse event was neutropenia (55% of patients, including the remission and maintenance phase), with 52% of infections occurring during an episode of neutropenia. There was no difference in renal outcomes between the groups, with renal failure occurring in only 3% of patients.

6.2. Methotrexate

A prospective, open-label, multicenter trial, comparing methotrexate and azathioprine for maintenance of remission in GPA and MPA (WEGENT) was designed to detect treatment tolerance [43]. Three-quarters of the patients had GPA. Sixty-three patients who had achieved remission with intravenous cyclophosphamide and corticosteroids received oral azathioprine (2 mg/kg/day) and 63 received methotrexate (initial 0.3 mg/kg/week, progressively increased to 25 mg per week) for 12 months. At the end of the scheduled maintenance therapy period, azathioprine and methotrexate were withdrawn over a period of 3 months at the discretion of the treating physician. T/S was recommended for 2 additional years for patients with GPA after discontinuation of the maintenance immunosuppressive agents. The primary end point was an adverse event requiring discontinuation of the study drug or causing death.

At the censoring date for analysis, the mean follow-up after randomization was 29 months. Adverse events leading to the primary end point (i.e., discontinuation of the study drug or death) occurred in 11% of the azathioprine group and 19% in the methotrexate group (p=0.21). After starting maintenance therapy, 46% of azathioprine recipients had at least one adverse event as compared with 56% of methotrexate recipients (p= 0.29). Thirty-six percent of azathioprine subjects and 33% of methotrexate subjects had a relapse (p=0.71). In 73% of the patients the relapse occurred after discontinuation of the drugs. This study demonstrated that the two agents were equivalent in safety and also efficacy. There was a trend toward a higher risk of adverse events with methotrexate, with a hazard ratio of 1.65 (95%CI, 0.65-4.18).

6.3. Mycophenolate mofetil

Mycophenolate mofetil is a prodrug of mycophenolic acid, which is a reversible inhibitor of inosine monophosphate dehydrogenase in guanosine nucleotide synthesis, upon which T and B cells are dependent, and has cytostatic effects on lymphocytes [44]. It has been proposed as a less toxic alternative to azathioprine and has been evaluated in one randomized trial. The IMPROVE study was an open-label trial to assess whether mycophenolate mofetil reduces the risk of relapse compared with azathioprine in patients with AAV in remission [45]. All patients received cyclophosphamide (daily oral or intermittent intravenous doses for a maximum of 6 months) and glucocorticoids (up to 3 g of methylprednisolone over 3 days was allowed for severe disease, then 1 mg/kg/day (maximum 80 mg) of oral prednisolone) for induction of remission. Plasma exchange could also be used for severe disease. Oral steroids were reduced according to a standardized schedule to 15 mg/day at the start of the remission regimen, tapered to 5 mg/day after 12 months, and were withdrawn after 24 months. One hundred and fifty six patients with a new diagnosis of GPA and MPA were enrolled after remission was achieved. The azathioprine group (n=80) initially received 2 mg/kg/day (maximum 200 mg), with dose reductions to 1.5 mg/kg/day after 12 months and 1 mg/kg/day after 18 months, with drug withdrawal after 42 months. Seventy-six patients assigned to the mycophenolate mofetil group received 2 g/day, which was reduced to 1500 mg/day after 12 months, 1000 mg/day after 18 months, and withdrawn after 42 months. The primary end point was relapse-free survival, defined as the time from remission to the first relapse (major or minor), withdrawal, death or loss to follow-up, or the end of the follow-up period.

Median follow-up for both treatment groups from start of maintenance therapy was 39 months. Relapses were more common in the mycophenolate mofetil group. In total, 55% of the mycophenolate mofetil recipients experienced relapses (18 major, 24 minor), as compared to 38% of azathioprine recipients (10 major, 20 minor), with an unadjusted hazard ratio for mycophenolate mofetil use of 1.69 (95%CI, 1.06-2.70; p=0.03) at 4 years. The risk of severe adverse events was not significantly different between groups, with a hazard ratio of 0.53 (95%CI, 0.23-1.18, p=0.12). Therefore mycophenolate mofetil should not be considered as a first

http://dx.doi.org/10.5772/54290

choice for maintenance of remission in AAV, but could be used in situations of intolerance or contraindication to azathioprine.

6.4. Leflunomide

Leflunomide is a disease-modifying agent commonly used in the treatment of rheumatoid arthritis as an alternative to methotrexate. A prospective randomized controlled trial of leflunomide compared to methotrexate in patients with generalized GPA for maintenance of remission was conducted in 5 German rheumatology centres [46]. The study was powered to find equivalence between the 2 drugs. Patients achieving complete or partial remission with daily oral cyclophosphamide (2mg/kg) and prednisolone and maintained remission for at least 3 months were enrolled in the study. Partial remission was defined as partial improvement of the disease persisting for at least 3 months represented by a constant disease extent index and BVAS. Complete remission was defined as the absence of pathological findings in clinical, radiological and serological investigations, irrespective of the ANCA titre. Twenty-eight subjects received oral methotrexate starting at a dose of 7.5 mg/week, increased over 9 weeks to 20 mg/week. Folic acid 10 mg weekly was taken the day after methotrexate. Twenty-six patients received leflunomide with a loading dose of 100 mg daily for 3 days, followed by 20 mg daily and then increased to 30 mg daily after 4 weeks. Prednisone was allowed at a dose of 10mg/day or less, and was tapered by 2.5mg/month in the absence of disease activity until a dose of 5 mg was reached, and then by 1 mg/month thereafter. The primary efficacy outcome was the number of major and minor relapses.

In the leflunomide group, 23% of subjects experienced a relapse, compared to 46% of methotrexate subjects (p=0.09), and the incidence of major relapses was significantly higher in the methotrexate group (p=0.037). The study was terminated prematurely in September 2003 after the advisory board had decided that the high rate of major relapses in the methotrexate group was not acceptable.

Safety: There was no significant difference in the number of adverse events between the groups. Thirty-four adverse events were observed in the leflunomide group and 17 in the methotrexate group (p=0.09). Leflunomide was stopped in two patients with intractable hypertension, one patient with peripheral neuropathy and one patient with leucopenia, whereas no patient stopped due to adverse events in the methotrexate group. Twenty-five infectious episodes, 13 in the leflunomide group and 12 in the methotrexate group were noted, all responding well to conventional antibiotic treatment on outpatient basis.

7. Refractory/relapsing disease

Some patients have disease that proves to be refractory to the therapies used for induction and maintenance of remission as above. Typically, patients with lung and upper airway involvement, positive PR3-ANCA and severe renal involvement have more resistant disease [47-49]. Relapse is also frequent in AAV, with an overall risk of 38% at 5 years seen in a large cohort of 535 patients from 70 European trial sites between 1995 and 2002 [32]. The presence of positive

PR3 ANCA, cardiac involvement and absence of severe renal disease at presentation was found to be a predictor of relapse in that group [9]. A variety of agents have been proposed to address these refractory cases.

7.1. Tumor necrosis factor inhibition

7.1.1. Etanercept

The "Wegener's Granulomatosis Etanercept Trial" (WGET) was a randomized, double blind, placebo controlled trial of etanercept as an adjunct to conventional therapy in patients with GPA [18]. The study enrolled 181 patients from 8 centres in the United States. Patients had newly diagnosed or relapsing GPA with a BVAS/WG of ≥3 and either limited or severe manifestations of their disease. Etanercept at the dose of 25 mg twice weekly subcutaneously or placebo was used simultaneously at the time of randomization with conventional therapy (corticosteroids along with methotrexate for limited disease and oral cyclophosphamide followed by methotrexate for severe disease induction and azathioprine for maintenance) and maintained as the conventional drugs were tapered over time. Prednisone was tapered by a specific protocol to be completely discontinued within six months, assuming that no relapse occurred.

The primary outcome measure was sustained disease remission, defined as a BVAS/WG of 0, for at least six months. The median duration of treatment was 25 months for etanercept and 19 months for placebo and the mean duration of follow-up was 27 months in the overall cohort. Seventy percent of subjects in the etanercept group met the primary outcome, as compared with 75% in the control group (p=0.39). There was no significant difference between groups in the time to sustained remission. The overall rate of sustained remission throughout follow-up was only 49.4%. Disease flares during treatment were not significantly different between the etanercept and control groups (relative risk, 0.89 (95%CI 0.62 to 1.28; p=0.54). The major concern arising from this study however was in the development of adverse events. Moderately severe to fatal infections occurred in 49% of subjects and were equal between treatment groups, however six solid cancers were identified during the trial, and all occurred in the etanercept group (standardized incidence ratio of 3.12 (95%CI 1.15–6.80, p=0.014)). An additional 3 other patients were subsequently diagnosed with a solid malignancy within 6 months of completion of the trial [50]. This study clearly demonstrated that etanercept was not effective, and the use of etanercept in combination with cyclophosphamide is associated with an increased risk of malignancy.

7.1.2. Infliximab and adalimumab

Infliximab has been studied as an adjuvant therapy for induction of remission in new, relapsing and refractory disease. A prospective, open label, multicenter study in the United Kingdom evaluated 2 small groups of patients with active disease [51]. In the new presentation or relapse group, infliximab (5 mg/kg) was given at 0, 2, 6 and 10 weeks as an adjuvant therapy to oral cyclophosphamide (2mg/kg/day) for 14 weeks and prednisolone. Once remission was achieved the cyclophosphamide was replaced by azathioprine (2 mg/kg/day, reduced to 1.5

mg/kg/day after 1 year) or mycophenolate mofetil if azathioprine wasn't tolerated. In patients with persistent disease despite the use of methotrexate, azathioprine, mycophenolate mofetil or T/S, infliximab (5 mg/kg) at 0, 2, 6 and 10 weeks was added. If remission was achieved infliximab was maintained every 6 weeks for 1 year. In both groups, 88% achieved remission (BVAS ≤1) within a mean of 6.4 weeks. During follow-up (mean 17 months), only 18% experienced a relapse of disease. Both groups were able to significantly reduce their glucocorticoid dose from a mean of 24 mg/day to 9 mg/day at week 14. There were 2 deaths in the newly diagnosed and relapsing group and 21% had severe infections. A second study has also examined infliximab use (5 mg/kg at 0, 2, 6 and 10 weeks) in addition to standard therapy and found no effect [52]. At 1 year, time to achieve remission, remission rates, adverse events, damage index scores, and relapse rates were similar between groups.

Adalimumab was used as an adjunctive therapy in a single centre, open label, prospective, uncontrolled study of newly diagnosed patients with GPA or MPA with renal involvement [53]. Seventy-nine percent of patients achieved remission (BVAS = 0) within the first 14 weeks of the study, and the mean oral prednisolone dose decreased from 37 to 8 mg/day, demonstrating potential efficacy but requiring further rigorous study.

7.2. Rituximab

Smith et al [54] reported a retrospective study of maintenance therapy with Rituximab in 73 patients with refractory or relapsing GPA and MPA. Twenty-eight received treatment with a single dose of rituximab (1000 mg) at the time of relapse. Of these, 19 were subsequently retreated at 6 months intervals. Another 45 patients were treated with rituximab (1000 mg twice at an interval of 2 weeks) and then received treatment (1000 mg) every 6 months for 24 months with ongoing follow-up for an additional 24 months. Of the patients treated with a single 1000 mg dose at relapse, 73% relapsed within 24 months. The frequency of relapse was lower in patients who received retreatment at 6 months at only 11% ($p<0.001$), and in those treated with the higher initial dose and ongoing retreatment at 12% ($p<0.001$). At 48 months, relapses had occurred in 81% of the single dose group, compared to 26% and 39% in the group with retreatment and the higher initial dose and retreatment. The median time to first relapse was 12 months (range 5-76) in the group receiving the single dose, compared to 29 months (range 5-48) in the group receiving retreatment and 34.5 months (range 5-53) in the group with the higher initial dose and retreatment. Retreatment was associated with a reduction in relapse rates compared to single rituximab courses and allowed early withdrawal of immunosuppression and glucocorticoid reduction or withdrawal. In this study B cell count and ANCA positivity didn't correlate with the time of relapse.

7.3. Intravenous immunoglobulin (IVIg)

IVIg consists of intact IgG molecules, representing all IgG subclasses, from the pooled plasma of donors [55]. Small amounts of IgM, IgA, HLA and cytokines are also present in the preparation. As such, IVIg contains a broad range of immune antibodies against pathogens and foreign antigens. Proposed mechanisms of action include modulation of the expression and function of Fc receptors, interference with the activation of complement and the cytokine network, provision of antiidiotypic antibodies (idiotypes are located in the variable region of autoantibodies in autoimmune conditions), and effects on the activation, differentiation and effector functions of both T and B cells [55]. In vasculitis, IVIG may reverse monocyte and neutrophil activation, reduce autoantibody production or effect the autoreactive T cell function [56]. In vitro, incubation of ANCA vasculitis patient sera with IVIg inhibited ANCA activity [57] which provided evidence to proceed with clinical use of this agent.

In the initial publication, 7 patients with long-standing ANCA vasculitis resistant to standard immunosuppressive therapy received IVIg at a dose of 0.4 g/kg/day for 5 days [58] with maintenance of steroids and cytotoxic drugs for at least 6 weeks following the infusions. All patients improved within 2 days to 3 weeks; 5 went into full remission, 1 had sustained improvement and 1 had a partial transient response within 8 weeks. Relapses occurred in 3 patients between 2 and 9 months after treatment, with no relapses documented in the others who were followed between 6 and 18 months. Other successful case reports, case series and open-label studies followed [59-64] describing positive treatment responses, however there is likely an element of publication bias and confounding due to the variety in disease presentations, prior and concomitant immunosuppressive therapies received, variable steroid doses and the lack of a control arm for comparison. Jayne et al reported on a prospective double-blind placebo-controlled multicentre randomized study targeting a reduction in the BVAS [65]. Patients had either GPA or MPA with active vasculitis despite 2 months of treatment with prednisolone and cyclophosphamide or azathioprine. The mean disease duration of subjects in this study was 52.5 months. Seventeen subjects were randomized to receive IVIg 0.4 g/kg/day for 5 days with no changes in immunosuppressive drugs for 3 months after the trial infusion, and 17 subjects were in the placebo arm. Patients were assessed 2 weeks following the infusion and then monthly until 12 months. A 50% reduction in the BVAS was observed in 14/17 of the IVIg group and 6/17 of the placebo group respectively (OR 8.56; 95%CI 1.74-42.2, p-0.015) and two subjects in the placebo group died within 3 months. The mean BVAS in the IVIg group at baseline was 6.1, with a BVAS reduction of 3.2 at 1 month and 4.1 at 3 months, compared to a baseline BVAS of 5.4 in the placebo group with reductions of 0.87 and 2.3 at 1 and 3 months. However, after 3 months there were no significant differences in the BVAS between groups or in the frequency of relapse (5/16 for IVIG and 4/15 for placebo), and no differences in the subsequent steroids or immunosuppressive doses in follow-up.

An open-label study enrolled 22 poor-prognosis patients experiencing a relapse of WG or MPA despite treatment or within 1 year of stopping corticosteroids and/or immunosuppressants (0.5 g/kg/day for 4 days) to monthly IVIg for 6 months [66]. Temporary increases in prednisone doses were allowed but other immunosuppressants had to be maintained during the 6 months of IVIg therapy but could then be reduced, discontinued or switched to maintenance agents if cyclophosphamide had been given. In this study, the mean disease duration was 27 months (range 7-109 months) and the median BVAS 2005 at study entry was 11 (range 3-25). All but 1 patient was receiving steroids and/or immunosuppressants. Between months 1 and 5, 21 subjects achieved remission, with complete remission in 73% at 6 months, partial remission in 9% and relapse in 14%. The effect seemed persistent, with 13/16 responders still in complete remission at 9 months, and with 12/16 in complete remission at month 24. In those achieving complete remission at month 9, steroids were stopped in 4 and reduced in 9, with reductions in other immunosuppressants in 4 subjects. The median BVAS 2005 was 0 (range 0-13) at month 9 and 0 (range 0-12) at month 24. Moderate and transient effects of IVIg were reported including nausea, headaches, fever, arthralgias, and 1 patient developed renal insufficiency and was deemed a treatment failure.

IVIg is a safe agent for use in particular clinical situations, such as pregnancy, those with a potential infection mimicking vasculitis, and for patients with refractory persistent disease despite traditional immunsuppressive agents. Adverse effects included headaches, rise in creatinine, aseptic meningitis, backache and fever/chills. Theoretical adverse effects include the transmission of blood-borne pathogens, although extensive screening of blood donors occurs. Randomized clinical trials are lacking, and the role in new-onset disease or specific ANCA vasculitis entities is unexplored. The current evidence base is considered poor given the open-label nature of the literature with a lack of a control arm data or control over concomitant treatments received in addition of IVIg.

7.4. 15-deoxyspergualin (DSG; 1-amino-19-guanidino-11-hydroxy-4,9,12-triazanona-decane-10,1-3-dione; gusperimus)

DSG is a synthetic analogue of spergualin, a natural product of the bacterium *Bacillus latero-sporus,* which possesses immunosuppressive properties [67, 68]. DSG has effects on B cell differentiation, blocks kappa light-chain expression at the transcriptional level and acts on T effector cells. A pilot study of DSG (0.5 mg/kg daily subcutaneously to target a leukocyte nadir of 3000/μ, 6 cycles with 2 week recovery periods) was performed in 20 subjects with refractory WG or MPA [68]. Steroids were dosed at the discretion of the treating physician but no other immunosuppressives were allowed. The primary endpoint was remission (either complete remission with no signs of disease activity, or partial remission defined as no new activity but with minor persistent activity) after 6 cycles of DSG. Response was noted in 14 subjects (6 complete, 8 partial, with the mean BVAS improving from 11 (SD 5.8) to 4 (2.9) in responders, and a reduction of oral steroids from 30 mg per day to 7.5 mg/day. Response was maintained out to 6 months for 11/14 of the responders. Side effects were largely infectious in nature, with diarrhea, headache, bronchitis, and anemia also reported. In a further open label-study, 44 patients with refractory WG received DSG (0.5 mg/kg/day in six cycles of 21 days with 7 days between cycles) followed by azathioprine [69]. In this study, 20 patients achieved remission (BVAS of 0 for 2 months) and 22 achieved partial remission (BVAS <50% of entry score).

7.5. Alemtuzumab (campath-1H)

The humanized monoclonal antibody, anti-CD52 (alemtuzumab, CAMPATH-1H) depletes circulating lymphocytes and macrophages. It has shown a promising effect in patients with multiple sclerosis and Behçet's disease. It has been studied in a group of patients with relapsing and refractory GPA or MPA in one UK centre [70]. Patients were eligible to receive CAM-PATH-1H if they had multiple relapses or life threatening disease despite the standard of care. Prednisolone was continued at 10 mg/day but all other immunosuppressants were discontin-ued. CAMPATH-1H was administered intravenously on consecutive days at doses of 4, 10,

40, 40 and 40 mg, for a total dose of 134 mg. CAMPATH-1H was readministered for relapsing disease if the initial treatment was tolerated. A total of 71 patients were treated and followed for a mean of 5 years. Sixty-five percent of patients achieved clinical remission, and an additional 20% had a clinically significant improvement in disease activity but still required greater than 10 mg of prednisolone per day or an additional immunosuppressive agent to control disease activity. Almost all subjects relapsed after 9 months, with better renal function and the absence of neurologic involvement protective for relapse. Unfortunately, 44% of the cohort died during the follow-up period, 5 patients were diagnosed with malignancy, and 11% developed Graves disease. These adverse events may limit the use of alemtuzumab in practice to highly selected patients or those with disease refractory to all other agents.

7.6. Antithymocyte globulin (ATG)

The SOLUTION protocol was an uncontrolled prospective open-label study of ATG in 15 subjects with refractory GPA [71]. ATG was given intravenously at a dose of 2.5 mg/kg for a mean of 2 doses. The authors describe partial remission in 9/15 subjects and complete remission in 4/15 with reduced prednisone requirements (mean 49 mg/day to 13 mg/day) and only experiencing relapse after 8 months. However, 2 patients died and 5 others developed severe infections.

8. Treatment of localized vasculitis

8.1. Trimethoprim/sulfamethoxazole (T/S)

There have been case reports and case series of patients with AAV limited to the upper and/or lower respiratory tract treated with T/S for induction of remission with a good outcome [72]. A study of 72 patients with GPA looked at the role of T/S for induction of remission in the localized stage, and maintenance of remission in the generalized stage [73]. Nineteen patients with localized disease received T/S (2×960 mg/day) with 58% achieving complete or partial remission for a median of 43 months. Patients with generalized disease in remission did poorly with T/S, with 42% of those treated with T/S alone relapsing after a median of 13 months compared to a relapse rate of 29% at a median of 23 months in the patients not receiving T/S.

T/S was found to be superior to placebo in maintaining remission in a prospective, placebo controlled study of 81 patients with GPA, 41 of whom received T/S after induction of remission of generalized disease [74]. At 24 months of follow-up 82% of patients in the T/S group were still in remission, as compared to only 60% in the placebo group, with a relative risk of relapse of 0.40 (95%CI 0.17 to 0.98). This reduction was especially evident with respect to relapses involving the upper airways.

Therefore, T/S can be considered for the induction of remission of localized GPA but patients should be monitored carefully for signs of progression to systemic disease. The efficacy of maintenance of remission in generalized disease is controversial and currently not the recommended standard of practice.

http://dx.doi.org/10.5772/54290

9. Treatment of eosinophilic granulomatosis with polyangiitis (Churg-Strauss syndrome)

Most of the studies in AAV include only a small number of patients with EGPA or exclude them altogether. We will discuss trials performed specifically in EGPA.

9.1. EGPA with poor prognosis

A prospective, multicenter, randomized trial of patients newly diagnosed with EGPA and at least 1 poor prognosis factor (creatinine >140 μmol/l (1.58 mg/dl); proteinuria >1 gm/day; or central nervous system, gastrointestinal, or myocardial involvement) was conducted to determine the shortest immunosuppressant duration able to limit the occurrence of side effects and still induce and maintain disease remission by comparing glucocorticoids and 6 compared to 12 intravenous cyclophosphamide pulses [75]. All patients received 3 consecutive intravenous pulses of methylprednisolone (15 mg/kg) followed by oral prednisone (1 mg/kg/day) for 3 weeks followed by a tapering regime. Intravenous cyclophosphamide (0.6 g/m^2) was given every 2 weeks for 1 month, then every 4 weeks, and patients were randomized to receive either 6 or 12 cyclophosphamide pulses. The cumulative cyclophosphamide dose was twice as high in the 12-pulse group than in the 6-pulse group (6.6 g/m^2 versus 3.48 g/m^2). There was a non-significant difference in the proportion of patients achieving complete remission, at 91% for the group receiving 6 pulses and 84% for the group receiving 12 pulses. Relapse frequency demonstrated a trend to significance at 74% for the group receiving 6-pulses compared to 62% in the 12-pulse group ($p=0.07$), and the mean time to first relapse was 268 days in the 12-pulse group compared to 222 days in the 6-pulse group, although this was not statistically different. Adverse events and deaths were equal between both groups.

9.2. EGPA without poor prognosis factor

One study examined treatment efficacy of corticosteroids as first-line treatment of EGPA without poor prognosis factors, and the use of azathioprine compared to intravenous cyclophosphamide for treatment failure or relapse [76]. Subjects could receive 1 intravenous pulse of methylprednisolone (15 mg/kg) and then oral prednisone (1 mg/kg/day for 3 weeks) followed by a tapering regimen. If the prednisone could not be tapered below 20 mg, or if the patient experienced a relapse, they were randomized to azathioprine (2 mg/kg/day for 6 months) or 6 cyclophosphamide doses (0.6 g/m^2 every 2 weeks for 1 month, then every 4 weeks). Ninety-three percent of subjects achieved remission, with a 1 year survival rate of 100% and 5 year survival rate of 97%. Of the subjects achieving remission, 37% relapsed, and 3% could not reduce their prednisone. A total of 19 subjects went onto randomization with 10 receiving cyclophosphamide and 9 receiving azathioprine. Fifty percent of the cyclophosphamide subjects achieved remission, compared to 78% of the azathioprine subjects. Low-dose corticosteroid therapy was required in 79% of subjects long-term, primarily due to lung disease.

10. Chapter summary

The treatment of AAV is directed at achieving disease control to prevent morbidity and mortality, while minimizing treatment toxicity. Corticosteroid use remains critical in rapidly achieving disease activity suppression, whereas cyclophosphamide and rituximab regimens should be reserved for induction of severe generalized disease, and plasma exchange for severe renal disease. In less severe cases of systemic disease methotrexate is suitable for remission induction. Maintenance of remission is achieved preferably with azathioprine or methotrexate, with leflunomide, mycophenolate mofetil and cyclophosphamide remaining as options. Finally, new discoveries and research will certify the role of alternative agents, such as monoclonal anti-tumor necrosis factor therapy, IVIg, DSG, ATG and CAMPATH-1, in refractory disease.

Author details

Aurore Fifi-Mah and Cheryl Barnabe

Department of Medicine, University of Calgary, Calgary, Canada

References

[1] A. T. Masi, G. G. Hunder, J. T. Lie, B. A. Michel, D. A. Bloch, W. P. Arend, L. H. Calabrese, S. M. Edworthy, A. S. Fauci, R. Y. Leavitt, and et al., "The American College of Rheumatology 1990 criteria for the classification of Churg-Strauss syndrome (allergic granulomatosis and angiitis)," *Arthritis and Rheumatism,* vol. 33, pp. 1094-100, Aug 1990.

[2] D. A. Bloch, B. A. Michel, G. G. Hunder, D. J. McShane, W. P. Arend, L. H. Calabrese, S. M. Edworthy, A. S. Fauci, J. F. Fries, R. Y. Leavitt, and et al., "The American College of Rheumatology 1990 criteria for the classification of vasculitis. Patients and methods," *Arthritis and Rheumatism,* vol. 33, pp. 1068-73, Aug 1990.

[3] R. Y. Leavitt, A. S. Fauci, D. A. Bloch, B. A. Michel, G. G. Hunder, W. P. Arend, L. H. Calabrese, J. F. Fries, J. T. Lie, R. W. Lightfoot, Jr., and et al., "The American College of Rheumatology 1990 criteria for the classification of Wegener's granulomatosis," *Arthritis and Rheumatism,* vol. 33, pp. 1101-7, Aug 1990.

[4] R. W. Lightfoot, Jr., B. A. Michel, D. A. Bloch, G. G. Hunder, N. J. Zvaifler, D. J. McShane, W. P. Arend, L. H. Calabrese, R. Y. Leavitt, J. T. Lie, and et al., "The American College of Rheumatology 1990 criteria for the classification of polyarteritis nodosa," *Arthritis and Rheumatism,* vol. 33, pp. 1088-93, Aug 1990.

[5] J. C. Jennette, R. J. Falk, K. Andrassy, P. A. Bacon, J. Churg, W. L. Gross, E. C. Hagen, G. S. Hoffman, G. G. Hunder, C. G. Kallenberg, and et al., "Nomenclature of systemic vasculitides. Proposal of an international consensus conference," *Arthritis and Rheumatism,* vol. 37, pp. 187-92, Feb 1994.

[6] F. J. van der Woude, N. Rasmussen, S. Lobatto, A. Wiik, H. Permin, L. A. van Es, M. van der Giessen, G. K. van der Hem, and T. H. The, "Autoantibodies against neutrophils and monocytes: tool for diagnosis and marker of disease activity in Wegener's granulomatosis," *Lancet,* vol. 1, pp. 425-9, Feb 23 1985.

[7] R. J. Falk and J. C. Jennette, "Anti-neutrophil cytoplasmic autoantibodies with specificity for myeloperoxidase in patients with systemic vasculitis and idiopathic necrotizing and crescentic glomerulonephritis," *The New England journal of medicine,* vol. 318, pp. 1651-7, Jun 23 1988.

[8] E. W. Walton, "Giant-cell granuloma of the respiratory tract (Wegener's granulomatosis)," *British medical journal,* vol. 2, pp. 265-70, Aug 2 1958.

[9] M. Walsh, O. Flossmann, A. Berden, K. Westman, P. Hoglund, C. Stegeman, and D. Jayne, "Risk factors for relapse of antineutrophil cytoplasmic antibody-associated vasculitis," *Arthritis and Rheumatism,* vol. 64, pp. 542-8, Feb 2012.

[10] L. Guillevin, F. Lhote, M. Gayraud, P. Cohen, B. Jarrousse, O. Lortholary, N. Thibult, and P. Casassus, "Prognostic factors in polyarteritis nodosa and Churg-Strauss syndrome. A prospective study in 342 patients," *Medicine,* vol. 75, pp. 17-28, Jan 1996.

[11] L. Guillevin, C. Pagnoux, R. Seror, A. Mahr, L. Mouthon, and P. Le Toumelin, "The Five-Factor Score revisited: assessment of prognoses of systemic necrotizing vasculitides based on the French Vasculitis Study Group (FVSG) cohort," *Medicine,* vol. 90, pp. 19-27, Jan 2011.

[12] C. Mukhtyar, L. Guillevin, M. C. Cid, B. Dasgupta, K. de Groot, W. Gross, T. Hauser, B. Hellmich, D. Jayne, C. G. Kallenberg, P. A. Merkel, H. Raspe, C. Salvarani, D. G. Scott, C. Stegeman, R. Watts, K. Westman, J. Witter, H. Yazici, and R. Luqmani, "EULAR recommendations for the management of primary small and medium vessel vasculitis," *Annals of the Rheumatic Diseases,* vol. 68, pp. 310-7, Mar 2009.

[13] D. R. Jayne and N. Rasmussen, "Treatment of antineutrophil cytoplasm autoantibody-associated systemic vasculitis: initiatives of the European Community Systemic Vasculitis Clinical Trials Study Group," *Mayo Clinic proceedings. Mayo Clinic,* vol. 72, pp. 737-47, Aug 1997.

[14] "TREATMENT of polyarteritis nodosa with cortisone: results after one year; report to the Medical Research Council by the collagen diseases and hypersensitivity panel," *British medical journal,* vol. 1, pp. 608-11, Mar 16 1957.

[15] "Treatment of Polyarteritis Nodosa with Cortisone: Results After Three Years: Report to the Medical Research Council by the Collagen Diseases and Hypersensitivity Panel," *British medical journal,* vol. 1, pp. 1399-400, May 7 1960.

[16] K. de Groot, L. Harper, D. R. Jayne, L. F. Flores Suarez, G. Gregorini, W. L. Gross, R. Luqmani, C. D. Pusey, N. Rasmussen, R. A. Sinico, V. Tesar, P. Vanhille, K. Westman, and C. O. Savage, "Pulse versus daily oral cyclophosphamide for induction of remission in antineutrophil cytoplasmic antibody-associated vasculitis: a randomized trial," *Annals of internal medicine,* vol. 150, pp. 670-80, May 19 2009.

[17] K. De Groot, N. Rasmussen, P. A. Bacon, J. W. Tervaert, C. Feighery, G. Gregorini, W. L. Gross, R. Luqmani, and D. R. Jayne, "Randomized trial of cyclophosphamide versus methotrexate for induction of remission in early systemic antineutrophil cytoplasmic antibody-associated vasculitis," *Arthritis and Rheumatism,* vol. 52, pp. 2461-9, Aug 2005.

[18] "Etanercept plus standard therapy for Wegener's granulomatosis," *The New England journal of medicine,* vol. 352, pp. 351-61, Jan 27 2005.

[19] J. H. Stone, P. A. Merkel, R. Spiera, P. Seo, C. A. Langford, G. S. Hoffman, C. G. Kallenberg, E. W. St Clair, A. Turkiewicz, N. K. Tchao, L. Webber, L. Ding, L. P. Sejismundo, K. Mieras, D. Weitzenkamp, D. Ikle, V. Seyfert-Margolis, M. Mueller, P. Brunetta, N. B. Allen, F. C. Fervenza, D. Geetha, K. A. Keogh, E. Y. Kissin, P. A. Monach, T. Peikert, C. Stegeman, S. R. Ytterberg, and U. Specks, "Rituximab versus cyclophosphamide for ANCA-associated vasculitis," *The New England journal of medicine,* vol. 363, pp. 221-32, Jul 15 2010.

[20] M. Walsh, P. A. Merkel, A. Mahr, and D. Jayne, "Effects of duration of glucocorticoid therapy on relapse rate in antineutrophil cytoplasmic antibody-associated vasculitis: A meta-analysis," *Arthritis care & research,* vol. 62, pp. 1166-73, Aug 2010.

[21] A. S. Fauci and S. M. Wolff, "Wegener's granulomatosis: studies in eighteen patients and a review of the literature," *Medicine,* vol. 52, pp. 535-61, Nov 1973.

[22] A. S. Fauci, B. F. Haynes, P. Katz, and S. M. Wolff, "Wegener's granulomatosis: prospective clinical and therapeutic experience with 85 patients for 21 years," *Annals of internal medicine,* vol. 98, pp. 76-85, Jan 1983.

[23] G. S. Hoffman, R. Y. Leavitt, T. A. Fleisher, J. R. Minor, and A. S. Fauci, "Treatment of Wegener's granulomatosis with intermittent high-dose intravenous cyclophosphamide," *The American journal of medicine,* vol. 89, pp. 403-10, Oct 1990.

[24] D. T. Boumpas, H. A. Austin, 3rd, E. M. Vaughn, J. H. Klippel, A. D. Steinberg, C. H. Yarboro, and J. E. Balow, "Controlled trial of pulse methylprednisolone versus two regimens of pulse cyclophosphamide in severe lupus nephritis," *Lancet,* vol. 340, pp. 741-5, Sep 26 1992.

[25] L. Harper, M. D. Morgan, M. Walsh, P. Hoglund, K. Westman, O. Flossmann, V. Tesar, P. Vanhille, K. de Groot, R. Luqmani, L. F. Flores-Suarez, R. Watts, C. Pusey, A.

Bruchfeld, N. Rasmussen, D. Blockmans, C. O. Savage, and D. Jayne, "Pulse versus daily oral cyclophosphamide for induction of remission in ANCA-associated vasculitis: long-term follow-up," *Annals of the Rheumatic Diseases,* vol. 71, pp. 955-60, Jun 2012.

[26] K. de Groot, D. Adu, and C. O. Savage, "The value of pulse cyclophosphamide in ANCA-associated vasculitis: meta-analysis and critical review," *Nephrology, dialysis, transplantation : official publication of the European Dialysis and Transplant Association - European Renal Association,* vol. 16, pp. 2018-27, Oct 2001.

[27] D. Adu, A. Pall, R. A. Luqmani, N. T. Richards, A. J. Howie, P. Emery, J. Michael, C. O. Savage, and P. A. Bacon, "Controlled trial of pulse versus continuous prednisolone and cyclophosphamide in the treatment of systemic vasculitis," *QJM : monthly journal of the Association of Physicians,* vol. 90, pp. 401-9, Jun 1997.

[28] L. Guillevin, J. F. Cordier, F. Lhote, P. Cohen, B. Jarrousse, I. Royer, P. Lesavre, C. Jacquot, P. Bindi, P. Bielefeld, J. F. Desson, F. Detree, A. Dubois, E. Hachulla, B. Hoen, D. Jacomy, C. Seigneuric, D. Lauque, M. Stern, and M. Longy-Boursier, "A prospective, multicenter, randomized trial comparing steroids and pulse cyclophosphamide versus steroids and oral cyclophosphamide in the treatment of generalized Wegener's granulomatosis," *Arthritis and Rheumatism,* vol. 40, pp. 2187-98, Dec 1997.

[29] M. Haubitz, S. Schellong, U. Gobel, H. J. Schurek, D. Schaumann, K. M. Koch, and R. Brunkhorst, "Intravenous pulse administration of cyclophosphamide versus daily oral treatment in patients with antineutrophil cytoplasmic antibody-associated vasculitis and renal involvement: a prospective, randomized study," *Arthritis and Rheumatism,* vol. 41, pp. 1835-44, Oct 1998.

[30] C. Heijl, L. Harper, O. Flossmann, I. Stucker, D. G. Scott, R. A. Watts, P. Hoglund, K. Westman, and A. Mahr, "Incidence of malignancy in patients treated for antineutrophil cytoplasm antibody-associated vasculitis: follow-up data from European Vasculitis Study Group clinical trials," *Annals of the Rheumatic Diseases,* vol. 70, pp. 1415-21, Aug 2011.

[31] G. S. Hoffman, G. S. Kerr, R. Y. Leavitt, C. W. Hallahan, R. S. Lebovics, W. D. Travis, M. Rottem, and A. S. Fauci, "Wegener granulomatosis: an analysis of 158 patients," *Annals of internal medicine,* vol. 116, pp. 488-98, Mar 15 1992.

[32] M. A. Little, P. Nightingale, C. A. Verburgh, T. Hauser, K. De Groot, C. Savage, D. Jayne, and L. Harper, "Early mortality in systemic vasculitis: relative contribution of adverse events and active vasculitis," *Annals of the Rheumatic Diseases,* vol. 69, pp. 1036-43, Jun 2010.

[33] R. Cartin-Ceba, F. C. Fervenza, and U. Specks, "Treatment of antineutrophil cytoplasmic antibody-associated vasculitis with rituximab," *Current Opinion in Rheumatology,* vol. 24, pp. 15-23, Jan 2012.

[34] R. B. Jones, J. W. Tervaert, T. Hauser, R. Luqmani, M. D. Morgan, C. A. Peh, C. O. Savage, M. Segelmark, V. Tesar, P. van Paassen, D. Walsh, M. Walsh, K. Westman,

and D. R. Jayne, "Rituximab versus cyclophosphamide in ANCA-associated renal vasculitis," *The New England journal of medicine,* vol. 363, pp. 211-20, Jul 15 2010.

[35] J. H. Stone, G. S. Hoffman, P. A. Merkel, Y. I. Min, M. L. Uhlfelder, D. B. Hellmann, U. Specks, N. B. Allen, J. C. Davis, R. F. Spiera, L. H. Calabrese, F. M. Wigley, N. Maiden, R. M. Valente, J. L. Niles, K. H. Fye, J. W. McCune, E. W. St Clair, and R. A. Luqmani, "A disease-specific activity index for Wegener's granulomatosis: modification of the Birmingham Vasculitis Activity Score. International Network for the Study of the Systemic Vasculitides (INSSYS)," *Arthritis and Rheumatism,* vol. 44, pp. 912-20, Apr 2001.

[36] K. Kessenbrock, M. Krumbholz, U. Schonermarck, W. Back, W. L. Gross, Z. Werb, H. J. Grone, V. Brinkmann, and D. E. Jenne, "Netting neutrophils in autoimmune small-vessel vasculitis," *Nature Medicine,* vol. 15, pp. 623-5, Jun 2009.

[37] C. G. Kallenberg, "Pathogenesis of PR3-ANCA associated vasculitis," *Journal of autoimmunity,* vol. 30, pp. 29-36, Feb-Mar 2008.

[38] D. R. Jayne, G. Gaskin, N. Rasmussen, D. Abramowicz, F. Ferrario, L. Guillevin, E. Mirapeix, C. O. Savage, R. A. Sinico, C. A. Stegeman, K. W. Westman, F. J. van der Woude, R. A. de Lind van Wijngaarden, and C. D. Pusey, "Randomized trial of plasma exchange or high-dosage methylprednisolone as adjunctive therapy for severe renal vasculitis," *Journal of the American Society of Nephrology : JASN,* vol. 18, pp. 2180-8, Jul 2007.

[39] M. Faurschou, K. Westman, N. Rasmussen, K. de Groot, O. Flossmann, P. Hoglund, and D. R. Jayne, "Long-term outcome of a clinical trial comparing methotrexate to cyclophosphamide for remission induction of early systemic ANCA-associated vasculitis," *Arthritis and Rheumatism,* May 21 2012.

[40] J. U. Holle, W. L. Gross, U. Latza, B. Nolle, P. Ambrosch, M. Heller, R. Fertmann, and E. Reinhold-Keller, "Improved outcome in 445 patients with Wegener's granulomatosis in a German vasculitis center over four decades," *Arthritis and Rheumatism,* vol. 63, pp. 257-66, Jan 2011.

[41] D. Jayne, N. Rasmussen, K. Andrassy, P. Bacon, J. W. Tervaert, J. Dadoniene, A. Ekstrand, G. Gaskin, G. Gregorini, K. de Groot, W. Gross, E. C. Hagen, E. Mirapeix, E. Pettersson, C. Siegert, A. Sinico, V. Tesar, K. Westman, and C. Pusey, "A randomized trial of maintenance therapy for vasculitis associated with antineutrophil cytoplasmic autoantibodies," *The New England journal of medicine,* vol. 349, pp. 36-44, Jul 3 2003.

[42] R. A. Luqmani, P. A. Bacon, R. J. Moots, B. A. Janssen, A. Pall, P. Emery, C. Savage, and D. Adu, "Birmingham Vasculitis Activity Score (BVAS) in systemic necrotizing vasculitis," *QJM : monthly journal of the Association of Physicians,* vol. 87, pp. 671-8, Nov 1994.

[43] C. Pagnoux, A. Mahr, M. A. Hamidou, J. J. Boffa, M. Ruivard, J. P. Ducroix, X. Kyndt, F. Lifermann, T. Papo, M. Lambert, J. Le Noach, M. Khellaf, D. Merrien, X. Puechal,

S. Vinzio, P. Cohen, L. Mouthon, J. F. Cordier, and L. Guillevin, "Azathioprine or methotrexate maintenance for ANCA-associated vasculitis," *The New England journal of medicine,* vol. 359, pp. 2790-803, Dec 25 2008.

[44] A. C. Allison, "Mechanisms of action of mycophenolate mofetil," *Lupus,* vol. 14 Suppl 1, pp. s2-8, 2005.

[45] T. F. Hiemstra, M. Walsh, A. Mahr, C. O. Savage, K. de Groot, L. Harper, T. Hauser, I. Neumann, V. Tesar, K. M. Wissing, C. Pagnoux, W. Schmitt, and D. R. Jayne, "Mycophenolate mofetil vs azathioprine for remission maintenance in antineutrophil cytoplasmic antibody-associated vasculitis: a randomized controlled trial," *JAMA : the journal of the American Medical Association,* vol. 304, pp. 2381-8, Dec 1 2010.

[46] C. Metzler, N. Miehle, K. Manger, C. Iking-Konert, K. de Groot, B. Hellmich, W. L. Gross, and E. Reinhold-Keller, "Elevated relapse rate under oral methotrexate versus leflunomide for maintenance of remission in Wegener's granulomatosis," *Rheumatology,* vol. 46, pp. 1087-91, Jul 2007.

[47] C. Pierrot-Deseilligny Despujol, J. Pouchot, C. Pagnoux, J. Coste, and L. Guillevin, "Predictors at diagnosis of a first Wegener's granulomatosis relapse after obtaining complete remission," *Rheumatology,* vol. 49, pp. 2181-90, Nov 2010.

[48] S. L. Hogan, R. J. Falk, H. Chin, J. Cai, C. E. Jennette, J. C. Jennette, and P. H. Nachman, "Predictors of relapse and treatment resistance in antineutrophil cytoplasmic antibody-associated small-vessel vasculitis," *Annals of internal medicine,* vol. 143, pp. 621-31, Nov 1 2005.

[49] C. Pagnoux, S. L. Hogan, H. Chin, J. C. Jennette, R. J. Falk, L. Guillevin, and P. H. Nachman, "Predictors of treatment resistance and relapse in antineutrophil cytoplasmic antibody-associated small-vessel vasculitis: comparison of two independent cohorts," *Arthritis and Rheumatism,* vol. 58, pp. 2908-18, Sep 2008.

[50] J. H. Stone, J. T. Holbrook, M. A. Marriott, A. K. Tibbs, L. P. Sejismundo, Y. I. Min, U. Specks, P. A. Merkel, R. Spiera, J. C. Davis, E. W. St Clair, W. J. McCune, S. R. Ytterberg, N. B. Allen, and G. S. Hoffman, "Solid malignancies among patients in the Wegener's Granulomatosis Etanercept Trial," *Arthritis and Rheumatism,* vol. 54, pp. 1608-18, May 2006.

[51] A. Booth, L. Harper, T. Hammad, P. Bacon, M. Griffith, J. Levy, C. Savage, C. Pusey, and D. Jayne, "Prospective study of TNFalpha blockade with infliximab in anti-neutrophil cytoplasmic antibody-associated systemic vasculitis," *Journal of the American Society of Nephrology : JASN,* vol. 15, pp. 717-21, Mar 2004.

[52] M. D. Morgan, M. T. Drayson, C. O. Savage, and L. Harper, "Addition of infliximab to standard therapy for ANCA-associated vasculitis," *Nephron. Clinical practice,* vol. 117, pp. c89-97, 2011.

[53] S. Laurino, A. Chaudhry, A. Booth, G. Conte, and D. Jayne, "Prospective study of TNFalpha blockade with adalimumab in ANCA-associated systemic vasculitis with

renal involvement," *Nephrology, dialysis, transplantation : official publication of the European Dialysis and Transplant Association - European Renal Association,* vol. 25, pp. 3307-14, Oct 2010.

[54] R. M. Smith, R. B. Jones, M. J. Guerry, S. Laurino, F. Catapano, A. Chaudhry, K. G. Smith, and D. R. Jayne, "Rituximab for remission maintenance in relapsing ANCA-associated vasculitis," *Arthritis and Rheumatism,* Jun 21 2012.

[55] M. D. Kazatchkine and S. V. Kaveri, "Immunomodulation of autoimmune and inflammatory diseases with intravenous immune globulin," *The New England journal of medicine,* vol. 345, pp. 747-55, Sep 6 2001.

[56] D. R. Jayne, V. L. Esnault, and C. M. Lockwood, "ANCA anti-idiotype antibodies and the treatment of systemic vasculitis with intravenous immunoglobulin," *Journal of autoimmunity,* vol. 6, pp. 207-19, Apr 1993.

[57] F. Rossi, D. R. Jayne, C. M. Lockwood, and M. D. Kazatchkine, "Anti-idiotypes against anti-neutrophil cytoplasmic antigen autoantibodies in normal human polyspecific IgG for therapeutic use and in the remission sera of patients with systemic vasculitis," *Clinical and Experimental Immunology,* vol. 83, pp. 298-303, Feb 1991.

[58] D. R. Jayne, M. J. Davies, C. J. Fox, C. M. Black, and C. M. Lockwood, "Treatment of systemic vasculitis with pooled intravenous immunoglobulin," *Lancet,* vol. 337, pp. 1137-9, May 11 1991.

[59] P. Tuso, A. Moudgil, J. Hay, D. Goodman, E. Kamil, R. Koyyana, and S. C. Jordan, "Treatment of antineutrophil cytoplasmic autoantibody-positive systemic vasculitis and glomerulonephritis with pooled intravenous gammaglobulin," *American journal of kidney diseases : the official journal of the National Kidney Foundation,* vol. 20, pp. 504-8, Nov 1992.

[60] C. Richter, A. Schnabel, E. Csernok, K. De Groot, E. Reinhold-Keller, and W. L. Gross, "Treatment of anti-neutrophil cytoplasmic antibody (ANCA)-associated systemic vasculitis with high-dose intravenous immunoglobulin," *Clinical and Experimental Immunology,* vol. 101, pp. 2-7, Jul 1995.

[61] D. R. Jayne and C. M. Lockwood, "Pooled intravenous immunoglobulin in the management of systemic vasculitis," *Advances in experimental medicine and biology,* vol. 336, pp. 469-72, 1993.

[62] Y. Levy, Y. Sherer, J. George, P. Langevitz, A. Ahmed, Y. Bar-Dayan, F. Fabbrizzi, J. Terryberry, J. Peter, and Y. Shoenfeld, "Serologic and clinical response to treatment of systemic vasculitis and associated autoimmune disease with intravenous immunoglobulin," *International archives of allergy and immunology,* vol. 119, pp. 231-8, Jul 1999.

[63] T. Ito-Ihara, T. Ono, F. Nogaki, K. Suyama, M. Tanaka, S. Yonemoto, A. Fukatsu, T. Kita, K. Suzuki, and E. Muso, "Clinical efficacy of intravenous immunoglobulin for

patients with MPO-ANCA-associated rapidly progressive glomerulonephritis," *Nephron. Clinical practice,* vol. 102, pp. c35-42, 2006.

[64] A. Hot, L. Perard, B. Coppere, M. Simon, F. Bouhour, and J. Ninet, "Marked improvement of Churg-Strauss vasculitis with intravenous gamma globulins during pregnancy," *Clinical rheumatology,* vol. 26, pp. 2149-51, Dec 2007.

[65] D. R. Jayne, H. Chapel, D. Adu, S. Misbah, D. O'Donoghue, D. Scott, and C. M. Lockwood, "Intravenous immunoglobulin for ANCA-associated systemic vasculitis with persistent disease activity," *QJM : monthly journal of the Association of Physicians,* vol. 93, pp. 433-9, Jul 2000.

[66] V. Martinez, P. Cohen, C. Pagnoux, S. Vinzio, A. Mahr, L. Mouthon, L. Sailler, C. Delaunay, A. Sadoun, and L. Guillevin, "Intravenous immunoglobulins for relapses of systemic vasculitides associated with antineutrophil cytoplasmic autoantibodies: results of a multicenter, prospective, open-label study of twenty-two patients," *Arthritis and Rheumatism,* vol. 58, pp. 308-17, Jan 2008.

[67] K. Maeda, Y. Umeda, and T. Saino, "Synthesis and background chemistry of 15-deoxyspergualin," *Annals of the New York Academy of Sciences,* vol. 685, pp. 123-35, Jun 23 1993.

[68] R. Birck, K. Warnatz, H. M. Lorenz, M. Choi, M. Haubitz, M. Grunke, H. H. Peter, J. R. Kalden, U. Gobel, J. M. Drexler, O. Hotta, R. Nowack, and F. J. Van Der Woude, "15-Deoxyspergualin in patients with refractory ANCA-associated systemic vasculitis: a six-month open-label trial to evaluate safety and efficacy," *Journal of the American Society of Nephrology : JASN,* vol. 14, pp. 440-7, Feb 2003.

[69] O. Flossmann, B. Baslund, A. Bruchfeld, J. W. Tervaert, C. Hall, P. Heinzel, B. Hellmich, R. A. Luqmani, K. Nemoto, V. Tesar, and D. R. Jayne, "Deoxyspergualin in relapsing and refractory Wegener's granulomatosis," *Annals of the Rheumatic Diseases,* vol. 68, pp. 1125-30, Jul 2009.

[70] M. Walsh, A. Chaudhry, and D. Jayne, "Long-term follow-up of relapsing/refractory anti-neutrophil cytoplasm antibody associated vasculitis treated with the lymphocyte depleting antibody alemtuzumab (CAMPATH-1H)," *Annals of the Rheumatic Diseases,* vol. 67, pp. 1322-7, Sep 2008.

[71] W. H. Schmitt, E. C. Hagen, I. Neumann, R. Nowack, L. F. Flores-Suarez, and F. J. van der Woude, "Treatment of refractory Wegener's granulomatosis with antithymocyte globulin (ATG): an open study in 15 patients," *Kidney International,* vol. 65, pp. 1440-8, Apr 2004.

[72] R. A. DeRemee, "The treatment of Wegener's granulomatosis with trimethoprim/sulfamethoxazole: illusion or vision?," *Arthritis and Rheumatism,* vol. 31, pp. 1068-74, Aug 1988.

[73] E. Reinhold-Keller, K. De Groot, H. Rudert, B. Nolle, M. Heller, and W. L. Gross, "Response to trimethoprim/sulfamethoxazole in Wegener's granulomatosis depends on

the phase of disease," *QJM : monthly journal of the Association of Physicians,* vol. 89, pp. 15-23, Jan 1996.

[74] C. A. Stegeman, J. W. Tervaert, P. E. de Jong, and C. G. Kallenberg, "Trimethoprim-sulfamethoxazole (co-trimoxazole) for the prevention of relapses of Wegener's granulomatosis. Dutch Co-Trimoxazole Wegener Study Group," *The New England journal of medicine,* vol. 335, pp. 16-20, Jul 4 1996.

[75] P. Cohen, C. Pagnoux, A. Mahr, J. P. Arene, L. Mouthon, V. Le Guern, M. H. Andre, M. Gayraud, D. Jayne, D. Blockmans, J. F. Cordier, and L. Guillevin, "Churg-Strauss syndrome with poor-prognosis factors: A prospective multicenter trial comparing glucocorticoids and six or twelve cyclophosphamide pulses in forty-eight patients," *Arthritis and Rheumatism,* vol. 57, pp. 686-93, May 15 2007.

[76] C. Ribi, P. Cohen, C. Pagnoux, A. Mahr, J. P. Arene, D. Lauque, X. Puechal, P. Letellier, P. Delaval, J. F. Cordier, and L. Guillevin, "Treatment of Churg-Strauss syndrome without poor-prognosis factors: a multicenter, prospective, randomized, open-label study of seventy-two patients," *Arthritis and Rheumatism,* vol. 58, pp. 586-94, Feb 2008.

Chapter 9

Treatment of ANCA-Negative Small Vessel Vasculitis

Christina G. Katsiari, Theodora Simopoulou and
Lazaros I. Sakkas

Additional information is available at the end of the chapter

http://dx.doi.org/10.5772/54272

1. Introduction

Small vessels refer to arterioles, capillaries and venules. According to an international consensus conference, small vessel vasculitides include, ANCA-associated vasculitis (granulomatosis with polyangitis [Wegener's], Churg-Strauss syndrome, microscopic polyangiitis), cryoglobulinaemic vasculitis, Henoch-Scholein purpura, and cutaneous leukocytoclastic angiitis [1].

2. ANCA-associated vasculitis

2.1. Cryoglobulinaemic vasculitis

Cryoglobulinaemia refers to circulating cryoglobulins. Cryoglobulins are immunoglobulins, which precipitate in temperatures below 37°C and dissolve upon rewarming [2]. Cryoglobulinaemia is classified in 3 types based on clonality and immunoglobulin class. In particular, type I consists of monoclonal IgM or IgG immunoglobulin, type II is a mixture of monoclonal IgM and polyclonal IgG, while type III is a mixture of polyclonal IgM and IgG. Type II and III are also called "mixed", since both contain a mixture of IgM and IgG immunoglobulins [3]. The IgM component of type II cryoglobulins has rheumatoid factor activity (can bind to the Fc portion of IgG). All 3 types of cryoglobulinaemia may or may not result from an underlying disorder. In the absence of an identifiable cause cryoglobulinaemia is characterized as "essential".

Circulating cryoglobulins induce damage through 2 mechanisms: type I monoclonal IgM cryoglobulins, due to the large size of IgM and their high concentration levels – usually associated with Waldenström disease– result in hyperviscosity-induced vascular damage. On the other hand, type II and III mixed cryoglobulins in combination with complement components form immune complexes, which deposit in capillaries and small arterioles leading to vascular inflammation [3]. Patients with symptomatic mixed cryoglobulinaemic vasculitis typically display low serum levels of complement C4, reflecting complement consumption via the classical, immune complexed-mediated activation pathway. Palpable purpura represents a typical clinical manifestation. Skin biopsy reveals small vessel leukocytoclastic vasculitis namely inflammation and destruction of the vessel wall along with polymorphonuclear leukocyte nuclear debris. Involvement of internal organs, most commonly peripheral nerves, kidneys and joints will dictate prognosis and treatment decisions. Clinical and laboratory features of cryoglobulinaemia are summarized in Table1.

Treatment of mixed cryoglobulinaemic syndrome depends essentially on two parameters: First the type and severity of manifestations and second the underlying disease. It is apparent that the identification and treatment of the underlying cause is of paramount importance. Mixed cryoglobulinaemic syndrome is typically divided as hepatitis virus C (HCV) – related or not.

CRYOGLOBULINAEMIA					
TYPE I monoclonal IgM or IgG		TYPE II monoclonal IgM + polyclonal IgG		TYPE III polyclonal IgM + polyclonal IgG	
Essential	**Secondary**	**Essential**	**Secondary**	**Essential**	**Secondary**
	Waldenström Myeloma Lymphoma		HCV Myeloma Lymphoma Autoimmune diseases		Autoimmune diseases Chronic Inflammatory diseases
HYPER – VISCOSITY Raynaud's Digital ischemia Hyperviscosity syndrome		CRYOGLOBULINAEMIC VASCULITIS Purpura, Arthritis, Raynaud's, Renal disease, Neuropathy			
CLINICAL SYNDROME					

Table 1. Clinical and laboratory characteristics of cryoglobulinaemia.

2.2. Treatment of HCV related cryoglobulinaemic vasculitis

2.2.1. Aiming the virus: Treatment of chronic HCV

The majority of cases with cryoglobulinaemia are considered to be induced by HCV. Evidence of HCV infection is usually displayed by serum antibodies against the virus or presence of HCV-RNA. It should be noted however that false negative results do occur. If

http://dx.doi.org/10.5772/54272

suspicion of HCV infection is strong further examination of the cryoprecipitate, where both antibodies and RNA are concentrated, should be performed. Management of patients in this category should take place in collaboration with a hepatologist

The role of interferon alpha (INFα) in the treatment of cryoglobulinaemic vasculitis has been examined approximately 2 decades ago. In an early study, among 53 patients with HCV – related cryoglobulinaemic vasculitis, only patients who displayed a drop in the virus RNA levels showed clinical improvement. Reduction of RNA levels was restricted to patients who received INFα in addition to conventional treatment [4]. Moreover, viremia, cryoglobulinaemia and clinical symptoms returned following INFα cessation. Apart from INFα therapeutic potential, this as well as similar studies showed that clinical response parallels the levels of viremia.

Addition of the broad spectrum anti-viral agent rivabirin proved to add therapeutic benefit to INFα monotherapy [5, 6]. More recently, PEGylated INFα combined with ribavirin was shown to have superior efficacy compared to non-pegylated INFα / ribavirin combination [7-9]. PEGylation is a process where polyethylene molecules (PEG) are covalently attached to, in this case, INFα producing a molecule with prolonged pharmacokinetics. A recent update of recommendations by the American Association for the Study of Liver Diseases is shown in Table 2 [10].

INFα (SC per week)	**plus**	Ribavirin (orally per day)
180 µg PEG-INFα-2a	+	BW<75kg: 1000mg, BW"/>75kg: 1200mg
	or	
1 – 5 µg PEG-INFα-2b	+	BW<65kg: 800mg, BW=65-85kg: 1000mg, BW=85-105kg: 1200mg BW"/>105kg: 1400mg

SC: subcutaneous, PEG-INFα: PEGylated interferon alpha, BW: body weight

Table 2. Antiviral combination treatment in HCV-related cryoglobulinaemic vasculitis

There are no definite guidelines regarding duration of treatment. Treatment of HCV infection is recommended to last from 24 weeks (for virus genotypes 2 and 3) to 48 weeks (genotypes 1 and 4). The rational behind this recommendation lies on the observation that if viral response has not been achieved within this time frame, it is highly unlikely that prolongation of treatment will lead to substantial and sustained viral response [10]. However, in the case of cryoglobulinaemic vasculitis accompanying HCV infection, a less strict approach is endorsed, where besides viral levels, clinical and immunologic features are also taken into account [7, 11]. Prolongation of antiviral therapies may be appropriate in a subset of patients who display clinical benefit and no drug intolerance [3].

2.2.2. *Downregulation of cryoglobulins: Rituximab*

Although many patients achieve virological response using INFα and ribavirin, several considerations still exist: only 50% patients carrying genotype 1, which is the most common genotype in Europe and Americas, respond. Also, pegylated form of INFα as well as ribavirin are contraindicated in patients with compromised renal function, which may prove puzzling when treating patients with severe renal involvement.

Rituximab is an anti-CD20 chimeric monoclonal antibody, which results in prompt depletion of circulating and tissue B cells. Cryoglobulins are produced by B cells. Hence, B-cell depleting biological therapy using Rituximab, holds theoretical promise of down-regulating the production and circulating levels of cryoglobulins. Following few cohort studies with promising results [12-16], a prospective randomized controlled trial to examine the role of rituximab in the treatment of patients non-responding to antiviral therapy has only recently been presented [17]. Twenty-four non-responders were included and followed for 12 months. Twelve patients were managed according to conventional strategies (maintain or increase immunosuppression) and twelve received rituximab (as administered in vasculitis: 375mg/m2 every week for 4 weeks). Following 6 months, 10 patients (83%) receiving rituximab achieved remission compared to 1 patient (8%) in the control group. At this point it appears that rituximab could be used in patients who did not respond to conventional treatment. In addition there is no restriction regarding renal function. However, the risk of serious infection remains an important consideration. Of note, in patients with high concentrations of IgM-k cryoglobulins with rheumatoid factor activity, complex formation with rituximab can occur resulting in severe systemic reactions.

A significant proportion of patients treated with conventional therapy despite sustained virological response relapsed during long-term follow-up, posing a significant question regarding the role of HCV on the pathophysiology of the disease [18]. Off label experience with rituximab to date may provide relevant insight: in patients receiving rituximab, relapses did not parallel virus load but coincided with the recovery of peripheral B cells. It has been proposed that B cell proliferation and thus subsequent cryoglobulin production can become independent of HCV overtime [3].

2.2.3. *Vasculitis treatment: Plasmapheresis and conventional immunosuppression*

Severe, life-threatening disease. Plasmapheresis is reserved for patients with acute, serious, life-threatening disease such as progressive renal failure, severe neuropathy, intestinal ischemia, alveolar hemorrhage and digital necrosis [19]. Removing cryoglobulins from the circulation presumably hinders immune-complex mediated vasculopathy leading to prompt improvement. However, following termination of plasma exchange a rebound overproduction of cryoglobulins may occur. Therefore, concomitant treatment aiming to mute cryoglobulin production is required. High dose glucocorticoids in conjunction with cyclophosphamide (CyP) represent the standard therapeutic regimen. Following the paradigm of ANCA-associated vasculitis, azathioprine and mycophenolate mofetil (MMF) are often used for remission maintenance or in the place of CyP when the disease is less severe (doses are presented in Table 2) [20]. Duration and efficacy of such treatment modalities

http://dx.doi.org/10.5772/54272

have not been assessed in controlled clinical trials. Consequently, therapeutic decisions are usually taken on an individual basis according to clinical response, personal history, comorbidity as well as the centre's experience to treat such patients.

Antiviral treatment is usually avoided until acute flare has been controlled [21, 22]. Exacerbation of the underlying vasculitis due to INFα and restrictions regarding ribavirin administration in patients with impaired renal function remain the main considerations. The same may apply to rituximab where monotherapy rather than combination with antiviral therapy is recommended by some authorities during the treatment of a severe disease [23]. Following remission of severe inflammatory phenomena, antiviral treatment should be administered.

Mild-to-moderate disease. Manifestations, such as purpura, arthralgias/arthritis, mild proteinuria/hematuria with normal serum creatinine or peripheral sensory neuropathy represent mild-to-moderate disease activity. In cases of HCV-related disease, viral clearance with combination therapy as described above is the initial treatment of choice.

Low-dose corticosteroids (<7.5–10 mg/day) can be administered for more efficient control of symptoms (arthritis/arthralgias, persisting purpura, etc.). Sequential or simultaneous administration [16, 24] of corticosteroids with IFNα did not influence the sustained virological response in treated patients. Nevertheless, whenever possible it is prudent to avoid corticosteroids during the initial course of antiviral therapy. Quick tapering of corticosteroids is also advised since long-term administration does not seem to grant a favorable effect on vasculitis, while can harm the liver function.

The use of immunosuppression in cyoglobulinaemic vasculitis is summarized in Table 3.

Drug	Dosage	Comments
Prednisolone	60 mg/day for 1 month tapered to 15 mg/day at 3 months	IV methylprednisolone 500-1,000 mg/day for 3 successive days in critical organ manifestations
Cyclophosphamide (CyP)	for 3-6 pulses	Oral CyP (2 mg/Kg/day) can be used
Rituximab IV	375 mg/m2/week for 4 pulses	In intolerance to CyP and in young patients with severe disease
Azathioprin	2 mg /kg/ day	
Mycophenolate Mofetil	2 g/day	In patients with moderate renal involvement who cannot take CyP
Plasmapheresis	three times weekly for two to three weeks	In critical organ manifestations

Table 3. Immunosuppressive treatment for cryoglobulinaemic vasculitis

2.3. Treatment of non-HCV mixed cryoglobulaenimic syndrome

According to current EULAR recommendations, patients presenting with mixed cryoglobulinaemic syndrome non-related to HCV or other disorder should be treated as patients with ANCA – associated vasculitis [8].

Although rare, cases associated to hepatitis B virus (HBV) have been documented. Antiviral therapy with lamivudine or entecavir has led to remission in isolated case reports. Myeloproliferative diseases and most commonly B cell lymphoma may also be the cause of mixed cryoglobulinaemia. Prompt diagnosis and appropriate treatments should be applied. Among autoimmune diseases, Sjogren's syndrome and systemic lupus erythematosus most commonly are associated with cryoglobulinaemia.

2.4. Special considerations

Patients with end Stage Renal Disease. Patients are treated with hemodialysis or peritoneal dialysis. Survival is comparable with with that of end stage renal diseases. Kidney transplantation can be performed. High rate of relapse has been recorded (up to 70%). However, recurrent disease does not lead to graft loss and thus relapse risk does not forbid transplantation in patients with end stage renal disease. Another concern in cases of HCV-related disease is that robust immunosuppression following transplantation may exacerbate HCV infection. Fortunately, this has proven to be the exception rather than the rule [25].

Cancer Risk. B-cell lymphoma has been reported in up to 25% of patients with mixed cryoglobulinaemic syndrome. Patients are usually diagnosed within 10 years. Low levels of gamma globulins may predate neoplastic transformation. Standard chemotherapy in combination with rituximab is usually required. HCV infection increases the B-cell lymphoma risk by 20-30% and is associated with increased frequency of liver cancer, which is diagnosed in up to 10% of patients [26].

2.5. Prognosis

Prognosis mainly depends on whether vital organ(s) are involved.

Most studies have examined glomerulonephritis (GN) where 10-year survival rate was reported to be 30-50%. However, therapeutic progress substantially improved prognosis since 10-year survival has recently been raised to almost 80%. Male gender, HCV infection, high cryocrit, low C3 and raised serum creatinine at baseline are considered bad prognostic factors. Intestinal ischaemia and alveolar haemorrhage have high mortality rates (>80%). In patients with HCV infection, carriers of genotype 2 and 3 along with early virological response have the best outcome. Of interest, changes of cryocrit level do not seem to correlate with clinical activity. It would be interesting, however, to examine whether the degree of solubility at 37°C or a decline in the temperature at which the cryoproteins precipitate might better correlate with response to treatment [27].

http://dx.doi.org/10.5772/54272

3. Henoch-Schonlein Purpura

Henoch-Schönlein purpura (HSP) is the most common vasculitis syndrome of childhood, although is also well described in adults. Clinical features include palpable non-thrombocytopenic purpura, particularly over the buttocks and lower extremities, arthritis (or arthralgia) affecting primarily large joints, diffuse abdominal pain and renal involvement with microscopic or gross haematuria, and/or proteinuria. There are also reports on the involvement of other organs, including lungs, brain and testes. Generally, it is a benign disorder that follows an intercurrent illness, usually an upper respiratory tract infection.

HSP is an immune complex-mediated small vessel vasculitis. Serologic studies document elevated levels of IgA and activation of the alternate pathway of the complement system. The characteristic histopathologic finding of HSP is leukocytoclastic vasculitis with IgA deposits with affected vessels.

Although prognosis is excellent in children with HSP, a small minority of patients develop long-term complications, and primarily renal disease. In adults, the risk of significant renal disease is increased. Management of HSP includes supportive care to ameliorate acute symptoms, as well as targeted treatment to decrease the risk of complications (usually due to gastrointestinal complications) and to prevent chronic renal insufficiency. Targeted treatment is summarized in Table 4.

3.1. Supportive management

Treatment of HSP is primarily supportive and includes adequate hydration and symptomatic relief of pain. Edema of the lower extremities and buttocks is improved with bed rest and/or elevating the affected area. Acetaminophen and non-steroidal anti-inflammatory drugs (NSAIDs) help with mild rash and arthritis. However, NSAIDs should be used cautiously in elderly persons due to increased risk of renal impairment and gastrointestinal bleeding.

3.2. Targeted treatment

3.2.1. Glucocorticosteroids

Oral steroids. Oral steroids are used in patients with painful cutaneous edema, severe rash, scrotal and testicular involvement, renal involvement and abdominal pain [28]. There is some supportive evidence for the use of corticosteroids in severe abdominal pain. In a systemic review that included three randomized trials and 12 retrospective studies, prednisolone at a dose of 1 mg/Kg/day for two weeks or 2 mg/Kg/day for one week may decrease the intensity and duration of abdominal pain and may decrease the frequency of bowel intussusceptions and thus surgical interventions [29-31] .

Renal involvement is a common finding in HSP. Although the prognosis of HSP is excellent in children, persistent renal disease can cause long-term morbidity. This risk of significant renal disease is greater in adults with HSP [32]

However, it is not clear if corticosteroids decrease the likelihood of renal disease [29;30;32-39]. A meta-analysis suggested that early use of corticosteroids reduced the odds of developing persistent renal disease [29]. However, concerns are raised over the validity of this analysis, which included studies with different treatment protocols and follow-up time [36]. A more recent meta-analysis of four randomized controlled trials showed no significant difference in the risk of persistent renal disease at 6 and 12 months in children treated with prednisone for 2-4 weeks after initial presentation compared with placebo or supportive treatment [34]. Thus there are no convincing data to support the routine use of oral steroids as a measure to prevent renal disease in patients with uncomplicated HSP.

High dose steroids. Steroid treatment with high intravenous doses (pulses) and/or long term oral administration are the treatment of choice in acute HSP glomerulonephritis in children [32]. Methylprednisolone pulse therapy was evaluated in a prospective study with 38 children with severe HSP nephritis, defined as nephrotic syndrome at presentation and/or 50% or more crescentic glomeruli on biopsy [37]. Clinical recovery was achieved in 20 children. Renal biopsy in these children showed a significant decrease of the activity index with a decrease or disappearance of IgA deposits.

Steroids can be used alone or in combination with immunosuppressive agents (i.e., cyclosporin A, cyclophosphamide, mycophenolate mofetil, and azathioprine) [32].

3.2.2. Cyclophosphamide

Cyclophosphamide (CyP) is widely used in the treatment for the majority of vasculitides. In HSP, CyP has been used mainly for rapidly progressive glomerulonephritis (GN), while case reports of successful management of pulmonary hemorrhage also exist [33].

In a randomized controlled trial, 56 children with severe HSP nephritis were treated with oral cyclophosphamide (90mg/m^2/day) without steroids for 42 days. At final follow-up, 48.2% of children had full recovery, 39.3% had persistent abnormalities and 12.5% ended up with end-stage renal failure or death. No patient with crescents in 50% or more of glomeruli went on to full recovery. The authors concluded that CyP had no significant efficacy [39].

The combination of CyP with steroids has provided better outcome. In a retrospective study, high dose corticosteroids plus oral CyP (2mg/kg/day for 12 weeks) significantly reduced proteinuria in children with HSP GN [35]. Oral prednisolone (1.5 mg/kg/day) combined with an 8-week course of CyP (2 mg/kg/day) in 9 children with severe HSP nephritis, resulted in remission of proteinuria in 7 children [38]. Triple therapy with oral CyP (2.5mg/kg/day), methylprednizolone (30 mg/kg/day [maximum 1g/day], for 3 days), and intravenous urokinase (5000 U/kg/day [max 180.000], for 7 days) reduced protein excretion and mesangial IgA deposition compared with the group that received the same therapeutic combination without CyP [40]. In another study, combined therapy with intravenous pulse methylprednisolone (for 3 days), oral CyP (for 2 months), oral dipyridamole (for 6 months) and oral prednisolone (for 3 months) resulted in normalization of glomerular filtration rate in all but 1 patient [41]. Combined therapy with prednisolone, CyP, heparin/warfarin, and dipyridamole, in 14 children with severe HSP nephritis, followed for 7.5 years, resulted in a significant improvement of histological grade of nephritis [42].

In adults, adding CyP to steroids provided no benefit in a 12-month, open-label trial of 54 patients with severe HSP GN [43].

3.2.3. *Cyclosporin A*

Cyclosporin A (CsA) is an effective immunosuppressive agent used for different immune-mediated glomerular diseases [32].

In a randomized study of of 24 children with nephrotic-range proteinuria or crescenting HSP nephritis, CsA was more efficacious compared to IV pulses of methylprednisolone [44]. In two retrospective studies by the same group, CsA plus steroids was found to be beneficial in HSP children with nephrotic syndrome [45,46]. In a retrospective study of 29 children with nephrotic-range proteinuria treated with CsA plus steroids, 23 achieved stable remission, while 6 patients became CsA-dependent [47]. In a clinical trial with a mean follow-up of 6 years all patients responded to CsA therapy (plus ACE inhibitors), however some patients developed CsA- dependent nephritis [48].

CsA plus steroids, either as initial treatment or after other immunosuppressive drugs in a small case series of 5 adult patients with HSP with nephrotic-range proteinuria showed beneficial effects on proteinuria and preservation of renal function, after a follow-up period of 5 years [49].

Overall, despite the data reporting proteinuria reduction by CsA in patients with HSP nephritis, this treatment is not supported by RCTs and cautiousness should be exercised for potential nephrotoxicity of CsA.

3.2.4. *Azathioprine*

Azathioprine is used in combination with steroids mostly in children with crescent HSP nephritis [32].

Azathioprine plus steroids showed beneficial effects in a clinical trial of 21 children with severe HSP GN. Treatment with either oral or intravenous (IV) corticosteroids led to comparable outcome [50]. Retrospective studies also support the use of combination of azathioprine with steroids for the treatment of severe HSP nephritis in children [51]. Early treatment with azathioprine plus steroids prevented progression of chronic kidney disease [52]. The combination was effective in improving histopathological changes [53]; however, 2 of the 10 patients treated with azathioprine showed definite tubulointerstitial nephritis at followup biopsy [54].

3.2.5. *Mycophenolate mofetil*

Mycophenolate mofetil (MMF) appears to be a promising therapeutic agent in many autoimmune diseases such as lupus nephritis, vasculitis and in IgA nephropathy.

There is limited evidence to support the use of MMF in HSP. Case reports [55-57] suggest a beneficial effect of MMF on HSP with complications. In six children in whom steroid therapy has failed, MMF was able to control complications and to sustain disease remission. MMF was well tolerated [58]. More recently, MMF along with ACE inhibitors reduced protein excretion and improved renal function in 12 children with HSP and nephrotic range proteinuria, who failed steroid treatment (20-25mg/kg/day) [59].

3.2.6. Rituximab

The efficacy of rituximab (RTX) in chronic HSP has been suggested by a case report. Three pediatric patients were treated with RTX for severe refractory chronic Henoch-Schönlein purpura, characterized mainly by neurologic and gastroenterological symptoms resistant to steroids and CyP. All 3 patients responded to 1 or 2 courses of RTX without serious adverse events [60]. In another case report one patient with moderate nephritis and severe skin HSP responded to RTX [61].

3.2.7. Plasma exchange

The addition of plasma exchange to common immunosuppressives and steroids have shown efficacy in patients with HSP and severe of extra-renal manifestations (alveolar and cerebral hemorrhage, haemorrhagic pancolitis, extensive vasculitic leg ulcers) [62-64]. Plasma exchange has also been used as sole treatment in patients with severe HSP nephritis with encouraging results [65,66].

3.2.8. Intravenous immunoglobulin

The clinical use of intravenous immunoglobulin (IVIg) has been extended beyond antibody-deficiency syndromes, to a wide variety of clinical conditions, such as neuroimmunological diseases, and systemic autoimmune diseases. Kawasaki disease was the first primary vasculitis in which IVIg had become the standard treatment of care. IVIg has also shown beneficial effects in patients with ANCA-associated vasculitis (AAV) refractory to standard therapy with prednisone and CyP [67]. In HSP, IVIg inhibited disease progression in isolated case reports [68,69].

3.3. Additional treatments

From a pathophysiological point of view, the removal of any source of chronic bacterial challenge, which may trigger HSP episodes, should theoretically be beneficial [70]. This is the reason why there are reports about tonsillectomy and periodontal therapy in children with HSP [71-73]. However, the therapeutic contribution of such approaches are difficult to evaluate since are commonly used in combination with other therapies.

Antithrombotic prophylaxis with warfarin, dipyridamole, and acetylsalicylic acid has been used along with immunosuppressive agents by several authors [70]. ACE inhibitors have been shown to be efficacious in reducing proteinuria and should be added at any level of proteinuria.

3.4. Emergencies

Patients with HSP may present with severe abdominal pain, gastrointestinal (GI) bleeding and renal insufficiency. Up to 50% of patients with HSP and GI manifestations have occult bleeding, but major hemorrhage occurs in only 5% and intussusceptions in 2% [74]. Other manifestations may include bowel infract, perforation and pancreatitis, which may require urgent surgical consultation.

Medication	Indication	Comments
Acetaminophen, NSAIDs	Arthritis, rash (mild)	Precautions: renal insufficiency and GI bleeding (for NSAIDs)
Oral steroids	painful cutaneous edema, severe rash, scrotal and testicular involvement, renal involvement and abdominal symptoms	Steroids may shorten the duration of abdominal pain and the risk of surgical interventions In few RCTs, short-course of oral prednisone does not prevent persistent renal disease
IV pulse steroids	Nephrotic range proteinuria, nephritic syndrome	
IV pulse steroids plus Immunosuppression	Rapidly progressive glomerulonephritis, pulmonary hemorrhage	CyP : no supporting RCT; serious side effects Azathioprine: no RCTs, cases of tubulointerstitial nephritis CsA: no RCTs, potential nephrotoxicity MMF: limited data Rituximab: limited data
Plasma exchange	Refractory HSP nephritis pulmonary and gastrointestinal hemorrhage, cerebral hemorrhage	
ACE inhibitors	Proteinuria	

Table 4. Medications used in the treatment of HSP

4. Idiopatic cutaneous vasculitis

Cutaneous vasculitis is a vasculitis confined to the dermis and is not a single disease. In fact, only less than 30% of cutaneous vasculitis can be defined as idiopathic. All other cases are systemic vasculitides, vasculitis associated with other rheumatic diseases (systemic lupus erythematosus, rheumatoid arthritis), or vasculitis induced by malignancy, infection or medication/toxin. Therefore, one should search carefully for extracutaneous manifestations of vasculitis and obtain a detailed medical history. Also mimics of vasculitis, such as antiphospolipid syndrome, should be ruled out. Even idiopathic cutaneous vasculitis is not a single entity. An international consensus conference defined cutaneous leukocytoclastic angiitis as isolated cutaneous leukocytoclastic angiitis without systemic vasculitis or glomerulonephritis [1]. This definition is controversial, since it requires biopsy for diagnosis and even biopsy is not diagnostic. Other terms used under the umbrella of idiopathic cutaneous vasculitis include hypersensitivity vasculitis, and urticarial vasculitis [75]. There are few points to consider in diagnosing cutaneous leukocytoclastic angiitis (CLA). First, CLA manifests with palpable purpura. On biopsy, cutaneous leukocytoclastic angiitis is characterized by leukocytoclastic vasculitis in upper to middle dermis (where small vessles are located), whereas necrotizing vasculitis in lower dermis and subcutaneous fat involves medium-sized vessels associated with cutaneous polyarteritis nodosa and other systemic vasculitides. Serum ANCA tests by immunofluorescence, with ELISA for MPO and PR3 to exclude ANCA-associated vasculitis, serum cryoglobulin test, to exclude cryoglobulinaemic vasculitis, and immunofluorescence for IgA deposits on skin biopsy, to exclude Henoch-Schonlein purpura, are necessary laboratory tests in diagnosing cutaneous leukocytoclastic angiitis.

Treatment of idiopathic cutaneous vasculitis depends on the severity of lesions and the extent of cutaneous involvement. For example, purpura is a manifestation of superficial dermal small vessel vasculitis with no serious consequences. Therefore any treatment should be with few if any side effects. However, it should be reminded that what initially appears to be isolated cutaneous vasculitis may be the presenting feature of an underlying disease, such as lymphoma or systemic vasculitis. Therefore, vigilance is required. Nodulal lesions and ulcers are caused by medium-sized vessels and suggest cutaneous polyarteritis nodosa or other systemic vasculitides Therefore, more intense treatment is required. It should be mentioned that there are no randomized controlled trials and treatment of idiopathic cutaneous vasculitis is based on case reports or small case series.

When cutaneous vasculitis is associated with a systemic disease one should treat the systemic disease. Also, any inciting agent, either drug or infective agent, should be removed. For instance, any infectious trigger should be treated with antibiotics. If food allergen is suspected, allergy testing is recommended, and if positive, elimination of the relevant food is tried, since low-antigen diet prevents recurrences of palpable purpura [76]. Drugs that are used with variable efficacy in idiopathic cutaneous vasculitis include non-steroidal anti-inflammatory drugs (NSAIDs), antihistamines (such as doxepin, loratadine, and cetirizine), colchicine, hydroxychloroquine (HCQ), dapsone, and prednisolone. However, no drug is universally efficacious. Colchicine inhibits neutrophil chemotaxis. Dapsone inhibits the alternative pathway of complement, and suppresses neutrophil chemotaxis. Hydroxychloroquine inhibits lysosomal enzyme release. The idiopathic leukocytoclastic cutaneous small vessel vasculitis is often self-limited and does not require specific treatment. Leg elevation, avoidance of excessive standing, and administration of

NSAIDs or antihistamines usually relieve symptoms, such as pruritus and burning sensation. For persistent disease, colchicine is considered a drug of first choice [77]. Colchicine is effective in 50% of patients with cutaneous leukocytoclastic vasculitis within 2 weeks, although in a randomized controlled trial colchicine (0.5 mg twice daily) for a month was no more efficacious than topical emollients [78]. Patients with chronic cutaneous venulitis are usually resistant to treatment. Dapsone (100-200 mg daily) may be very effective in leukocytoclastic vasculitis and urticarial vasculitis. Dapsone appears to have synergistic effects with colchicine or pentoxifylline [79]. HCQ is more often used in urticarial vasculitis associated with connective tissue diseases. Prednisolone, at the initial dose of 0.5-1 mg/Kg/day for 2 weeks with rapid tapering, can be very effective in acute severe episodes. However, Idiopathic Cutaneous Small Vessel Vasculitis can be active for 10 years and prednisolone monotherapy is not recommended for chronic use. In difficult to treat cases, azathioprine may be used with low-dose prednisolone. Other medications that have been used include CsA (2.5-5 mg/kg/day, in two doses).

4.1. Urticarial vasculitis

Urticarial vasculitis(UV) is characterized by persistent (greater than 24 hours) urticarial skin lesions and leukocytoclastic vasculitis on histology. It is associated with low serum complement (hypocomplementaemic urticarial vasculitis, HUV) or normal serum complement levels (normocomplementaemic urticarial vasculitis, NUV). HUV is usually a systemic disease and associated with systemic lupus erythematosus (SLE) with autoantibodies against C1q. NUV is usually confined to the skin and rarely associated with SLE. Nearly 50% of patients with idiopathic UV have autoantibodies against IgE or IgE receptor.

Treatment of UV is based on manifestations. For mild skin lesions antihistamines, colchicines, dapsone, HCQ and prednisolone are used. The addition of reserpine (0.3-0.4 mg/day) to antihistamines may improve UV symptoms [80]. For extracutaneous disease or chronic necrotizing skin lesions prednisolone is used, often in association with azathioprine, mycophenolate mofetil (MMF), CsA, or CyP. IVIg and plasmapheresis have been used in difficult to treat urticarial vasculitis [76]. Rituximab, a monoclonal antibody against CD20, present on mature B cells, was successfully tried in a patient with UV with angioedema unresponsive to prednisolone, CsA and plasmapheresis [8].

4.2. Cutaneous polyarteritis nodosa

In mild cases, colchicine or NSAIDs may suffice. In moderate to severe cases, prednisolone is administered at an initial dose of 1 mg/kg/day, usually in conjunction with HCQ, dapsone, methotrexate, azathioprine, CyP, or intravenous immunoglobulin [81]. Mizoribine, an inhibitor of inosine monophosphate and guanosine monophosphate synthetase, which inhibits T and B cell proliferation, is also efficacious. Warfarin or clopidogrel are helpful adjuvant treatment [82].

5. Precautions

Certain precautions should be observed to reduce side effects of drugs used. CyP dose should be adjusted for renal function and age.

Patients should be checked for tuberculosis with chest x-rays and PPD skin test, and patients with latent tuberculosis should receive prophylaxis with isoniazid plus vitamin B6. Patients on IV pulse CyP, receive antiemetic drug (ondaserton) immediately prior to and 8 hours after the CyP pulse. On the day of IV CyP pulse, patients receive oral or IV hydration with 2-3 liters of fluid. They also receive IV 2-mercaptoethanesulfonate (mesna) (20% of CyP dose) immediately before and at 2, 4 and 8 hours after the CyP pulse to reduce irritation of urinary bladder. The dose of next IV CyP pulse is adjusted to keep nadir white blood cell (WBC) count (12-14 days after the IV pulse) >3,000/μL. The rate of leucopenia, infections, and gonadal toxicity is reduced in the IV pulse CyP compared to oral CyP regimen [83,84]. Oral mesna is also beneficial for patients on oral CyP.

According to a recent study ever-tobacco smoking and previous episode of hemorrhagic cystitis were strong predictors for the development of cancer in the urinary tract. Thus patients with these characteristics need close surveillance with urine cytology tests.

All patients receiving CyP are advised to take prophylaxis against Pneumocystis jiroveci with trimethoprime/sulphamethoxazole (800/160 mg thrice weekly).

Gonadal failure is a common side effect in patients treated with CyP, where the risk increases in parallel with the increase of the cumulative dose received. No standard care to preserve gonadal function has been proposed for patients with small vessel vasculitis under CyP. For similar issues encountered in female patients with systemic lupus erythematosus (SLE) two protocols exist: administration of leuprolide acetate with or without transdermal estrogen and depo-progesterone for contraception. Leuprolide should be administered 10-14 days prior to each CyP infusion. In men with SLE, administration of intramuscular monthly injections of testosterone has been proposed. Analogous approaches should probably be adopted for young patients with small vessel vasculitis at risk.

Patients on immunosuppression should not be vaccinated with live attenuated vaccines. They can and should be vaccinated with dead pathogens. Patients with granulomatosis with polyangiitis(Wegener's granulomatosis) exhibit adequate antibody [85] and cell-mediated immune response to influenza vaccines [86].

INFα may cause hepatic dysfunction and extreme caution is advised in patients with cirrhosis. PEG-INFα and ribavirin are contraindicated in renal impairment (creatinine clearance [ClCr] <50ml). Ribavirin can cause haemolytic anaemia.

Colchicine can induce gastrointestinal upset (diarrhoea, vomiting) and rarely cytopenia. Dapsone can cause granulopenia and severe haemolysis in patients with glucose-6-phosphate dehydrogenase (G6PD) deficiency. Therefore, before initiation of dapsone, G6PD should be measured, and then full blood count regularly. Side effects of HCQ are rare and include retinopathy and cytopenias.

http://dx.doi.org/10.5772/54272

6. Conclusion

Small vessel vasculitis may be a manifestation of systemic vasculitis or may be confined to the skin. Therefore, biopsy of skin lesion with immunofluorescence and careful search for systemic disease are mandatory for the correct diagnosis. The treatment of cryoglobulinaemic vasculitis is based on the underlining aetiology. In HCV positive patients with severe vasculitic manifestations, immunosuppressives with plasmapheresis is the modality of choice. Anti-HCV treatment is administered after the control of inflammatory manifestations. In HCV-associated cryoglobulinaemic vasculitis with mild disease, anti-HCV treatment may suffice. HSP is usually a self limited disease. In patients with HSP complications, corticosteroids remain the main treatment. In severe refractory cases, plasmapheresis in conjunction with immunosuppressives have been tried. Idiopathic cutaneous leukocytoclastic vasculitis is most of the time a mild disease and does not require toxic medications. Rituximab is a promising new treatment for systemic or refractory small vessel vasculitis.

Author details

Christina G. Katsiari[1], Theodora Simopoulou[1] and Lazaros I. Sakkas[1,2*]

*Address all correspondence to: lsakkas@med.uth.gr

1 Rheumatology Clinic, School of Medicine, Faculty of Health Sciences, University of Thessaly, Larissa, Greece

2 Center of Molecular Medicine,Old Dominion University, Norfolk, VA, USA

References

[1] Jennette JC, Falk RJ, Andrassy K, Bacon PA, Churg J, Gross WL, Hagen EC, Hoffman GS, Hunder GG, Kallenberg CG. Nomenclature of systemic vasculitides. Proposal of an international consensus conference. Arthritis and Rheumatism 1994; 37: 187-192

[2] Tedeschi A, Barate C, Minola E, Morra E. Cryoglobulinemia. Blood Review 2007; 21: 183-200.

[3] Ramos-Casals M, Stone JH, Cid MC, Bosch X. The cryoglobulinaemias. Lancet 2012; 379: 348-360.

[4] Misiani R, Bellavita P, Fenili D, Vicari O, Marchesi D, Sironi PL, Zilio P, Vernocchi A, Massazza M, Vendramin G. Interferon alfa-2a therapy in cryoglobulinemia associated with hepatitis C virus. The New England Journal of Medicine 1994; 330: 751-756.

[5] Alric L, Plaisier E, Thebault S, Peron JM, Rostaing L, Pourrat J, Ronco P, Piette JC, Cacoub P. Influence of antiviral therapy in hepatitis C virus-associated cryoglobulinemic MPGN. American Journal of Kidney Diseases 2004; 43: 617-623.

[6] Zuckerman E, Keren D, Slobodin G, Rosner I, Rozenbaum M, Toubi E, Sabo E, Tsykounov I, Naschitz JE, Yeshurun D. Treatment of refractory, symptomatic, hepatitis C virus related mixed cryoglobulinemia with ribavirin and interferon-alpha. The Journal of Rheumatology 2000; 27: 2172-2178.

[7] Saadoun D, Resche-Rigon M, Thibault V, Piette JC, Cacoub P. Antiviral therapy for hepatitis C virus--associated mixed cryoglobulinemia vasculitis: a long-term follow-up study. Arthritis and Rheumatism 2006; 54: 3696-3706.

[8] Mukhtyar C, Guillevin L, Cid MC, Dasgupta B, De Groot K, Gross W, Hauser T, Hellmich B, Jayne D, Kallenberg CG. EULAR recommendations for the management of primary small and medium vessel vasculitis. Annals of the Rheumatic Diseases 2009; 68: 310-317.

[9] Cacoub P, Saadoun D, Limal N, Sene D, Lidove O, Piette JC. PEGylated interferon alfa-2b and ribavirin treatment in patients with hepatitis C virus-related systemic vasculitis. Arthritis and Rheumatism 2005; 52: 911-915.

[10] Ghany MG, Strader DB, Thomas DL, Seeff LB. Diagnosis, management, and treatment of hepatitis C: An update. Hepatology 2009; 49: 1335-1374.

[11] Joshi S, Kuczynski M, Heathcote EJ. Symptomatic and virological response to antiviral therapy in hepatitis C associated with extrahepatic complications of cryoglobulimia. Digestive Diseases and Sciences 2007; 52: 2410-2417.

[12] Zaja F, De Vita S, Mazzaro C, Sacco S, Damiani D, De Marchi G, Michelutti A, Baccarani M, Fanin R, Ferraccioli G. Efficacy and safety of rituximab in type II mixed cryoglobulinemia. Blood 2003; 101: 3827-3834.

[13] Sansonno D, De Re V, Lauletta G, Tucci FA, Boiocchi M, Dammacco F. Monoclonal antibody treatment of mixed cryoglobulinemia resistant to interferon alpha with an anti-CD20. Blood 2003; 101: 3818-3826.

[14] Saadoun D, Resche RM, Sene D, Terrier B, Karras A, Perard L, Schoindre Y, Coppere B, Blanc F, Musset L. Rituximab plus Peg-interferon-alpha/ribavirin compared with Peg-interferon-alpha/ribavirin in hepatitis C-related mixed cryoglobulinemia. Blood 2010; 116: 326-334.

[15] Quartuccio L, Soardo G, Romano G, Zaja F, Scott CA, De Marchi G, Fabris M, Ferraccioli G, De Vita S. Rituximab treatment for glomerulonephritis in HCV-associated mixed cryoglobulinaemia: efficacy and safety in the absence of steroids. Rheumatology (Oxford) 2006; 45: 842-846.

[16] Dammacco F, Tucci FA, Lauletta G, Gatti P, De Re V, Conteduca V, Sansonno S, Russi S, Mariggio MA, Chironna M. Pegylated interferon-alpha, ribavirin, and rituximab

combined therapy of hepatitis C virus-related mixed cryoglobulinemia: a long-term study. Blood 2010; 116: 343-353.

[17] Sneller MC, Hu Z, Langford CA. A randomized controlled trial of rituximab following failure of antiviral therapy for hepatitis C-associated cryoglobulinemic vasculitis. Arthritis and Rheumatism 2012; 64: 835-842.

[18] Landau DA, Saadoun D, Halfon P, Martinot-Peignoux M, Marcellin P, Fois E, Cacoub P. Relapse of hepatitis C virus-associated mixed cryoglobulinemia vasculitis in patients with sustained viral response. Arthritis and Rheumatism 2008; 58: 604-611.

[19] Guillevin L, Pagnoux C. Indications of plasma exchanges for systemic vasculitides. Therapeutic apheresis and dialysis: official peer-reviewed journal of the International Society for Apheresis, the Japanese Society for Apheresis, the Japanese Society for Dialysis Therapy 2003; 7: 155-160.

[20] Ramos-Casals M, Font J. Mycophenolate mofetil in patients with hepatitis C virus infection. Lupus 2005; 14: s64-s72.

[21] Lamprecht P, Gause A, Gross WL. Cryoglobulinemic vasculitis. Arthritis and Rheumatism 1999; 42: 2507-2516.

[22] Vassilopoulos D, Calabrese LH. Hepatitis C virus infection and vasculitis: implications of antiviral and immunosuppressive therapies. Arthritis and Rheumatism 2002; 46: 585-597.

[23] De Vita S, Quartuccio L. Rituximab monotherapy, rather than rituximab plus antiviral drugs, for initial treatment of severe hepatitis C virus-associated mixed cryoglobulinemia syndrome: comment on the article by Terrier et al. Arthritis and Rheumatism 2009; 60: 2531-2540.

[24] Guilera M, Forns X, Torras X, Enriquez J, Coll S, Solá R, Morillas R, Planas R, Ampurdanes S, Soler M. Pre-treatment with prednisolone does not improve the efficacy of subsequent alpha interferon therapy in chronic hepatitis C. Journal of Hepatology 2000; 33: 135-141.

[25] Tarantino A, Moroni G, Banfi G, Manzoni C, Segagni S, Ponticelli C. Renal replacement therapy in cryoglobulinaemic nephritis. Nephrology, dialysis, transplantation: official publication of the European Dialysis and Transplant Association-European Renal Association 1994; 9: 1426-1430.

[26] Saadoun D, Landau DA, Calabrese LH, Cacoub PP. Hepatitis C-associated mixed cryoglobulinaemia: a crossroad between autoimmunity and lymphoproliferation. Rheumatology (Oxford, England) 2007; 46: 1234-1242.

[27] Valbonesi M, Florio G, Montani F, Mosconi L. A method for the study of cryoglobulin solubilization curves at 37 degrees C. Preliminary studies and application to plasma exchange in cryoglobulinemic syndromes. The International Journal of Artificial Organs 1983; 6: 87-90.

[28] Sohagia AB, Gunturu SG, Tong TR, Hertan HI. Henoch-Schonlein Purpura-a case report and review of the literature. Gastroenterology Research and Practice 2010; 2010 DOI: 10.1155/2010/597648.

[29] Weiss PF, Feinstein JA, Luan X, Burnham JM, Feudtner C. Effects of corticosteroid on Henoch-Schonlein purpura: a systematic review. Pediatrics 2007; 120: 1079.

[30] Ronkainen J, Koskimies O, Ala-Houhala M, Antikainen M, Merenmies J, Rajantie J, Ormala T, Turtinen J, Nuutinen M. Early prednisone therapy in Henoch-Schonlein purpura: a randomized, double-blind, placebo-controlled trial. The Journal of Pediatrics 2006; 149: 241-7.

[31] Huber AM, King J, McLaine P, Klassen T, Pothos M. A randomized, placebo-controlled trial of prednisone in early Henoch Schonlein Purpura. BMC Medicine 2004; 2: 7.

[32] Zaffanello M, Brugnara M, Franchini M. Therapy for children with henoch-schonlein purpura nephritis: a systematic review. The Scientific World Journal 2007; 7: 20.

[33] Besbas N, Duzova A, Topaloglu R, Gok F, Ozaltin F, Ozen S, Bakkaloglu A. Pulmonary haemorrhage in a 6-year-old boy with Henoch-Schonlein purpura. Clinical Rheumatology 2001; 20: 293-6.

[34] Chartapisak W, Opastiraku S, Willis NS, Craig JC, Hodson EM. Prevention and treatment of renal disease in Henoch-Schonlein purpura: a systematic review. Archives of Disease in Childhood 2009; 94: 132-7.

[35] Flynn JT, Smoyer WE, Bunchman TE, Kershaw DB, Sedman AB. Treatment of Henoch-Schonlein Purpura glomerulonephritis in children with high-dose corticosteroids plus oral cyclophosphamide. American Journal of Nephrology 2001; 21: 128-133.

[36] Gibson KL, Amamoo MA, Primack WA. Corticosteroid therapy for Henoch Schonlein purpura. Pediatrics 2008; 121: 870-1.

[37] Niaudet P, Habib R. Methylprednisolone pulse therapy in the treatment of severe forms of Schonlein-Henoch purpura nephritis. Pediatric Nephrology (Berlin, Germany) 1998; 12: 238-43.

[38] Tanaka H, Suzuki K, Nakahata T, Ito E, Waga S. Early treatment with oral immuno suppressants in severe proteinuric purpura nephritis. Pediatric Nephrology (Berlin, Germany) 2003; 18: 347-50.

[39] Tarshish P, Bernstein J, Edelmann Jr CM. Henoch-Schonlein purpura nephritis: course of disease and efficacy of cyclophosphamide. Pediatric Nephrology (Berlin, Germany) 2004; 19: 51-6.

[40] Kawasaki Y, Suzuki J, Suzuki H. Efficacy of methylprednisolone and urokinase pulse therapy combined with or without cyclophosphamide in severe Henoch-Schoenlein nephritis: a clinical and histopathological study. Nephrology, dialysis, transplanta-

tion: official publication of the European Dialysis and Transplant Association-European Renal Association 2004; 19: 858-64.

[41] Oner A, Tinaztepe K, Erdogan O. The effect of triple therapy on rapidly progressive type of Henoch-Sch+¦nlein nephritis. Pediatric nephrology (Berlin, Germany) 1995; 9: 6-10.

[42] Lijima K, Ito- Kariya S, Nakamura H, Yoshikawa N. Multiple combined therapy for severe Henoch- Schonlein nephritis in children. Pediatric Nephrology 1998; 12(3): 244-248

[43] Pillebout E, Alberti C, Guillevin L, Ouslimani A, Thervet E, LESAR study group. Addition of cyclophosphamide to steroids provides no benefit compared with steroids alone in treating adult patients with severe Henoch Scholein purpura. Kidney International 2010; 78(5):495- 502

[44] Jauhola O, Ronkainen J, Autio-Harmainen H, Koskimies O, Ala-Houhala M, Arikoski P, Holtta T, Jahnukainen T, Rajantie J, Ormala T. Cyclosporine A vs. methylprednisolone for Henoch-Schonlein nephritis: a randomized trial. Pediatric Nephrology (Berlin, Germany) 2011;26 (12):2159-66.

[45] Shin JI, Park JM, Shin YH, Kim JH, Kim PK, Lee JS, Jeong HJ. Cyclosporin A therapy for severe Henoch-Schonlein nephritis with nephrotic syndrome. Pediatric Nephrology (Berlin, Germany) 2005; 20: 1093-7

[46] Shin JI, Park JM, Shin YH, Kim JH, Lee JS, Jeong HJ. Henoch-Schonlein purpura nephritis with nephrotic-range proteinuria: histological regression possibly associated with cyclosporin A and steroid treatment. Scandinavian Journal of Rheumatology 2005; 34: 392-395.

[47] Park JM, Won SC, Shin JI, Yim H, Pai KS. Cyclosporin A therapy for Henoch-Sch+¦nlein nephritis with nephrotic-range proteinuria. Pediatric Nephrology (Berlin, Germany) 2011; 26: 411-7

[48] Ronkainen J, Autio-Harmainen H, Nuutinen M. Cyclosporin A for the treatment of severe Henoch-Schonlein glomerulonephritis. Pediatric Nephrology (Berlin, Germany) 2003; 18: 1138-42.

[49] Kalliakmani P, Benou E, Goumenos DS. Cyclosporin A in adult patients with Henoch-Schonlein purpura nephritis and nephrotic syndrome; 5 case reports. Clinical Nephrology 2011; 75: 380-3.

[50] Bergstein J, Leiser J, Andreoli SP. Response of crescentic Henoch-Schoenlein purpura nephritis to corticosteroid and azathioprine therapy. Clinical Nephrology 1998; 49: 9.-14

[51] Singh S, Kumar L, Joshi K, Minz RW, Datta U. Severe Henoch-Schonlein nephritis: resolution with azathioprine and steroids. Rheumatology International 2002; 22: 133-7.

[52] Foster BJ, Bernard C, Drummond KN, Sharma AK. Effective therapy for severe Henoch-Schonlein purpura nephritis with prednisone and azathioprine: a clinical and histopathologic study. The Journal of Pediatrics 2000; 136: 370-5.

[53] Shin JI, Park JM, Shin YH, Kim JH, Lee JS, Kim PK, Jeong HJ. Can azathioprine and steroids alter the progression of severe Henoch-Schonlein nephritis in children? Pediatric Nephrology (Berlin, Germany) 2005; 20: 1087-92.

[54] Shin JI, Lee JS, Jeong HJ. Azathioprine and tubulointerstitial nephritis in HSP. The Journal of Rheumatology 2006; 33: 2551.

[55] Muzaffar M, Taj A, Sethi N, Kaw D. Rapidly progressing glomerulonephritis secondary to Henoch-Schonlein purpura treated with mycophenolate mofetil: a case report with atypical etiology and presentation. American Journal of Therapeutics 2010; 17: e163-e166.

[56] Martin S, Cramer CH, Heikenen J, Gitomer JJ. Gastrointestinal symptoms of Henoch-Schonlein purpura treated with mycophenolate mofetil. Journal of Pediatric Gastroenterology and Nutrition 2006; 43: 245-7.

[57] Dede F, Onec B, Ayli D, Gonul II, Onec K. Mycophenolate mofetil treatment of crescentic Henoch-Schonlein nephritis with IgA depositions. Scandinavian Journal of Urology and Nephrology 2008; 42: 178-80.

[58] Nikibakhsh AA, Mahmoodzadeh H, Karamyyar M, Hejazi S, Noroozi M, Macooie AA, Gholizadeh A, Gholizadeh L. Treatment of Complicated Henoch-Schonlein Purpura with Mycophenolate Mofetil: A Retrospective Case Series Report. International Journal of Rheumatology 2010; 2010 DOI:10.1155/2010/254316.

[59] Du Y, Hou L, Zhao C, Han M, Wu Y. Treatment of children with Henoch-Schonlein purpura nephritis with mycophenolate mofetil. Pediatric Nephrology (Berlin, Germany) 2012;27(5):765-71.

[60] Donnithorne KJ, Atkinson TP, Hinze CH, Nogueira JB, Saeed SA, Askenazi DJ, Beukelman T, Cron RQ. Rituximab therapy for severe refractory chronic Henoch-Schonlein purpura. The Journal of Pediatrics 2009; 155: 136-9.

[61] Pillebout E, Rocha F, Fardet L, Rybojad M, Verine J, Glotz D. Successful outcome using rituximab as the only immunomodulation in Henoch-Schonlein purpura: case report. Nephrology, dialysis, transplantation 2011;26(6):2044-6.

[62] Donghi D, Schanz U, Sahrbacher U, Recher M, Tr++eb RM, M++llhaupt B, French LE, Hafner J. Life-threatening or organ-impairing Henoch-Schonlein purpura: plasmapheresis may save lives and limit organ damage. Dermatology (Basel, Switzerland) 2009; 219(2): 167-70.

[63] Wen YK, Yang Y, Chang CC. Cerebral vasculitis and intracerebral hemorrhage in Henoch-Sch+¦nlein purpura treated with plasmapheresis. Pediatric Nephrology (Berlin, Germany) 2005; 20(2): 223-5.

[64] Wortmann SB, Fiselier TJ, Van De Kar NC, Aarts RA, Warris A, Draaisma JM. Refractory severe intestinal vasculitis due to Henoch-Sch+¦nlein purpura: successful treatment with plasmapheresis. Acta Paediatrica (Oslo, Norway: 1992) 2006; 95(5): 622-3.

[65] Hattori M, Ito K, Konomoto T, Kawaguchi H, Yoshioka T, Khono M. Plasmapheresis as the sole therapy for rapidly progressive Henoch-Schonlein purpura nephritis in children. American journal of kidney diseases: the official journal of the National Kidney Foundation 1999; 33(3): 427-33

[66] Shenoy M, Ognjanovic MV, Coulthard MG. Treating severe Henoch-Schonlein and IgA nephritis with plasmapheresis alone. Pediatric Nephrology (Berlin, Germany) 2007; 22: 1167-71.

[67] Aries PM, Hellmich B, Gross WL. Intravenous immunoglobulin therapy in vasculitis: speculation or evidence? Clinical Reviews in Allergy & Immunology 2005; 29: 237-45.

[68] Kusuda A, Migita K, Tsuboi M, Degawa M, Matsuoka N, Tominaga M, Kawakami A, Kawabe Y, Taguchi T, Eguchi K. Successful treatment of adult-onset Henoch-Schonlein purpura nephritis with high-dose immunoglobulins. Internal Medicine (Tokyo, Japan) 1999; 38: 376-9.

[69] Rostoker G, Desvaux-Belghiti D, Pilatte Y, Petit-Phar M, Philippon C, Deforges L, Terzidis H, Intrator L, Andre C, Adnot S. Immunomodulation with low-dose immunoglobulins for moderate IgA nephropathy and Henoch-Schonlein purpura. Preliminary results of a prospective uncontrolled trial. Nephron 1995; 69: 327-334.

[70] Davin JC. Henoch-Schonlein Purpura Nephritis: Pathophysiology, Treatment, and Future Strategy. Clinical journal of the American Society of Nephrology: CJASN 2011;6(3):67-89.

[71] Inoue CN, Matsutani S, Ishidoya M, Homma R, Chiba Y, Nagasaka T. Periodontal and ENT Therapy in the Treatment of Pediatric Henoch-Schonlein Purpura and IgA Nephropathy. Advances in Oto-rhino-laryngology 2011; 72: 53-6.

[72] Kanai H, Sawanobori E, Kobayashi A, Matsushita K, Sugita K, Higashida K. Early Treatment with Methylprednisolone Pulse Therapy Combined with Tonsillectomy for Heavy Proteinuric Henoch-Schonlein Purpura Nephritis in Children. Nephron Extra 2011; 1: 101-111.

[73] Ohara S, Kawasaki Y, Matsuura H, Oikawa T, Suyama K, Hosoya M. Successful therapy with tonsillectomy for severe ISKDC grade VI Henoch-Schonlein purpura nephritis and persistent nephrotic syndrome. Clinical and ExperimentalNephrology 2011;15(5):749-53

[74] Szer IS, Pierce H. Henoch-Schonlein purpura. In Rheumatology, Hochberg ed. Elsevier; 2011: 1587-1595.

[75] Carlson JA. The histological assessment of cutaneous vasculitis. Histopathology 2010; 56: 3-23.

[76] Russell JP, Gibson LE. Primary cutaneous small vessel vasculitis: approach to diagnosis and treatment. International Journal of Dermatology 2006; 45: 3-13.

[77] Chen KR, Carlson JA. Clinical approach to cutaneous vasculitis. American Journal of Clinical Dermatology 2008; 9: 71-92.

[78] Sais G, Vidaller A, Jucgl+á A, Gallardo F, Peyr+¡ J. Colchicine in the treatment of cutaneous leukocytoclastic vasculitis. Results of a prospective, randomized controlled trial. Archives of Dermatology 1995; 131: 1399-402.

[79] Nurnberg W, Grabbe J, Czarnetzki BM. Synergistic effects of pentoxifylline and dapsone in leucocytoclastic vasculitis. Lancet 1994; 343: 491.

[80] Demitsu T, Yoneda K, Kakurai M, Sasaki K, Hiratsuka Y, Azuma R, Yamada T, Umemoto N. Clinical efficacy of reserpine as" add-on therapy" to antihistamines in patients with recalcitrant chronic idiopathic urticaria and urticarial vasculitis. The Journal of Dermatology 2010; 37: 827-9.

[81] Morgan AJ, Schwartz RA. Cutaneous polyarteritis nodosa: a comprehensive review. International Journal of Dermatology 2010; 49: 750-6.

[82] Kawakami T. New algorithm (KAWAKAMI algorithm) to diagnose primary cutaneous vasculitis. The Journal of Dermatology 2010; 37: 113-24.

[83] De Groot K, Harper L, Jayne DR, Flores SLF, Gregorini G, Gross WL, Luqmani R, Pusey CD, Rasmussen N, Sinico RA. Pulse versus daily oral cyclophosphamide for induction of remission in antineutrophil cytoplasmic antibody-associated vasculitis: a randomized trial. Annals of Internal Medicine 2009; 150: 670-80.

[84] Haubitz M, Schellong S. Intravenous pulse administration of cyclophosphamide versus daily oral treatment in patients with antineutrophil cytoplasmic antibody-associated vasculitis and renal involvement: a prospective, randomized study. Arthritis and Rheumatism 1998; 41: 1835-44.

[85] Holvast A, Stegeman CA, Benne CA, Huckriede A, Wilschut JC, Palache AM, Kallenberg CG, Bijl M. Wegener's granulomatosis patients show an adequate antibody response to influenza vaccination. Annals of the Rheumatic Diseases 2009; 68: 873-8.

[86] Holvast A, de Haan A, van Assen S, Stegeman CA, Huitema MG, Huckriede A, Benne CA, Westra J, Palache A, Wilschut J. Cell-mediated immune responses to influenza vaccination in Wegener's granulomatosis. Annals of the Rheumatic Diseases 2010; 69: 924-7.

Chapter 10

Recent Advances in the Management of Refractory Vasculitis

Reem Hamdy A. Mohammed

Additional information is available at the end of the chapter

http://dx.doi.org/10.5772/54517

1. Introduction

Systemic necrotizing vasculitides are a broad family of conditions characterized by injury or destruction of the blood vessel walls by inflammatory cells with subsequent vessel occlusion and ischemic tissue injury with high rates of morbidity and mortality. [1] The heterogeneous nature of the involved etio-pathogenetic mechanisms together with the diversities in clinical presentations poses a great challenge to successful induction and maintenance therapy in vasculitis. Untreated, these diseases can be devastating. Treatment strategy in vasculitis depends entirely upon the type of vasculitis, the pattern and severity of organ involvement. High dose corticosteroids and cytotoxic drugs remain the cornerstones in the management of vasculitis that dramatically improved the prognosis with increasing chances for remission. However, despite such aggressive therapy the relapse rate in systemic vasculitis ranges from 30-50%. With the increasing relapses in some cases, refractoriness to standard care measures in others together with the toxicities associated with the use of long term high dose corticosteroids and cytotoxic drugs there is an increasing demand for an alternative effective therapy.

The pathogenetic background in human autoimmune diseases remains poorly understood. The recent advances in the understanding of epigenetics of autoimmune rheumatic diseases have revealed a variety of disease specific pathways responsible for immune-mediated inflammatory and destructive events. In most of these situations including vasculitis the initial trigger is mostly an infectious trigger. It is mostly an antigen driven response that involves activation of the antigen presenting cells (dendritic cells, macrophages, monocytes, B lymphocytes), priming of T lymphocytes towards a Th1, Th17 response. The primed Th1, Th17 lymphocytes initiates a cascade of pro-inflammatory events involving the release of pro-inflammatory cytokines (TNF alpha, IL-1 β,IL-6, TGF- β, IFN-γ, IL-17, IL-23) with subsequent priming of neutrophils, overexpression of adhesion molecules, activation of co-stimulatory signals with further release of pro-inflammatory mediators and autoantibody production. Figure 1

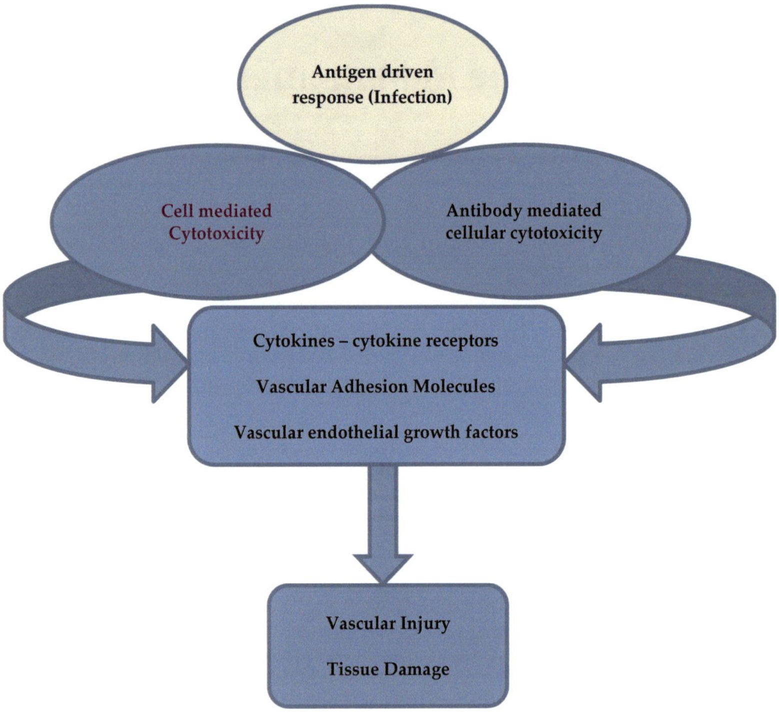

Figure 1. Basic pathogenic theory of autoimmunity in vasculitis.

Advances in the understanding of the pathogenesis of autoimmune diseases, allow increasingly specific, targeted therapies to be developed for clinical use. These therapies are nominated as biologic disease modifying drugs that fall under two categories: anti-cytokine strategies, and drugs that target specific subsets of immune cells. The ultimate goal of these therapies is to target pathogenetic pathways that contribute to disease initiation and progression. The recent attempts to use biologic disease modifying drugs in refractory systemic vasculitis has revolutionized the therapeutic landscape with promising observable outcome. [2]

2. Tumor necrosis factor alpha in vasculitis

TNF-α, with its' brother lymphotoxin TNF-β, represent a family of pro-inflammatory cytokines produced by a variety of immune cells, primarily by lipopolysaccharide-stimulated macrophages and monocytes, as well as by T lymphocytes. TNF exists in both cell membrane-bound and soluble forms with TNF receptors (TNF- R1, TNF- R2) on many cells, including macrophages and monocytes, thereby allowing it to stimulate its own production and release. It has been shown to be a key cytokine in the host inflammatory response. Its actions are modulated through various mechanisms, which include adhesion molecule expression, pro-inflammatory cytokine release, synthesis of chemokines, inhibition of regulatory T cells and activation of a variety of immune cells. [3, 4]

http://dx.doi.org/10.5772/54517

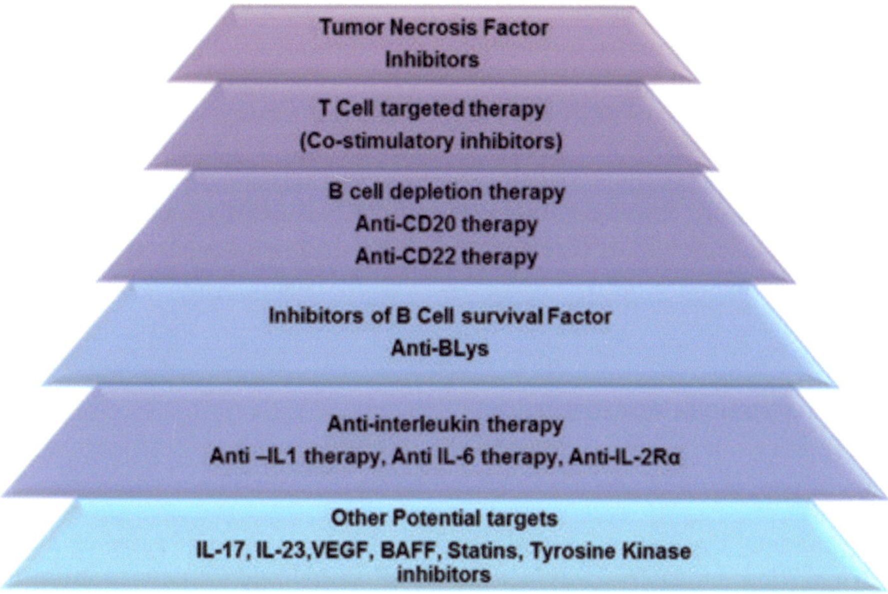

Figure 2. The Role of Tumor necrosis Factor Targeted Biologic Therapy in Primary Systemic Vasculitides.

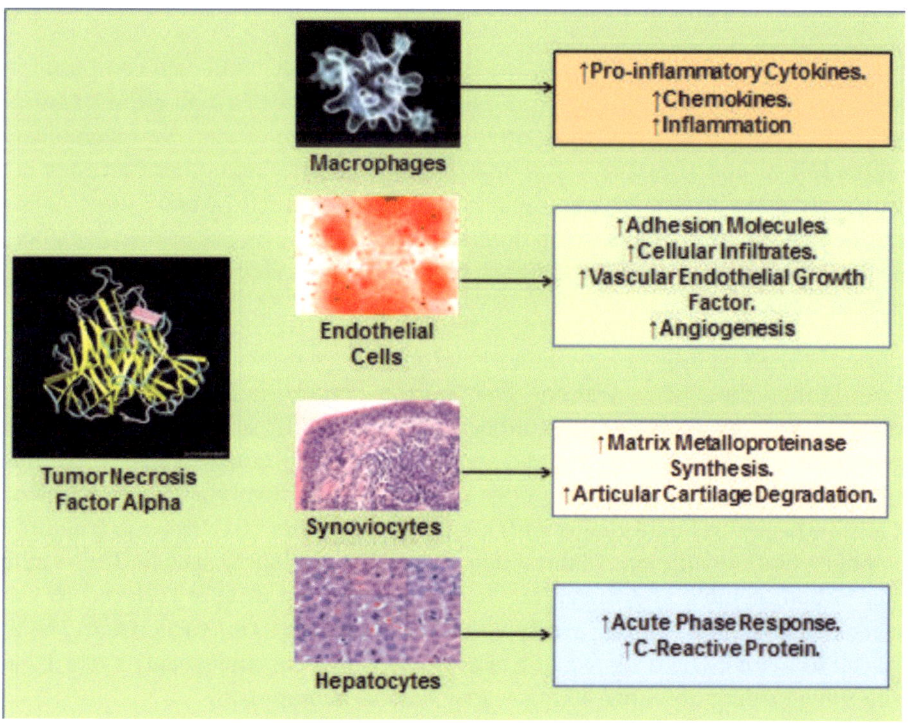

Figure 3. Role of Tumor Necrosis Factor in Inflammatory Response.

The primary immunopathogenic events that initiate the process of vascular inflammation and blood vessel damage remain largely unknown. Granulomatous inflammation involving the vessel itself, the adjacent tissue, or distant sites is a feature of several systemic vasculitic syndromes and tumor necrosis factor is being identified as a major contributor to granulomatous tissue inflammation via its' stimulatory effects on tissue macrophages. The unopposed actions of TNF via its' receptors highly potentiates and sustains inflammatory granuloma formation and integrity. The recognition of the role of this pro-inflammatory cytokine sets it as a potential therapeutic target. Tumor necrosis factor inhibitors have been approved for the treatment of rheumatoid arthritis as well as sero-negative spondylo-arthropathies.

3. Tumor necrosis factor inhibitors

3.1. Classification of tumor necrosis factor inhibitors

There are presently five TNF-α inhibitors available. They are classified based on their mechanism of inhibition of tumor necrosis factor into TNF neutralizing monoclonal antibodies that are capable of neutralizing the soluble as well as the tissue bound TNF and TNF receptor fusion protein that is capable of neutralizing the effects of the soluble TNF in circulation.

3.2. Tumor necrosis factor monoclonal antibodies

Infliximab: A chimeric human/mouse monoclonal anti-TNF antibody composed of the constant regions of human (Hu) IgG1κ, coupled to the Fv region of a high-affinity neutralizing murine anti-Hu TNF-α antibody. The antibody exhibits high affinity for recombinant and natural hu TNF-α, and neutralizes TNF-mediated cytotoxicity and other functions in vitro. The drug is given at a dose of 3-10mg/ Kg intravenous infusion at 0-2-6 and 8 weeks then every 8 weeks. Because of the potential for an immune reaction to the mouse protein components of a chimeric antibody, an alternate strategy has been to develop a fully human anti-TNF monoclonal antibody. [4]

Adalimumab: The first fully human monoclonal anti-tumor necrosis factor (TNF)-α antibody approved in the year 2002 as a second line anti-tumor necrosis factor for the treatment of refractory rheumatoid arthritis. Such antibody, known as D2E7, also known as adalimumab, was generated by phage display technology. A high affinity murine anti-TNF monoclonal antibody was used as a template for guided selection, which involves complete replacement of the murine heavy and light chains with human counterparts and subsequent optimization of the antigen-binding affinity. Adalimumab is considered a highly specific TNF-a inhibitor. It binds to both soluble and membrane-bound TNF-a. The drug is believed to exert its pharmacological effect by binding to soluble TNF-a preventing its interaction with TNFR1 and TNFR2 cell receptors. The drug is given at a dose of 40mg subcutaneously every 1-2 weeks (initially 80mg loading dose then 40 mg as maintenance therapy). [5]

Golimumab: is a human immunoglobulin (Ig) G1-kappa monoclonal antibody (mAb) that is specific for TNF-alpha. Golimumab binds to both the soluble and transmembrane forms

http://dx.doi.org/10.5772/54517

of human TNF-alpha. The drug is given in a dose of 50 mg subcutaneously every 4 weeks. Golimumab is approved for the treatment of rheumatoid arthritis, and seronegative arthropathies. [6]

Certolizumab: Certolizumab is a PEGylated recombinant, humanized antibody Fab' fragment specific for human tumor necrosis factor alpha (TNFα) that is indicated for treatment of moderately to severely active Rheumatoid Arthritis (RA), treatment and maintenance of remission of moderate to severe active Crohn's disease (CD) in adult patients who have an inadequate response to conventional therapy. [7]

The latest two new monoclonal antibody TNF inhibitors, certolizumab and golimumab have been genetically engineered recently aiming to improve affinity and specificity to TNF with better tolerability and less autoimmunity. Neither golimumab nor certolizumab have been tried in patients with vasculitis.

3.3. Tumor necrosis factor receptor block

Etanercept: Etanercept: is a dimeric fusion protein composed of two extracellular TNF-receptor domains bound to the Fc portion of human IgG and is injected once or twice weekly at a dose of 50mg. It effectively binds soluble TNF, thereby blocking TNF-receptor activation. [5]

3.4. Tumor necrosis factor inhibitors in vasculitis

TNF-α is increasingly being implicated in the etio-pathogenesis of several autoimmune diseases, including systemic vasculitis, featuring an interesting therapeutic target. Several case series studies and case reports addressing the role of suppressing tumor necrosis factor in vasculitis have been issued. Such studies have shown that anti TNF therapy might provide a promising therapeutic alternative in the management of refractory systemic vasculitides [8, 9, 10] especially of granulomatous inflammatory nature including; Takayasu's arteritis, probably in giant cell arteritis (GCA) and granulomatous polyangiitis (GPA) amongst other forms of vasculitis.

3.4.1. Takayasu vasculitis — TAK

Takayasu's arteritis is a rare, chronic, systemic panarteritis of unknown etiology characterized by granulomatous inflammation of the aorta and its major branches (occasionally including the pulmonary arteries as well) with progressive fibrosis and stenosis of the affected vessel wall and, less commonly, aneurysm formation. [11, 12, 13] The disease typically presents in women before the age of 40 years old. Glucocorticoids and methotrexate are the mainstays of treatment.[] Amongst the identified pathogenic targets in Takayasu arteritis displayed in (Figure 2), TNF alpha is the only cytokine under evaluation. There have been several case series [14, 15, 16] and case reports [17, 18, 19] that have shown clinical benefit of TNF inhibition for refractory cases with TAK. The use of TNF blockade therapy was associated with significant improvement in BVAS, successful reduction in the dose of oral corticosteroids and longer glucocorticoid drug free remission in cases with refractory Takayasu arteritis. In a case series study by Hoffman et al. including 15 patients with treatment-resistant TAK, patients were

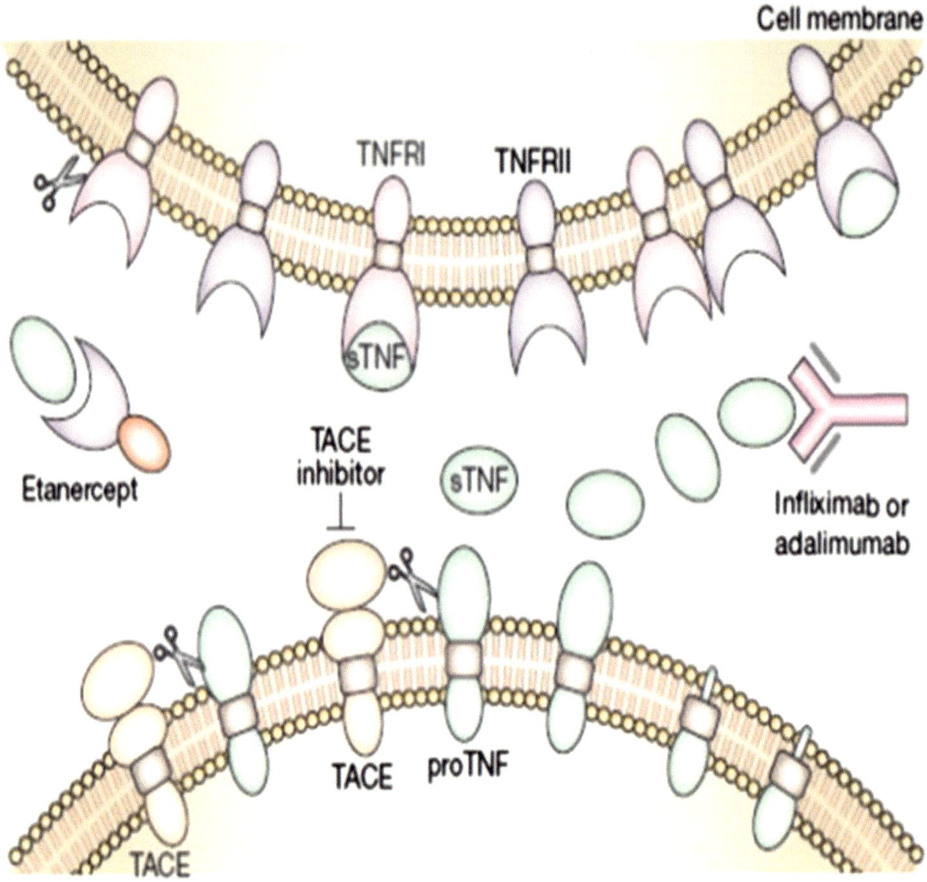

Figure 4. Mode of action of Tumor necrosis factor inhibitors.

treated with either infliximab or etanercept for disease relapse with 93% of patients showing marked improvement with significant reduction in the dose of oral corticosteroids from a median dose of 20mg/day to 0 mg/day and 67% of patients sustaining up to 3 years glucocorticoid drug free remission. The need for randomized, controlled trials remains necessary to further characterize the effectiveness of TNF inhibition in Takayasu arteritis. [20,21]

3.4.2. Giant Cell Arteritis — GCA

Giant cell arteritis is a granulomatous vasculitis that affects predominantly large- to medium-sized arteries, including the aorta and its major branches with advancing concentric intimal hyperplasia and subsequent vascular occlusion. Figure 5 Experimental data support the concept that the disease is initiated in the most outer layer of the arterial wall, the adventitia. CD4 T cells are recruited to the adventitia, undergo local activation and subsequently orchestrate macrophage differentiation. T cells and macrophages infiltrate into all wall layers and acquire different effector functions dependent on cues in their immediate microenvironment.

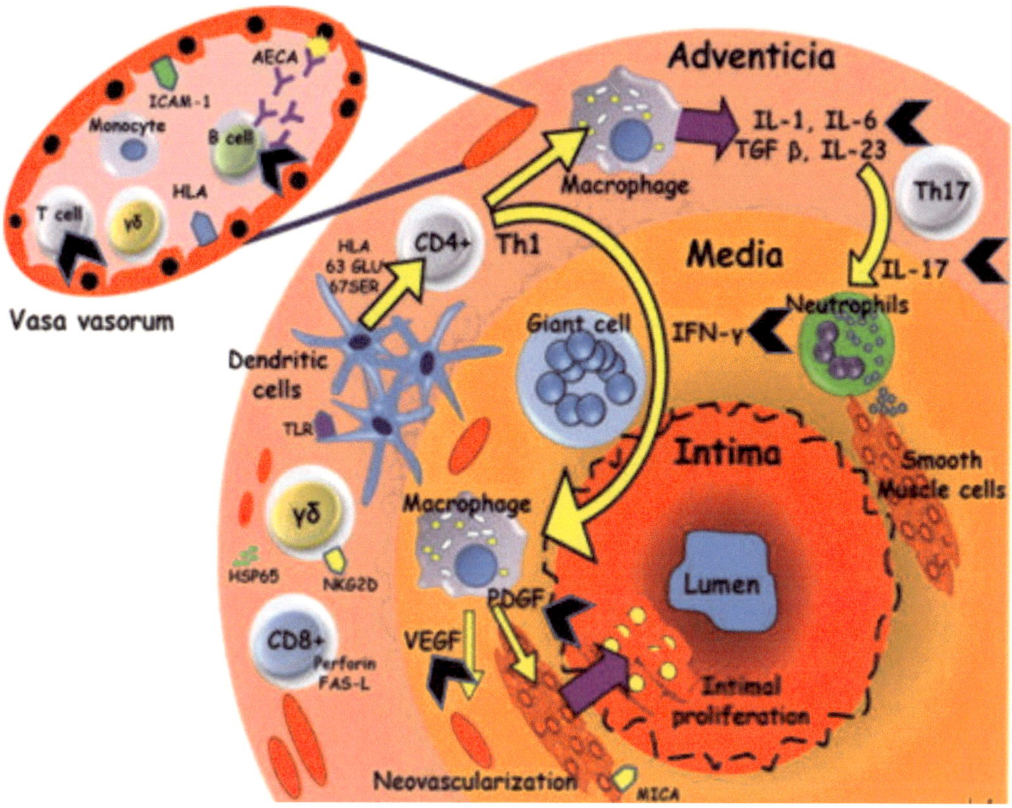

Figure 5. Identified Pathogenic Targets (black arrows) in Takayasu Arteritis.

The end result is myofibroblastic proliferation, luminal stenosis, and tissue ischemia. Adaptive immune responses in the adventitia are triggered by a population of indigenous dendritic cells (DC) placed at the adventitia-media junction. These arterial DCs have a unique surface receptor profile, including a series of Toll-like receptors (TLR). These adventitial DCs produce chemokines (TNF alpha, IL-1B), recruit T cells and support their local activation. TNF is one of several cytokines linked to vascular injury in giant cell arteritis.

The standard treatment for GCA is glucocorticoids, methotrexate might be used in some cases as a steroid sparing drug. Up to 60- 80% of treated patients ultimately develop serious adverse effects related to glucocorticoid therapy necessitating an alternative therapy. Tumor necrosis factor alpha inhibitors have been proposed as a therapeutic alternative. Randomized controlled trials studying the efficacy of infliximab in GCS revealed infliximab to be non-superior to conventional therapy with insignificant difference in the percentage of patients successfully tapered off glucocorticoids (71-56%). Infliximab therapy was associated with significanlty higher rates of infections. The use of TNF-αI in GCA remains a pit controversial awaiting further studies. [22-27]

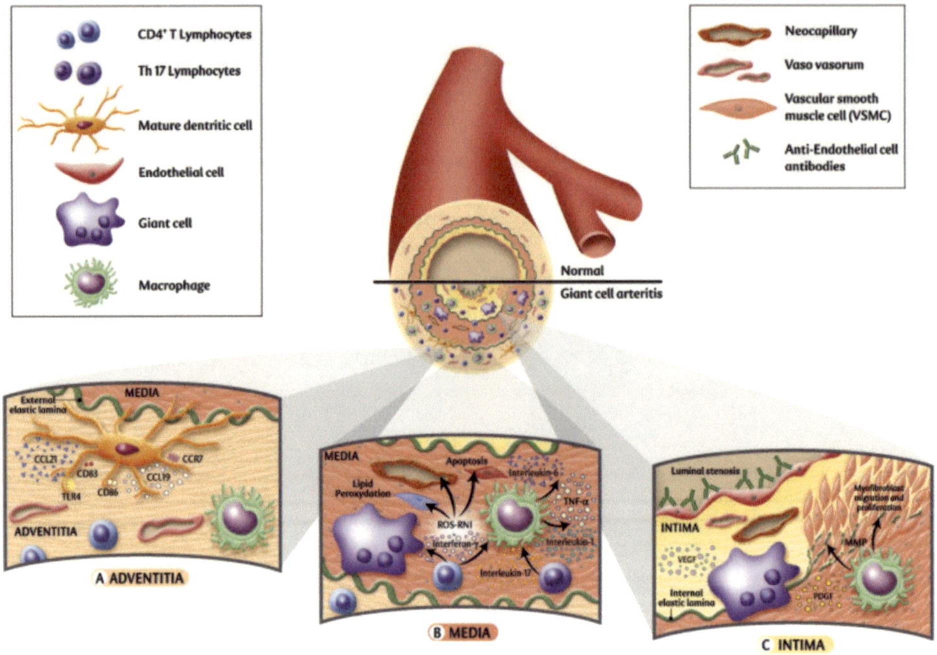

Figure 6. Pathogenesis of Giant Cell Arteritis. [22]

3.4.3. Granulomatosis with polyangiitis GPA-(Wegener's granulomatosis)

Granulomatosis with polyangiitis (Wegener's Granulomatosis) is a systemic inflammatory disorder characterized predominantly by the presence of a small vessel vasculitis with necrotizing granulomatous inflammation, primarily of the upper and lower respiratory tract. The pathogenetic pathways in ANCA associated vasculitis primarily involves neutrophil activation secondary to an infectious trigger. *S. aureus*-derived products (superantigens and peptidoglycans) stimulate APCs to produce IL-23, which induces proliferation of T_H17 cells. IL-17 secretion from T_H17 cells activates macrophages that, in turn, produce pro-inflammatory cytokines (IL-1β and TNF), which results in the priming of neutrophils. PR3 produced by neutrophils is processed by APCs, followed by presentation to T_H cells. These cells provide help to B cells for the production of PR3-ANCAs, which interact with PR3 on the surface of primed neutrophils that are rolling on the endothelium. These neutrophils become firmly adhesive and produce ROS and NETs that cause necrotizing vasculitis. T_H cells also differentiate into T_{EM} cells that interact with the endothelium and participate in granuloma formation, resulting in granulomatous vasculitis. Figure 7

Infection is the identified initial trigger with subsequent priming of neutrophils. Priming of neutrophils leads to a cascade of events including: (a) Up-regulation of adhesion molecules on endothelial cells, and expansion of circulating effector T cells. Primed neutrophils show increased surface expression of ANCA antigens and adhesion molecules. ANCA binding activates the neutrophil in the following ways: [1] enhancing vessel wall adherence and transmigration capacity; [2] production and release of oxygen radicals, and [3] degranulation

http://dx.doi.org/10.5772/54517

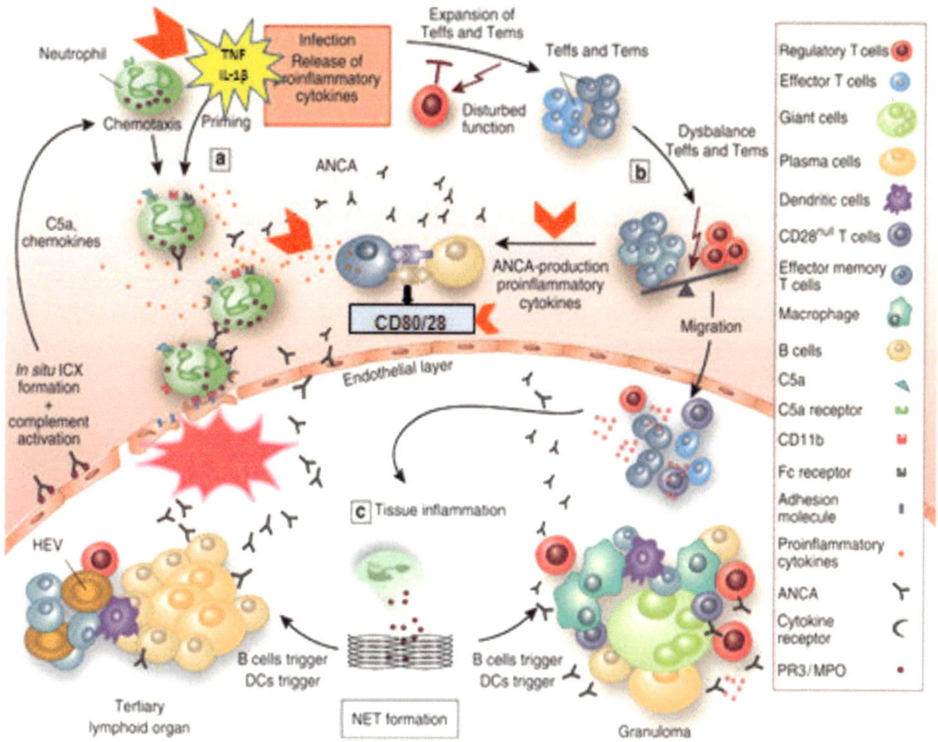

Figure 7. Identified Pathogenic targets (red arrow heads) contributing to inflammation and tissue damage in anti-neutrophil cytoplasmic antibody (ANCA)-associated vasculitis (AAV).

and release of enzymes including myeloperoxidase (MPO) and proteinase-3 (PR3) (a). Transient immune complexes are formed locally by binding of ANCA to PR3/MPO sticking to endothelial cells. Subsequently, complement is activated, which further promotes neutrophil degranulation. This all adds to the development of necrotizing vasculitis. Whether this specific cascade is also applicable to disease pathogenesis in ANCA-negative AAV patients remains unclear. The expanded effector memory T cells (Tems) are not sufficiently regulated by regulatory T cells (Tregs, b). This virtually leads a state of imbalance between Tregs and Tems, resulting in further release of pro-inflammatory cytokines promoting neutrophil priming (a); moreover, ANCA production is enhanced by further T-cell/B-cell interaction. (c) Expanded circulating Tems migrate into target organs such as the lungs or the kidney. Within tissues, Tems drive granuloma formation, which is considered an 'executioner' of tissue destruction. Granulomas are composed of numerous cell types such as T cells, B cells, giant cells, and dendritic cells (DCs) with local ANCA production. [28]

Randomized controlled trials studying the outcome of tumor necrosis factor inhibitors in ANCA associated vasculitis proved that anti TNF-α therapy was non-superior to conventional therapy in remission induction. The addition of infliximab to standard therapy did not confer clinical benefit for patients with active AAV [29, 30]

The WGET (The Wegener Granulomatosis Etanercept Trial) was a double-blind study that aimed to assess the role of etanercept in the induction and maintenance of remission in 180 patients with GPA. In this trial the use of etanercept showed no impact on the rate of achieving sustained remission compared to placebo (69% for etanercept vs 75% for placebo) with a slight increase in the rate of solid tumors among patients receiving a combination therapy of cyclophosphamide and etanercept. A risk that proved to be insignificant. [31] Another open label phase II prospective study including 14 patients with acute flares of AASV either as first manifestation of disease or relapse demonstrated that the addition of adalimumab to prednisolone and cyclophosphamide for the treatment of severe ANCA associated systemic vasculitis (AASV) was associated with response rates and adverse events similar to standard therapy alone but with a reduced prednisolone exposure. [32]

4. TNF-α inhibitors in other forms of systemic vasculitis

4.1. Behcet's syndrome

Infliximab at a dose of 5mg/kg, showed efficacy in cases with refractory uveo-retinitis with improvement of visual acuity, healing of oro-genital ulcers, healing of intestinal lesions and remission. It has also been disclosed that infliximab is a rapid and effective therapy for sight-threatening panuveitis in Behçet's disease. Infliximab administration thus leads to a rapid and effective suppression of acute ocular inflammation, and the remission of the uveitis remained for as long as 28 days after infliximab administration in all five patients. Etanercept is also now being used in refractory Behçet's disease. [33, 34, 35, 36, 37] Despite that Tumor necrosis factor therapy is not an approved therapeutic alternative in Behcet's syndrome due to lack of randomized controlled studies, yet TNF inhibition might provide a valuable alternative in Behçet's syndrome patients who were proven refractory to more commonly used treatments.

4.2. Kawasaki disease

TNF has been suggested as an important cytokine in the active phase of coronary disease in mouse models of Kawasaki disease.However, the current use of anti TNF therapy in Kawasaki remains restricted only to cases with immunoglobulin resistant disease. [38,39]

4.3. Deep idiopathic small vessels cutaneous vasculitis

Cutaneous vasculitis, is a disease with an annual incidence rate ranging from 39.6 to 59.8 per million, can be classified as primary or idiopathic; or secondary, when it presents as a manifestation of connective tissue diseases, infections, drug reactions or malignancies. [41, 42] Most of the idiopathic cases are self-limited and responsive to supportive measures (limb elevation, warming, avoid standing) and nonsteroidal anti-inflammatory drugs, potent immune-suppressants are sometimes required for the management of the refractory situations. [42]

The high serum levels of the pro-inflammatory cytokines TNF-α, IL-1β observed in sera of patients with small vessels cutaneous vasculitis supports a potential role of these cytokines in the pathogenesis of such forms of vasculitis. [43] Reports support the benefit of infliximab in the treatment of some cases of deep cutaneous vasculitis as well as in difficult to treat cases who failed to respond to cyclophosphamide pulse therapy with successful tapering of oral corticosteroids [44, 45, 46] Cases of deep cutaneous vasculitis following infliximab therapy have also been reported. [47]

5. B cell targeted therapy in systemic vasculitis

5.1. The role of B cells in vasculitis

B lymphocytes are key players in immune mediated vasculitis representing the the humoral arm of the immune response. B cells produce pathogenic autoantibodies and because they have multiple effector functions, including antigen uptake and transport, antigen presentation and costimulation of T cells via membrane associated molecules, production of cytokines and chemokines migration to sites of inflammation. B lymphocytes arise from hematopoietic stem cells in the bone marrow. These cells mature independently of an antigen first into pro-B cells, then into pre-B cells and immature B cells. They subsequently enter the antigen-dependent phase in the peripheral lymphoid tissues, where mature-but-naive B cells, after encountering their antigen in the extrafollicular regions of the lymphoid organs, become activated B cells and migrate to the follicular regions. B lymphocytes then exit the follicular regions to differentiate into memory B cells, late plasmablasts and plasma cells. Specific markers, such as CD20, CD27, BAFF-R (B-cell-activating factor receptor), CD38 and CD138, identify the transitional phases of B cells from stem cells to plasma cells. (Figure 7) [48, 49, 50]

5.2. B cells surface target molecules in vasculitis

5.2.1. CD-20 cell surface molecule

CD20 is a 297-amino acid activated glycosylated trans-membrane phosphoprotein specifically expressed on the surface of B cells, starting at the early pre-B cell stage and persists until the differentiation of B cells into plasma cells. CD-20 is not expressed on hematopoietic stem cells, pro-B cells, or normal plasma cells. Plasma-blasts and stimulated plasma cells may express CD20. CD20 is co-expressed on B cells with CD19, another B cell differentiation marker. CD20 appears to play a crucial role in B cell development, differentiation, proliferation and cell-cycle regulation events. B cell mediated disorders with clonal B cell expansion including lymphomas, leukemias, autoimmune diseases were found to be associated with increasing expression of the CD-20 antigen in variable densities. [51, 52, 53, 54]

5.2.2. CD-22 cell surface molecule

CD22 is a 135-kDa trans-membrane sialoglycoprotein, a member of the immunoglobulin superfamily. Its expression is restricted to lymphocytes of the B cell lineage and is highly developmentally regulated.

CD22 is present in the cytoplasm of pro- and pre-B cells and becomes detectable on the cell surface only at mature stages of B cell differentiation. Cell surface expression is lost during terminal differentiation into plasma cell and after B cell activation. CD22 is also expressed by the vast majority of B cell NHLs. The CD22 molecule has multiple ligands because it binds to α2–6-linked sialic acid residues present on glycoproteins expressed by activated T and B cells, monocytes, neutrophils, erythrocytes, and activated endothelial cells. Although its function is not yet well understood, CD22 appears to be involved in the regulation of B cell activation through BCR signaling, (demonstrating both positive and negative roles in vitro) as well as in cell adhesion. In vivo, the important biological functions of this receptor have been demonstrated by genetic disruption of CD22. CD22-deficient mice have a shorter life span, a reduced number of mature B cells in the bone marrow and in circulation, and a chronic exaggerated antibody response to antigen and develop elevated levels of autoantibodies, suggesting a key role for CD22 in B cell development, survival, and function. [55-60]

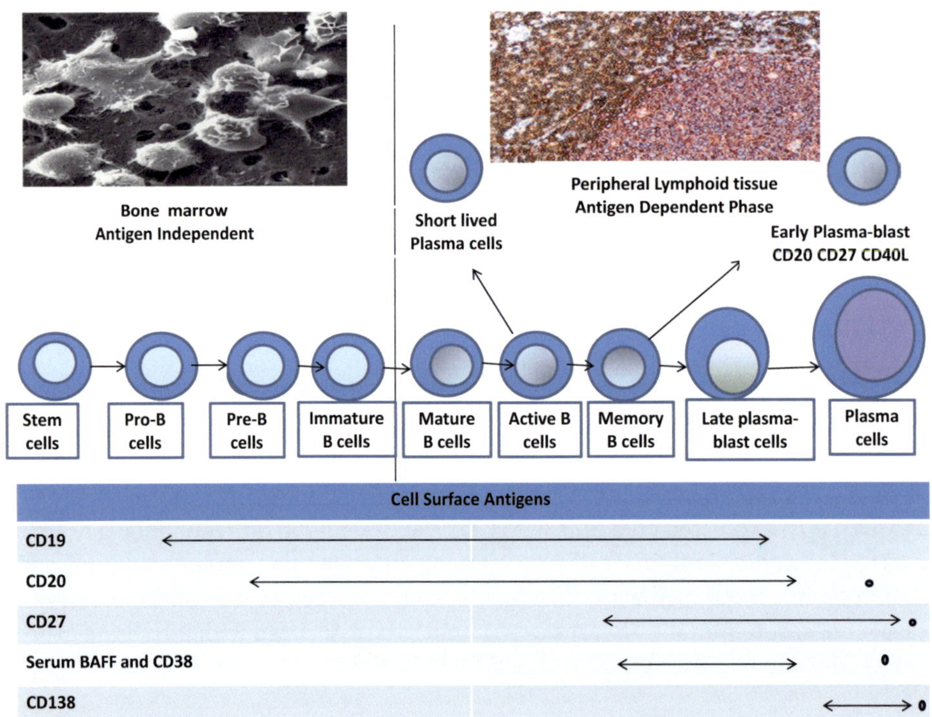

Figure 8. Surface molecules and receptors involved in B cell Maturation, the black bullet refers to identified therapeutic targets [51]

http://dx.doi.org/10.5772/54517

5.3. B-cell targeted therapy

Currently available B cell targeted biologic drugs can be classified into two different mechanisms, the first mechanism is the B cell depletion therapy, the second mechanism acts via inhibition of B cell maturation. Different trials and case reports showed promising results with the use of B cell depletion therapy in vasculitis.

5.3.1. The B-cell depletion therapy

5.3.1.1. Rituximab

A chimeric human/mouse IgG1 antibody directed at human CD20, which is found on only pre-B and mature B cells. B-cell depletion with rituximab might be useful for patients with autoimmune diseases driven by autoantibody production. Rituximab (anti-CD-20 therapy) showed efficacy in autoimmune disorders including refractory systemic lupus with nephritis and vasculitis. The types of vasculitis investigated in this regard include cryoglobulinemic vasculitis, ANCA associated vasculitis, cutaneous vasculitis with connective tissue diseases like rheumatoid arthritis, systemic lupus erythematosus and Sjogren's syndrome. [51, 52, 53, 54] Figure 9.

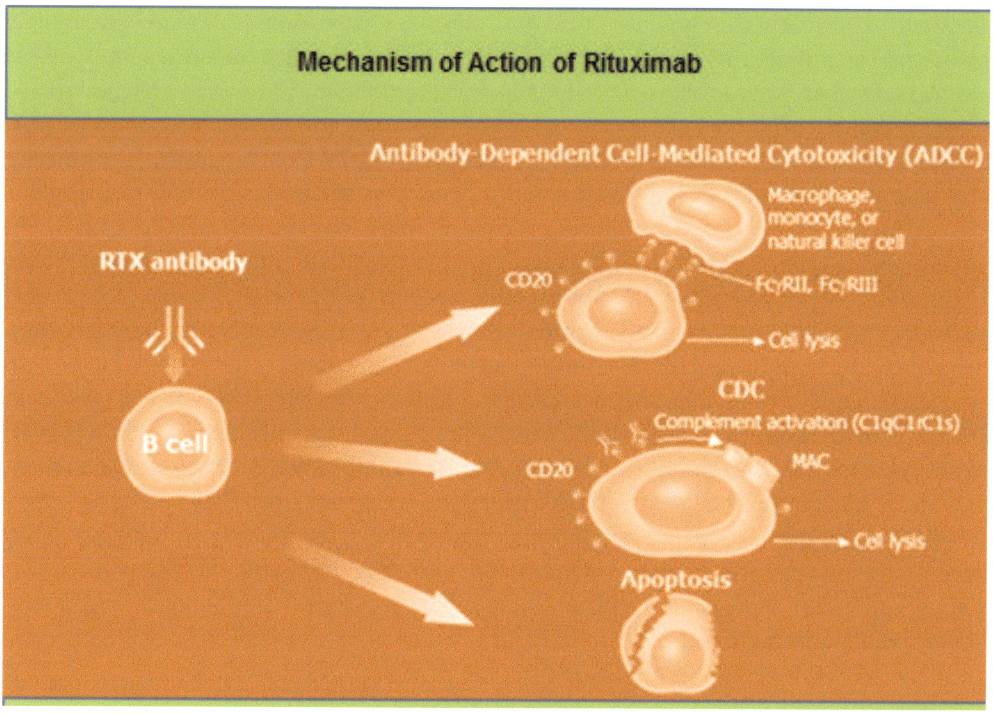

Figure 9. Mechanism of B cell depletion with anti-CD20 therapy [54]

5.3.1.2. Epratuzumab

Epratuzumab is a humanized monoclonal antibody targeting CD22 receptors on B lymphocytes. Two multicenter, placebo-controlled, randomized, double-blind studies (EMBODY™ 1 and EMBODY™ 2), designed to evaluate the efficacy, safety, tolerability, and immunogenicity of Epratuzumab in patients with moderate to severe SLE, are being designed and processed, each will enroll 780 subjects and will last a maximum of 54 weeks. Ongoing experimental studies addressing the role of anti-CD22 in ANCA vasculitis are being run with promising results, whilst randomized controlled trials are still lacking. [61-65]

5.3.2. The role of B cells targeted therapy in systemic vasculitis

5.3.2.1. Cryoglobulinemic vasculitis

Mixed cryoglobulinemia (MC) is a chronic immune complex (IC) mediated systemic small vessel vasculitis, characterized by immune complex deposits (cryo-deposits) and frequent visceral involvement. A frequent synonym of this disease is "cryoglobulinemic vasculitis". [66] The term cryoglobulinemia refers to the presence of a single or monoclonal immunoglobulin Ig or more polyclonal immunoglobulins. Cryoglobulins are classified on the basis of their Ig components. These cryoglobulins precipitate at temperatures below 37°C giving rise to high molecular weight aggregates and re-dissolve on rewarming. Cryoglobulins are found in small quantities in normal serum and are present in variable concentrations in many pathological conditions, including myeloproliferative disorders, autoimmune disorders and several infectious diseases. They are classified into: Type I cryoglobulins (10-15% of cryoglobulins) is comprised simply of monoclonal immunoglobulins, typically IgM but less frequently IgG, IgA, or serum light chains. Individuals with Type I cryos typically have a paraproteinemia (e.g., myeloma, Waldenstrom's macroglobulinemia). Type II cryoglobulins (50-60% of cryoglobulins) occurs when a monoclonal Ig M recognizes and binds to polyclonal IgG's, accordingly, type II cryos are typically IgM-IgG complexes.Type III cryoglobulins (30-40% of cryoglobulins) are composed of polyclonal Ig M that binds to polyclonal IgG. Type II & III cryoglobulinemia are referred to as "Mixed Cryoglobulinemia", these two types are most commonly associated with hepatitis C virus infection. [67]. The term essential cryoglobulinemia was used to describe cryoglobulinemia without identifiable underlying disease, currently it is clear that most of the patients with essential mixed cryoglobulinemia are chronically infected with HCV [68] The classic pathology in cryoglobulinemic vasculitis is leukocytoclastic vasculitis. The disease presents by Meltzer triad which is a triad of purpura, weakness, arthralgia and/or arthritis in 25-30% of cases, thereafter, a series of multisystem pathologies follow involving peripheral nervous system and the kidneys. Widespread vasculitis involving medium-small sized arteries, capillaries and venules with multiple organ involvement may develop in a small proportion of patients [69-72].

The incidence of hepatitis C infection in mixed cryoglobulinemia ranges from 40 to 90%. [69, 73, 74] The hepatitis C virus infects B cells, resulting in clonal expansion and stimulation of autoantibody production. Eradication of hepatitis C with interferon and ribavirin has been tried, but is often ineffective for controlling extra-hepatic disease,[45] particularly with genotype 1, and interferon induced many side effects. On the other hand, treatments such as cyclophosphamide and plasmapheresis are generally reserved for life- or organ-threatening disease.

Rituximab showed efficacy in cases of HCV-mixed cryoglobulinemia. The rationale behind anti-B-cell therapy in mixed cryoglobulinemic vasculitis includes the presence immune complex deposition as the cause of symptoms in hepatitis C virus extra-hepatic syndrome, in which chronic stimulation by hepatitis C virus induces the production of cryoglobulins by infected B cells. [75, 76] Rituximab was successfully used in combination with antiviral agents as well as mono-therapy in HCV cryoglobulinemic vasculitis. Rituximab combined with Peg-IFN-α/ribavirin delete both virus-dependent and -independent B-cell clones. Antiviral therapy alone decreased the memory B cells; whereas in association with rituximab, naive B cells are the main depleted population. The observable delay in B-cell reconstitution after rituximab plus Peg-IFN-α/ribavirin stresses the synergistic action of rituximab and antiviral therapy at the immunologic level. Rituximab shortens the therapeutic interval required for achieving a complete clinical response. Clonal expansion of marginal zone–like IgM+ CD27+ B cells (VH1-69 clonal B) has been recently observed in certain HCV-MC patients. Rituximab with Peg-IFN and ribavirin exerts a synergistic effect on polyclonal B lymphocyte expansion. Rituximab plus Peg-IFN-α/ribavirin was more efficient to suppress both memory and VH1-69 clonal B cells compared with Peg-IFN-α/ribavirin alone. A standard therapeutic dose of 375 mg/m2 weekly for 4 weeks is effective, well tolerated and induces a significant and rapid improvement of clinical signs (purpura, arthralgia, peripheral neuropathy) with a decline of cryocrit in most patients with mixed cryoglobulinemia even in cases resistant to IFN therapy. Rituximab trials emphasized the benefit of the drug in inducing remission in cutaneous vasculitis, cryoglobulinemic glomerulonephritis, cryoglobulinemic neuropathy and in underlying malignant lymphoproliferative disorder. [74, 76, 77, 78]

Complete clinical remission was associated with a significant reduction of RF activity and anti-HCV antibody titers. Relapse might occur in up to 36.1%.Complete immunologic response was higher with the combination of rituximab plus Peg-IFN-α/ribavirin. Rituximab treatment of a renal-transplant patient with de novo HCV-related type III cryoglobulinemic MPGN resulted in clearance of cryoglobulinemia, a decrease in proteinuria without a change in serum creatinine or HCV RNA. [69, 77, 78, 79] Rituximab can cause serum sickness, serum sickness like disease, neutropenia and increased risk of infections, pneumopathy, varicella zoster infection, erysipelas, thrombosis of the retinal artery and cold agglutinin disease, occasional flare of vasculitis. Factors that were found to be associated with increased risk of side effects include high complement activation, higher rituximab doses and elevated levels of cryoglobulins. An increase of viremia might be observed in responders with rituximab monotherapy with insignificant variation of transaminases or deterioration of liver disease. [80, 81] Table 1

5.3.2.2. ANCA-Associated Systemic Vasculitis (AASV)

Standard treatment of ANCA-associated vasculitic syndromes (AAVS) is composed of remission induction regimen that involves the use of cyclophosphamide and high-dose glucocorticoids, followed by a remission maintenance regimen using methotrexate, azathio-

Study	Patients (number with nephritis)	Rituximab dose	Other treatments	Remission overall (nephritis)	Remission Purpura Neuropathy	Side effects	HCV viral load	Relapse (number of cases)
Sansonno *et al. 2003*	20 (1)	375 mg/m^2 weekly × 4 weeks	S (low doses)	16/20 (1/1)	12/14 (6/12)	Septic fever (1)	↑ responders = nonresponders	4/16 (>7 months)
Zaja *et al.* 2003	15 (2)	375 mg/m^2 weekly × 4 weeks	S (<0.5 mg/kg/day)	13/14 (1/2)	12/12 (5/5)	Retinal thrombosis (1)	↑ 2/8 ↑ 1/8 = 5/8	6 (3–6 months)
Roccatello *et al.* ,2004	6 (5)	375 mg/m^2 weekly × 4 weeks; 375 mg/m^2 monthly × 2 months		5/5	4/4 (5/6)	Transient bradycardia (2)	4 unchanged	2 (>12 months)
Quartuccio *et al.*, 2006	5 (5)	375 mg/m^2 weekly × 4 weeks	S (one case)	5/5 (5/5)	4/4 (1/2)	Transient neutropenia (1)	NR	3 (>5, >7 and >12 months)
Basse *et al.* 2005	7 (7) (post-kidney transplant)	375 mg/m^2 weekly × 2–4 weeks	CNI, MMF and S	7/7		Lethal infection (2, fungal and HSV)	NR	NR
Visentini *et al.* 2007	6 (2)	250 mg/m^2 weekly × 2 weeks	S	4/6 (1/2)	4/5 (2/2)	Lethal intestinal infarction	↓ 2/5 = 3/5	NR

Table 1. Rituximab treatment in Patients with HCV cryoglobulinemic vascultis.CNI = Calcineurin inhibitor; HCV = Hepatitis C virus; HSV = Herpes simplex virus; MMF = Mycophenolate mofetil; NR = Not reported; S = Steroids.↑: Increase; ↓: Decrease; =: No change. [69]

prine or other antimetabolite therapy. Patients who develop undetectable ANCA titers after treatment are less likely to experience disease relapse than patients who remain ANCA positive. Conventional immunosuppression led to a dramatic improvement in the prognosis of patients with increasing remission reaching up to 70%. Conventional immunosuppression might fail to achieve remission in a substantial minority of patients (25-30%). [82] With the tumor necrosis factor inhibition therapy clearly proven to be non-superior to conventional lines of therapy alternative biologic targets are being extensively investigated in AAVS. [31]

B-cell activation is believed to play an important role in the pathogenesis of the ANCA-associated vasculitis concerning antigen presentation, activation of T cell differentiation to Th1 and Th17 cell types and activating TNF-primed neutrophils, leading to premature degranulation and resultant endothelial damage. [83] Given the role of B cells in the pathogenesis of this disease, B cell depletion and interruption of B cell dependent T cell regulator function with rituximab represents a potentially attractive treatment alternative. [84] Open label and cohort studies demonstrated successful treatment of the ANCA-associated vasculitides with rituximab. [85-88] These early successes led to two landmark studies that support the use of B-cell therapies for these diseases. The efficacy of rituximab in ANCA associated vasculitis was further studied in 2010 in two randomized controlled trials. Both trials examined the use of rituximab for patients with ANCA-associated vasculitis.

5.3.2.2.1. The Rituximab for ANCA-associated Vasculitis (RAVE) trial

A multicentered randomized, double-blind, non-inferiority study of patients with severe GPA and microscopic polyangiitis. In this trial, 197 patients with either new or relapsing disease were randomized in a 1:1 ratio to receive remission-induction therapy with either oral cyclophosphamide (2 mg/kg/day) or rituximab (375 mg/m^2 weekly for 4 weeks). Both groups received the same glucocorticoid regimen (i.e., up to 3 pulses of 1 g of intravenous methylprednisolone, and then prednisone 1 mg/kg/day, followed by a protocolized taper). Approximately 50% of subjects enrolled in this trial had significant renal disease and 28% had alveolar hemorrhage at trial entry, although patients were not eligible for this trial if their serum creatinine exceeded 4 mg/dl or if the patient required mechanical ventilation during the study period. The primary end point of this study was achievement of remission at 6 months in the absence of glucocorticoids.

The RAVE trial showed that rituximab was non-inferior to cyclophosphamide in inducing remission especially in cases with alveolar haemorrhage and/or glomerulonephritis. Rituximab was proven superior to cyclophosphamide in the treatment of relapsing disease in AASV. Rituximab therapy was associated with sustained remission over a period of 6 months with encouraging steroid sparing effect. In general, the frequency of adverse events was the same and correlated significantly with the early use of high doses of glucocorticoids in both groups.

5.3.2.2.2. The Randomized Trial of Rituximab versus Cyclophosphamide in ANCA-Associated Vacsulitis (RITUXVAS) Trial

A randomized open-label study that looked at the effectiveness of rituximab for the treatment of 44 patients with newly diagnosed ANCA-associated glomerulonephritis. Subjects were randomized in a 3:1 ratio, stratified by age, diagnosis and baseline renal function. The rituximab group (33 patients) received standard dosing of rituximab (375 mg/m^2 weekly for 4 doses) as well as two intravenous cyclophosphamide pulses (15 mg/kg) with the first and third rituximab doses. A third dose of cyclophosphamide was permitted if remission had not been achieved after 6 months of therapy. No maintenance therapy was given in this group. The control group (11 patients) received intravenous cyclophosphamide monthly for 3–6 months followed by azathioprine for remission maintenance. Some subjects also underwent plasmapheresis. Remission was defined as the absence of disease activity for 2 months and relapse was defined as any disease activity after remission had been attained. In this trial, 76% of patients in the rituximab group had a sustained remission at 12 months as opposed to 82% in the cyclophosphamide group. Severe adverse effects were noted 42% of the rituximab patients and 36% of patients in the control group. A total of eight patients died, six of whom had been randomized to receive rituximab therapy. Adverse events were not lower in the rituximab group as had been expected. [90]

	RAVE	RITUXVAS
Median age (years)	54	68
Male (%)	46	52
Disease process		
Granulomatosis with polyangiitis (%)	75	55
Microscopic polyangiitis (%)	24	36
Renal involvement (%)	66	100
ANCA positivity		
PR3-ANCA (%)	66	61
MPO-ANCA (%)	33	39

Abbrevaitions: Antineutrophil cytoplasmic autoantibodies; RAVE: Rituximab for ANCA-associated vasculitis; RITUXVAS: Rituximab versus cyclophosphamide in ANCA-associated vasculitis. [55,56]

Table 2. Demographics of patients enrolled in RAVE and RITUXVAS.

Rituximab may be an effective alternative treatment in newly diagnosed as well as refractory ANCA-associated vasculitis. Wegener's Granulomatosis (granulomatosis with polyangiitis) patients with retro-orbital granulomas tend to be less responsive to rituximab therapy. [91] The great limitation of rituximab is some cases with GPA or microscopic polyangiitis may need to be retreated following initial treatment. New anti-CD20 agents, or agents that attack different B-cell precursors, may overcome this hurdle, and may enable even longer periods of remission.

6. Future perspectives in the management of systemic vasculitis

6.1. Inhibitors of B cell maturation

BAFF (B lymphocyte survival Factor, BLyS) is a member of the tumor necrosis factor (TNF) family and is expressed on the surface of monocytes, dendritic cells (DC), neutrophils, stromal cells, activated T cells, malignant B cells and epithelial cells. BAFF binds to three different receptors, BAFF-R, TACI (transmembrane activator and calcium modulator and cyclophilin ligand interactor) and BCMA (B cell maturation protein), that are expressed differentially at various times during B cell maturation. BAFF enhances long-term B cell survival primarily by up-regulating anti-apoptotic proteins provoking a prompt response

http://dx.doi.org/10.5772/54517

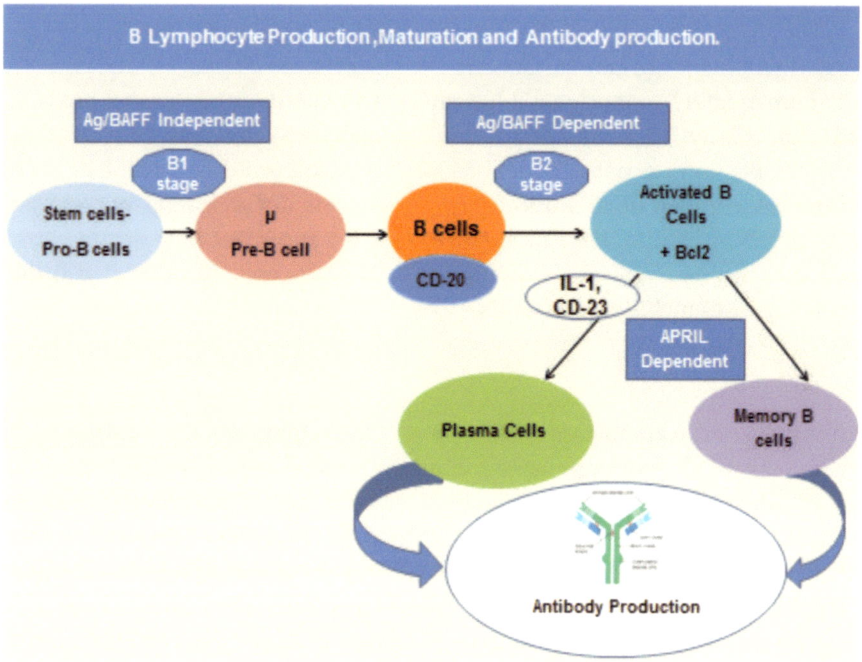

Figure 10. B cells maturation and antibody production in autoimmune diseases.

of B cells to BCR activation. TACI and BCMA signal through the classic NF-κB pathway and through the Mek (mitogen-activated protein extracellular signal-related kinase) pathway to up-regulate anti-apoptotic and down-regulate pro-apoptotic pathways, and through JNK/p38 (c-Jun N-terminal kinase) to drive class-switching. Survival and reactivation of B cell memory is BAFF-independent. Plasma cells express TACI and/or BCMA and their survival can be supported by either BAFF or APRIL. In contrast, B1 cells do not require BAFF or APRIL for survival. BAFF plays an important role in humoral immunity. T cell-independent type II responses require the interaction of BAFF 60-mer or membrane BAFF with TAC. This interaction is vital for T cell-dependent immunoglobulin (Ig)M responses. BAFF is also an essential component of the innate immune response and is induced in myeloid DC by type I interferons (IFNs). BAFF up-regulates Toll-like receptor (TLR) expression, promotes B cell survival and, together with IL-6, promotes Ig class-switching and plasma cell differentiation. Soluble BAFF and APRIL are expressed at high levels in the serum and in the target organs of individuals with established antibody dependent autoimmune diseases. Therapeutic antagonism of BAFF and its homologue APRIL (a proliferation-inducing ligand) targets an important homeostatic signal for B cell survival and selection (Figure 10). Belimumab and atacicept are two potential therapeutic anatgonists to the BAFF-APRIL pathway for B cell activation that are currently being investigated. [92-105]

6.1.1. Belimumab

Belimumab (LymphoStat-B; Human Genome Sciences, Inc., Rockville, MA, USA) is a recombinant, fully human IgG1λ monoclonal B-lymphocyte stimulator inhibitor that binds to soluble BLyS with high affinity. The drug exerts its biologic activity by preventing the binding of BLyS to its receptors. Belimumab potently inhibits BLyS-induced proliferation of B cells *in vivo and vitro* and prevents human BLyS-induced increases in splenic B-cell numbers and serum IgA titers. Belimumab is the only biologic approved for the treatment of systemic lupus erythematosus. Experimental evidences support the possible benefit in other B cell dependent autoimmune diseases including vasculitis. [106]

6.1.2. Atacicept

Atacicept is a human recombinant fusion protein that comprises the binding portion of a receptor for both BLyS (B-Lymphocyte Stimulator) and APRIL (A PRoliferation-Inducing Ligand), two cytokines that have been identified as important regulators of B-cell maturation, function and survival. Atacicept has shown selective effects on cells of the B-cell lineage, acting on mature B cells and blocking plasma cells and late stages of B-cell development while sparing B-cell progenitors and memory cells. Experimental studies demonstrated the efficacy of atacicept in animal models of autoimmune disease and the biological activity of atacicept in patients with systemic lupus erythematosus (SLE) and rheumatoid arthritis (RA) has been demonstrated. [107] The use of atacicept as an alternative B cells targeted therapy in refractory vasculitis remains to be investigated.

6.2. Inhibition of T cell co-stimulation

T cells require at least two signals for activation. The first is an antigen driven signal delivered when the antigen binds to the T-cell receptor. The second is a co-stimulatory signal delivered by receptor ligand interactions between the T cell and the antigen-presenting cell (eg, CD28 and B7.1). Binding of CD28 to B7.1 upregulates the production of multiple cytokines by CD8+ and CD4+ cells especially interleukin2 (IL-2) and interferon-gamma. The potential role of this approach is just beginning to be explored for patients with systemic vasculitis. (Figure 11)

6.2.1. Abatacept

Soluble, recombinant, fully-human fusion protein, comprising the extracellular domain of CTLA-4 linked to the Fc (hinge, CH2 and CH3 domains) portion of immunoglobulin G1. Abatacept is an inhibitor of T-cell co- stimulation, is being explored as a potential treatment for GPA, TAK, and GCA. [108, 109]

6.3. Other potential suppressors of T cells effector functions [Anti-cytokine therapy]

6.3.1. Tocilizumab

The first humanized monoclonal antibody that targets and inhibits the human interleukin-6. Tocilizumab binds both soluble and membrane-bound IL-6 receptors (sIL-6R and mIL-6R),

http://dx.doi.org/10.5772/54517

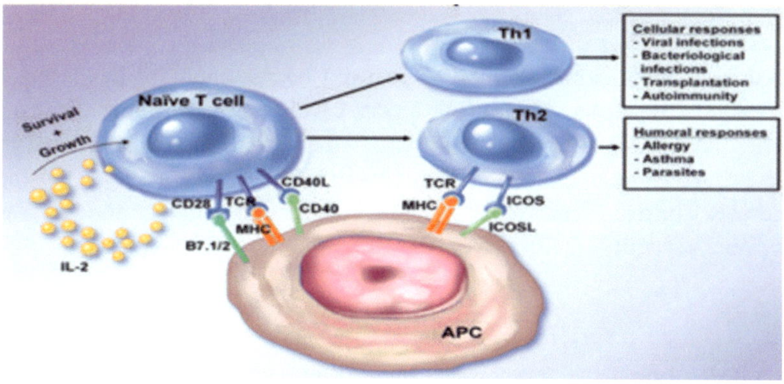

Figure 11. T cells targeted biologic therapy. T cells require two signals to become fully activated. A first signal which is antigen-specific is provided through the T cell receptor which interacts with peptide MHC molecules on the membrane of the antigen presenting cells (APC). A second signal, the co-stimulatory signal, is antigen non-specific and is provided by the interaction between co-stimulatory molecules expressed on the membrane of the APC and the T cell. One of the best characterized co-stimulatory molecules expressed by the T cells is CD-28, which interacts with CD80 (B7.1) and CD86 (B7.2) on the membrane of APC. MHC: major histocompatibility complex, APC: antigen presenting cells.

thereby preventing the signalling associated with IL-6 binding to its receptor. Tocilizumab is currently being investigated as a possible remission induction alternative in old aged patients with active Giant cell arteritis who are intolerable to high doses of steroid and as asteroid sparing agent that might provide substantial long term benefit for these patients. [110, 111] Figure 12

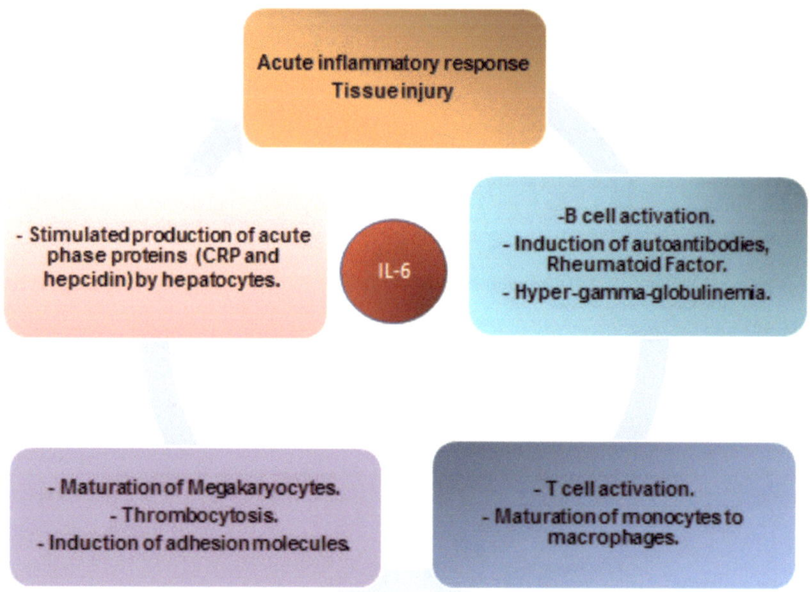

Figure 12. The role of interleukin-6 in autoimmunity.

6.3.2. Dacilizumab

A humanized IgG1 monoclonal antibody produced by recombinant DNA technology that binds specifically to the alpha subunit (p55 alpha, CD25, or Tac subunit) of the human high-affinity interleukin-2 (IL-2) receptor that is expressed on the surface of activated lymphocytes. Dacilizumab proved to be an effective alternative in interferon refractory relapsing remitting multiple sclerosis. The drug is currently being investigated in autoimmune diseases including ANCA associated vasculitis. [112]

6.3.3. Basiliximab

A chimeric (murine/human) monoclonal antibody (IgG1K), produced by recombinant DNA technology, that functions as an immunosuppressive agent, specifically binding to and blocking the interleukin-2 receptor α-chain (IL-2Rα, also known as CD25 antigen) on the surface of activated T-lymphocytes, inhibiting the binding of IL-2 to it's receptor on target T cells. The drug is being currently used for treatment of allograft rejection and potentially under consideration for the ANCA associated vasculitis. [113, 114]

Principle	Mechanism	Agent	Evidences
Depletion of effector T cells	Antibodies directed to CD25 cell surface antigen on activated T cells	Basiliximab Daclizumab	Randomized controlled trials in AAV
Regulation of effector T cells	Blockade of CD28/CD80 co-stimulatory signal for T cell activation	Abatacept Belatacept (CTLA-4 fusion proteins)	Randomized controlled trials in AAV
Interference with granuloma formation	Tumor necrosis factor blockade	Infliximab Adalimumab	Experimental and clinical evidences in AAV
Depletion of B lymphocytes	B lymphocyte depletion by antibodies directed to CD20/ CD22 cell surface molecule	Rituximab Epratezumab (both are anti-CD20)	Experimental and clinical evidences in AAV
Inhibition of B cell maturation	Neutralization of BLys and blockade of BLys receptor on B cells	Belimumab Atacicept	Experimental evidence
Antimicrobial treatment	Reduction of microbial flora that might provoke disease flares	cotrimoxazole	Experimental and clinical evidences in AAV
Inhibition of migration	Blockade of a-4integrins on T cells	Natalizumab	Experimental and clinical evidences in MS Evidences in AAV are lacking
Enhance vascular repair	Promote epithelial progenitor cell (EPC) function and repair	Erythropoietin (EPO) Statins	Experimental and clinical evidence

Table 3. Current and future considerations in treat to target strategy in systemic vasculitis.[116]

7. Secondary vasculitis

The role of biologic therapy in the management of leukocytoclastic vasculitis secondary to rheumatoid arthritis, systemic lupus erythematosus and Sjogren's syndrome has not been fully explored. Anti-tumor necrosis factor (TNF) treatment proved to be effective in rheumatoid arthritis patients with refractory systemic rheumatoid vasculitis after failure of conventional therapy including cyclophosphamide and corticosteroids with successful tapering of corticosteroids. The use of anti-TNF therapy and other biologic drugs might be considered in refractory secondary vasculitis to induce remission and as steroid sparing therapy for maintenance of remission. [115]

8. Special considerations in ANCA Associated Small vessels Vasculitis AASV

Therapeutic targets that are currently being considered in ANCA associated vasculitis include: (a) Inhibition of adhesion and activation of neutrophils aiming to dampen vascular injury. (b) Boosting vascular repair via endothelial progenitor cells (EPCs) which are regarded as an important factor of vascular repair. EPC mobilization and function might be enhanced by additional treatment with erythropoietin (EPO) or statins. (c) The use of antibiotics (cotrimoxazole) might prevent disease flares triggered by bacteria.

9. Hazards of biologic therapy

The development of recombinant technology represented the single biggest advance leading to humanized products with minimal or no contaminants in comparison to products purified from animal tissues. Nevertheless, the type of manufacturing process including choice of cell type, culture medium, and purification method can result in changes to the protein. Monoclonal antibodies represent a major class of successful biologics. Toxicities associated with these agents include those associated with the binding of the complementary determining region (CDR) with the target biologic molecule. [117, 118] Most of the concerns about safety of biologic therapy are related to the use of biologic agents particularly TNFi in the treatment of rheumatoid arthritis.

9.1. Infections

Bacterial, mycobacterial and fungal infections might occur during biologic therapy especially with tumor necrosis factor inhibitors. Infections usually occur in first year of treatment, including life threatening serious infections and mostly caused by intracellular pathogens (tubercle bacillus, listeria, histoplasma, atypical mycobacteria, coccidioidomycosis and legionella). Infection risk with biologic therapy in patients with autoimmune diseases significantly correlated to the dose of glucocorticoids given in such patients.

An analysis of Medicare beneficiaries enrolled in the Pharmaceutical Assistance Contract for the Elderly in Pennsylvania, USA demonstrated that among almost 16,000 patients with rheumatoid arthritis over the age of 65 years old, treatment with TNF inhibitors didn't increase the risk of serious bacterial infections when compared with patients who had received treatment with methotrexate. Another review of three European registries suggested an increased risk of several types of infections among patients treated with TNF inhibitors, including tuberculosis. Therapy with biologic agents especially TNFi carries a potential risk for reactivation of latent TB, reactivation of dormant hepatitis B or C infection. [117-121]

Biologic	Lymphoma SIR (95% CI)	Malignancy SIR (95% CI)	Malignancy Rate Biologic Vs Placebo
Abatacept	3.5	0.9(0.6-1.3)	1.3%vs 1.1%
Adalimumab	4.35 (2.6-10)	1 (0.7-1.3)	0.6vs 0.5/100 PY
Anakinra	3.6(0.12/100 PY)	ND	0.83
Certolizumab	2.06(0.42-6.02)	0.86 (0.59-1.22)	0.5 vs 0.6/100 PY
Etanercept	3.47 (1.6-6.59)	0.9821	ND
Golimumab	3.8	50mg: 1.46 (0.87-2.3) 100mg: 0.72 (0.4-1.2)	ND
Infliximab	6.4 (1.7-16.3)	0.91 (0.53-1.46)	1.31vs 0.46/100 PY
Rituximab	ND	1.05#(0.76-1.42)	Not increased
Tocilizumab	ND	0.80 (0.77-0.83)	1.32 vs 1.37/ 100 PY

Table 4. Standardized Incidence Ratios (SIR) for Lymphoma and Malignancies in RA on Biologics versus the Population Rate from Package Insert or Registration RCTs* [126]

9.2. Malignancy

Lymphomas: Increased risk for lymphoma (with anti-TNF therapy). Concern regarding a potential relationship between use of biologic agents and lymphoma arose in 2003 when the FDA noted 6 lymphomas among the first 6303 RA patients treated with etanercept, infliximab and adalimumab, but none in the control subjects treated with placebo during the first six months of exposure. [122, 123]

Hepatosplenic T cell lymphomas (HSTCL): There are over 200 documented HSTCL cases in literature. This is a very rare, aggressive and often fatal malignancy that may be associated with IBD (25%), immunosuppression or immunosuppressive drugs. HSTCL primarily affects children and young adults (< 30 yrs) who are receiving azathioprine or 6-mercaptopurine treatment for Crohn's colitis. This lymphoma also has been reported in a few adults (over age 60 yrs.) receiving TNFi for RA. [122, 123]

Melanoma and non-melanoma skin cancer (NMSC): have been reported to occur more commonly among patients with RA, especially in those receiving TNF inhibitors (TNFi).

Solid tumors: Increased rates of other solid tumors have been observed among patients treated with TNFi for inflammatory diseases other than RA. Three RCTs have described more solid tumors among patients receiving TNFi in studies of: [1] infliximab in COPD; [2] etanercept in granulomatosis polyangiitis (formerly Wegener's granulomatosis); and [3] golimumab in severe asthma. The finding of greater numbers of solid tumors among TNFi-treated patients in these relatively small RCTs was unexpected and remains of uncertain significance.

Data from recent multiple registries and randomized controlled trials RCTs showed no increase in overall malignancy risk among RA patients treated with biologic agents (with the possible exception of an increased risk of melanoma recurrence with TNFi). Over 40,000 patients participating in numerous large databases and RA registries worldwide (CORRONA, National Databank for Rheumatic Diseases, ARTIS, BSRBR, BIOBADASER,LORHEN), have shown consistent cancer incidence rates (~1%), both among TNFi- and non-biologic DMARD treated patients. The noticed increase in the risk of hematological cancers in patients with autoimmune diseases particularly among males over the age of 65 years old should be balanced against the increased risk of lymphoma in rheumatoid arthritis. [124, 125, 126](Table 3)

9.3. Cardiac complications

The risk of aggravation of heart failure has been a major concern with TNF inhibition therapy particularly in patients classified as class III-IV according to the American heart Association. An analysis of the cardiovascular risk in rheumatoid arthritis patients treated with TNF inhibitors demonstrated no difference in cardiovascular events when compared with patients treated with conventional disease-modifying anti-rheumatic drugs. Increase in the risk of dyslipidemia was observed with anti IL-6 therapy. [120]

9.4. Autoimmune phenomena

–Drug induced lupus.

–Sarcoidosis.

–Human anti-chimeric antibodies with or without autoimmune phenomena.

–Vasculitis: cases of TAK arteritis, ANCA associated vasculitis (Wegener's granulomatosis) and deep cutaneous vasculitis have been reported in rheumatoid arthritis patients treated with tumor necrosis factor inhibitors. [47, 127-133].

Demyelinating diseases demyelinating neuropathies, and flare of multiple sclerosis and other diseases of the central nervous system have been reported with tumor necrosis factor inhibition therapy. [134]

9.5. Pulmonary complications

Flare and progression of interstitial lung disease, allergic pneumonitis, new onset interstitial lung disease, culture-negative pneumonitis have been reported in cases treated with tumor necrosis factor inhibitors, tocilizumab, rituximab and golimumab. Flare of chronic obstructive pulmonary disease was reported in patients treated with abatacept. [135]

9.6. Infusion reactions

Biologics encompass a broad range of therapeutics that include proteins and other products derived from living systems. First dose reactions or infusion reactions are generally thought to be mediated via the Fc region of the antibody activating cytokine release, and have been observed with several antibodies. Usually, these effects (flu-like symptoms, etc.) are transient with subsequent dosing. Although biologics can have nonpharmacologic toxicities, these are less common than with small molecule drugs. Fever, shivering, chest pain, blood pressure oscillation, dyspnea, pruritus and/or urticaria, injection site reactions have been reproted. [118]

9.7. Hematological complications: Neutropenias and thrombocytopenias

The use of biologics as targeted therapies not only targets the currently identified pathogenic targets even more it might also improve the understanding of the pathophysiology of inflammation with autoimmunity. While the advent of biologics heralds a new era in the therapeutic armamentarium of the systemic vasculitis, evidences for their efficacy and safety in vasculitis is still in its infancy and are not yet superior to conventional immune-suppressants [136] with the exception of anti-CD20 B cell targeted therapy.

Author details

Reem Hamdy A. Mohammed

Faculty of Medicine Cairo University, Cairo, Egypt

References

[1] John, H. Stone. The Classification and Epidemiology of Systemic Vasculitis. Chapter 80. In Kelley's Textbook of Rheumatology by Gary S. Firestein, Ralph C. Budd, Edward D. Harris Jr., Iain B. McInnes, Shaun Ruddy. 8th edition, (2008).

[2] Chung, S. A, & Seo, P. Advances in the use of biologic agents for the treatment of systemic vasculitis. Curr. Opin. Rheumatol. ((2009).

[3] 3- Vassalli P. The pathophysiology of tumor necrosis factors. Annu. Rev. Immunol. (1992),10, 411-452.

[4] Aries, P. M, Lamprecht, P, & Gross, W. L. Biological therapies: new treatment options for ANCA-associated vasculitis? Expert Opin. Biol. Ther. 7(4), 521-533 ((2007).

[5] Cush, J, & Kavanaugh, A. TNF-α blocking therapies, in Rheumatology. 4th ed. Hochberg M, editor. Philadelphia, PA: Mosby Elsevier; (2008). , 501-517.

[6] Shealy, D. Characterization of golimumab (CNTO 148), a novel monoclonal antibody specific for human TNFα. (2007). ACR Poster Pres.

[7] Nesbitt, A, Fossati, G, Bergin, M, et al. Mechanism of action of certolizumab pegol (CDP870): in vitro comparison with other anti-tumor necrosis factor agents. Inflamm. Bowel Dis. 13, 1323-1332 ((2007).

[8] Booth, A. D, Jefferson, H. J, Ayliffe, W, Andrews, P. A, & Jayne, D. R. Safety and efficacy of TNF α blockade in relapsing vasculitis. Ann. Rheum. Dis. 61, 559 ((2002).

[9] Josselin, L, Mahr, A, Cohen, P, et al. Infliximab efficacy and safety against refractory systemic necrotising vasculitides: long-term follow-up of 15 patients. Ann. Rheum. Dis. 67, 1343-1346 ((2008).

[10] Bartolucci, P, Ramanoelina, J, Cohen, P, et al. Efficacy of the anti-TNF-α antibody infliximab against refractory systemic vasculitides: an open pilot study on 10 patients. Rheumatology 41, 1126-1132 ((2002).

[11] Pariser, K. M. Takayasu's arteritis. Curr. Opin. Cardiol. 9, 575-580 ((1994).

[12] Johnston, S. L, Lock, R. J, & Gompels, M. M. Takayasu arteritis: a review. J. Clin. Pathol. 55, 481-486 ((2002).

[13] Mason, J. C. Takayasu arteritis- advances in diagnosis and management. Nat. Rev. Rheumatol. 6, 406-415 ((2010).

[14] Kerr, G. S, Hallahan, C. W, Giordano, J, et al. Takayasu arteritis. Ann. Intern. Med. 120(11), 919-929 ((1994).

[15] Rossa, A. D, Tavoni, A, Merlini, G, et al. Two Takayasu arteritis patients successfully treated with infliximab: a potential disease-modifying agent? Rheumatology (Oxford) 44, 1074-1075 ((2005).

[16] Karageorgaki, Z. T, Mavragani, C. P, Papathanasiou, M. A, & Skopouli, F. N. Infliximab in Takayasu arteritis: a safe alternative? Clin. Rheumatol. 26, 984-987 ((2007).

[17] Tanaka, F, Kawakami, A, Iwanaga, N, et al. Infliximab is effective for Takayasu arteritis refractory to glucocorticoid and methotrexate. Intern. Med. 45, 313-316 ((2006).

[18] Jolly, M, & Curran, J. J. Infliximab-responsive uveitis and vasculitis in a patient with Takayasu arteritis. J. Clin. Rheumatol. 11, 213-215 ((2005).

[19] Tato, F, Rieger, J, & Hoffmann, U. Refractory Takayasu's arteritis successfully treated with the human, monoclonal antitumor necrosis factor antibody adalimumab. Int. J. Angiol. 24, 304-307 ((2005).

[20] Hoffman, G. S, Merkel, P. A, Brasington, R. D, Lenschow, D. J, & Liang, P. Anti-tumor necrosis factor therapy in patients with difficult to treat Takayasu arteritis. Arthritis Rheum. 50(7), 2296-2304 ((2004).

[21] Katoh, N, Kubota, M, Shimojima, Y, et al. Takayasu's arteritis in a patient with Crohn's disease: an unexpected association during infliximab therapy. Intern. Med. 49(2), 179-182 ((2010).

[22] Kim-Heang LyaAlexis Régenta, Mathieu C. Tambya, Luc Mouthona. Pathogenesis of giant cell arteritis: More than just an inflammatory condition?.Autoimmunity Reviews; August ((2010)., 9(10), 635-645.

[23] Martinez-taboada, V. M, & Alvarez, L. RuizSoto M, Marin-Vidalled MJ, Lopez-Hoyos M. Giant cell arteritis and polymyalgia rheumatica: role of cytokines in the pathogenesis and implications for treatment. Cytokine 44, 207-220 ((2008).

[24] Hoffman, G. S, Cid, M. C, Rendt-zagar, K. E, et al. Infliximab for maintenance of glucocorticosteroid-induced remission of giant cell arteritis. Ann. Intern. Med. 146, (621-630), ((2007).

[25] Cantini, F, Niccoli, L, Salvarani, C, Padula, A, & Olivieri, I. Treatment of longstanding active giant cell arteritis with infliximab: report of four casses. Arthritis Rheum. 44(12), 2932-2935 ((2001).

[26] Andonopoulos, A. P, Meimaris, N, Daoussis, D, Bounas, A, & Giannopoulos, G. Experience with infliximab (anti-TNFα monoclonal antibody) as monotherapy for giant cell arteritis. Ann. Rheum. Dis. 62;1116 ((2003).

[27] Tan, A, Holdsworth, J, Pease, C, Emery, P, & Mcgonagle, D. Successful treatment of resistant giant cell arteritis with etanercept. Ann. Rheum. Dis. 62, 373-374 ((2003).

[28] Wilde, B, Van Paassen, P, Witzke, O, & Tervaert, J. W C. New pathophysiological insights and treatment of ANCA-associated vasculitis. Kidney International (2011). March (2);, 79, 599-612.

[29] Morgan, M. D, Drayson, M. T, Savage, C. O, & Harper, L. Addition of infliximab to standard therapy for ANCA-associated vasculitis.Nephron Clin Pract. (2011). c Epub 2010 Aug 6., 89-97.

[30] Lamprecht, P, Voswinkel, J, Lilienthal, T, et al. Effectiveness of TNF-α blockade with infliximab in refractory Wegener's granulomatosis. Rheumatology 41, 1303-1307 ((2002).

[31] Wegener's Granulomatosis Etanercept Trial (WGET) Research GroupEtanercept plus standard therapy for Wegener's granulomatosis. N. Engl. J. Med. 352(4), 351-361 ((2005).

[32] Laurino S, Chaudhry A, Booth A, Conte G, Jayne D. Prospective study of TNFalpha blockade with adalimumab in ANCA-associated systemic vasculitis with renal involvement. Nephrol Dial Transplant. 2010 Oct;25(10):3307-14.

[33] Keino, H, Okada, A. A, Watanabe, T, & Taki, W. Decreased ocular inflammatory attacks and background retinal and disc vascular leakage in patients with Behçet's disease on infliximab therapy. Br. J. Ophthalmol. (2010). doi:bjo.2010.194464 (2010) (Epub ahead of print).

[34] Hirohata, S, & Kikuchi, H. Behcet's Disease: review article. Arthritis Res Ther (2003).

[35] Sfikakis, P. P, Theodossiadis, P. G, Katsiari, C. G, & Kaklamanis, P. Markomichelakis NN: Effect of infliximab on sight-threatening panuveitis in Behcet's disease. Lancet (2001).

[36] Gulli, S, Arrigo, C, Bocchino, L, Morgante, L, Sangari, D, Castagna, I, & Bagnato, G F. Remission of Behcet's disease with anti-tumor necrosis factor monoclonal antibody therapy: a case report. BMC Musculoskeletal Disorders (2003).

[37] Lee, J H, Kim, T N, Choi, S T, Jang, B I, Shin, K, Lee, S B, & Shim, Y R. Remission of intestinal Behçet's disease treated with anti-tumor necrosis factor α monoclonal antibody (Infliximab). Korean J Intern Med. (2007). March; , 22(1), 24-27.

[38] Hui-yuen, J. S, & Duong, T. T. Yeung RSM. TNF-α is necessary for induction of coronary artery inflammation and aneurysm formation in an animal model of Kawasaki disease. J. Immunol. 176(10), 6294-6301 ((2006).

[39] Son MBFGauvreau K, Ma L et al. Treatment of Kawasaki disease: analysis of 27 US pediatric hospitals from 2001 to 2006. Pediatrics 124, 1-8 ((2009).

[40] J. A. Carlson, B. T. Ng, and K.-R. Chen, "Cutaneous vasculitis update: diagnostic criteria, classification, epidemiology, etiology, pathogenesis, evaluation and prognosis," American Journal of Dermatopathology, vol. 27, no. 6, pp. 504-528, 2005.

[41] Carlson, J. A, Cavaliere, L. F, & Grant-kels, J. M. Cutaneous vasculitis: diagnosis and management," Clinics in Dermatology, (2006). , 24(5), 414-429.

[42] Russell, J. P, & Gibson, L. E. Primary cutaneous small vessel vasculitis: approach to diagnosis and treatment," International Journal of Dermatology, (2006). , 45(1), 3-13.

[43] Papi, M, Didona, B, De Pit, O, et al. Livedo vasculopathy vs small vessel cutaneous vasculitis: cytokine and platelet P selectin studies," Archives of Dermatology, (1998). , 134(4), 447-452.

[44] Mang, R, Ruzicka, T, & Stege, H. Therapy for severe necrotizing vasculitis with infliximab," Journal of the American Academy of Dermatology, (2004). , 51(2), 321-322.

[45] Uthman, I. W, Touma, Z, Sayyad, J, & Salman, S. Response of deep cutaneous vasculitis to infliximab," Journal of the American Academy of Dermatology, (2005). , 53(2), 353-354.

[46] Marcelo Derbli Schafranski and Giuliano Doretto CampanariInfliximab for Idiopathic Deep Cutaneous Vasculitis Refractory to Cyclophosphamide. International Journal of Vascular Medicine, , 2010

[47] Mccain, M. E, Quinet, R. J, & Davis, W. E. Etanercept and infliximab associated with cutaneous vasculitis," Rheumatology, (2002). , 41(1), 116-117.

[48] Hasler, P, & Zouali, M. B lymphocytes as therapeutic targets in systemic lupus erythematosus. Expert Opin Ther Targets, (2006). , 10, 803-815.

[49] Shlomchik, M. J, et al. From T to B and back again: positive feedback in systemic autoimmune disease. Nat Rev Immunol. ((2001). , 1, 147-153.

[50] Browning, J. L. B cells move to centre stage: novel opportunities for autoimmune disease treatment. Nat Rev Drug Discov. ((2006). , 5, 564-576.

[51] Dalakas, M. C. Invited article: inhibition of B cell functions: implications for neurology. Neurology, (2008). , 70, 2252-2260.

[52] Yang, O. Huh, Michael J. Keating, Helene L. Saffer. Higher Levels of Surface CD20 Expression on Circulating Lymphocytes Compared With Bone Marrow and Lymph Nodes in B-Cell Chronic Lymphocytic LeukemiaAm J Clin Pathol (2001). , 116, 437-443.

[53] Plosker, G. L, & Figgitt, D. P. Rituximab: a review of its use in non-hodgkin's lymphoma and chronic lymphocytic leukaemia. Drugs ((2003).

[54] Silverman, G. J, & Carson, D. A. Role of B cells in rheumatoid arthritis. Arthritis Res Ther. (2003). Suppl 4:S , 1-6.

[55] Engel, P, Nojima, Y, Rothstein, D, Zhou, L. J, Wilson, G. L, Kehrl, J. H, & Tedder, T. F. The same epitope on CD22 of B lymphocytes mediates the adhesion of erythrocytes, T and B lymphocytes, neutrophils, and monocytes. J Immunol., (1993). , 150, 4719-4732.

[56] Cyster, J. G, & Goodnow, C. C. Tuning antigen receptor signaling by CD22: integrating cues from antigens and the microenvironment. Immunity, (1997). , 6, 509-517.

[57] Otipoby, K. L, Andersson, K. B, Draves, K. E, Klaus, S. J, Farr, A. G, Kerner, J. D, Perlmutter, R. M, Law, C, & Clark, L. E. A. CD22 regulates thymus-independent responses and the lifespan of B cells. Nature, (1996). , 384, 634-637.

[58] Keefe, O, Williams, T. L, Daives, G. T, Neuberger, S. L, Hyperresponsive, M. S, Cells, B, & In, C. D. deficient mice. Science, (1996). Wash. DC), , 274, 798-801.

[59] Sato, S, Miller, A. S, Inaoki, M, Bock, C. B, Jansen, P. J, Tang, M. L, & Tedder, T. F. CD22 is both a positive and negative regulator of B lymphocyte antigen receptor signal transduction: altered signaling in CDdeficient mice. Immunity ((1996). , 22.

[60] Tuscano, J. M, Agostino, R, Toscano, S. N, Tedder, T. F, Kehrl, J. H, & Cross-linking, C. D. generates B-cell antigen receptor-independent signals that activate the JNK/SAPK signaling cascade. Blood ((1999).

[61] Kalunian, K. C, Wallace, D. J, Petri, M. A, Houssiau, F. A, Pike, M. C, Kilgallen, B, Kelley, L, & Gordon, C. P. BILAG-measured improvement in moderately and severely affected body systems in patients with systemic lupus erythematosus (SLE) by Epratuzumab: Results from EMBLEM™, a phase IIb study. Ann Rheum Dis. ((2010). Suppl3):553.

[62] Wallace, D. J, Kalunian, K. C, Petri, M. A, Strand, V, Kilgallen, B, Kelley, L, & Gordon, C. P. Epratuzumab demonstrates clinically meaningful improvements in patients with moderate to severe systemic lupus erythematosus (SLE): Results from EMBLEM™, a phase IIb study. Ann Rheum Dis. ((2010). Suppl3):558.

[63] Daridon, C, Blassfeld, D, Reiter, K, Mei, H. E, Giesecke, C, Goldenberg, D. M, Hansen, A, Hostmann, A, Frölich, D, & Dörne, T. Epratuzumab targeting of CD22 affects adhesion molecule expression and migration of B-cells in systemic lupus erythematosus. r. Arthritis Res Ther. ((2010). R204, PMID: 21050432.

[64] Jacobi, A. M, Goldenberg, D. M, Hiepe, F. T, Radbruch, A, Burmester, G. R, & Dörner, T. Differential effects of Epratuzumab on peripheral blood B cells of SLE patients versus normal controls. Ann Rheum Dis. ((2008).

[65] Dörner, T, Kaufman, J, Wegener, W. A, Teoh, N, Goldenberg, D. M, & Burmester, G. R. Initial clinical trial of Epratuzumab (humanized anti-CD22 antibody) for immunotherapy of systemic lupus erythematosus. Arthritis Res Ther. ((2006). R74.PMID 16630358.

[66] Agnello, V. The etiology of mixed cryoglobulinaemia associated with hepatitis C virus infection. Scand J Immunol (1995). , 42, 179-84.

[67] Dammaco, F, & Sansonno, D. Mixed cryoglobulinemia as a model of systemic vasculitis. Clin Rev Allergy Immunol (1997). , 15, 97-119.

[68] Sansonno, D, Carbone, A, De Re, V, & Dammacco, F. Hepatitis C virus infection, cryoglobulinaemia, and beyond. Rheumatology (2007). , 46, 572-578.

[69] Mohammed, R H, & El Makhzangy, H I. Chapter 16: Hepatitis C related Vasculitides. In Textbook: Advances in the etiology, pathogenesis and pathology of vasculitis. (2011). 978-9-53307-334-7

[70] Meltzer, M, Franklin, E. C, Elias, K, et al. (1996). Cryoglobulinemia--a clinical and laboratory study. II. Cryoglobulins with rheumatoid factor activity. Am J Med. Jun 1996; , 40(6), 837-56.

[71] Ferri, C, Sebastiani, M, & Giuggioli, D. Zignego AL: Mixed cryoglobulinemia: demographic, clinical, and serological features, and survival in 231 patients. Sem Arthritis Rheum (2004).

[72] Ferri, C, Zignego, A. L, & Pileri, S. A. Cryoglobulins (review). J Clin Pathol. (2002).

[73] Ferri, C. and Mascia MT: Cryoglobulinemic vasculitis: Review. Curr Opin Rheumatol (2006).

[74] Sansonno, D, De Re, V, Lauletta, G, et al. Monoclonal antibody treatment of mixed cryoglobulinemia resistant to interferon alpha with an anti-CD20. Blood. (2003). , 101(10), 3818-3826.

[75] Roccatello, D, Baldovino, S, Rossi, D, et al. Longterm effects of anti-CD20 monoclonal antibody treatment of cryoglobulinemic glomerulonephritis. Nephrol Dial Transplant. (2004)., 19(12), 3054-3061.

[76] Roccatello, D, Fornasieri, A, Giachino, O, et al. Multicenter study on hepatitis C virus-related cryoglobulinemic glomerulonephritis. Am. J. Kidney Dis. 49(1), 69-82 ((2007).

[77] Roccatello, D, Baldovino, S, Rossi, D, et al. Rituximab as a therapeutic tool in severe mixed cryoglobulinemia. Clin. Rev. Allergy Immunol. ((2008).

[78] Zaja, F, De Vita, S, Mazzaro, C, et al. Efficacy and safety of rituximab in type II mixed cryoglobulinemia. Blood. (2003)., 101, 3827-3834.

[79] Saadoun, D, Rosenzwajg, M, Landau, D, et al. Restoration of peripheral immune homeostasis after rituximab in mixed cryoglobulinemia vasculitis. Blood. (2008). , 111(11), 5334-5341.

[80] Saadoun, D, Rigon, M R, Sene, D, et al. Rituximab plus Peg interferon-alpha/ribavirin compared with Peg interferon-alpha/ribavirin in hepatitis C related mixed cryoglobulinemia. Blood, (2010)., 116, 326-334.

[81] Pereira, P F, Lemos, L B, Uehara, S, et al. Long-term eYcacy of rituximab in hepatitis C virus-associated cryoglobulinemia. Rheumatol Int ((2010).

[82] Sanders JSFHuitma MG, Kallenberg CGM, Stegeman CA. Prediction of relapses in PRANCA associated vasculitis by assessing responses of ANCA titres to treatment *Rheumatology (Oxford)* 45, 724-729 ((2006)., 3.

[83] Popa, E, Stegeman, C, Bos, N. A, Kallenberg, C. G, Tervaert, J. W, & Differential, B. and T-cell activation in Wegener's granulomatosis. J. Allergy Clin. Immunol. 103, 885-894 ((1999).

[84] Falk, R. J, & Jennette, J. C. Rituximab in ANCA-associated disease. N. Engl. J. Med. 363(3), 285-286 ((2010).

[85] Keogh, K. A, Wylam, M. E, Stone, J. H, & Specks, U. Induction of remission by B lymphocyte depletion in eleven patients with refractory antineutrophil cytoplasmic antibody-associated vasculitis. Arthritis Rheum. 52(1), 262-268 ((2005).

[86] Smith KGCJones RB, Burns SM, Jayne DRW. Long-term comparison of rituximab treatment for refractory systemic lupus erythematosus and vasculitis: remission, relapse, and re-treatment. Arthritis Rheum. 54, 2970-2982 ((2006).

[87] Keogh, K. A, Ytterberg, S. R, Fervenza, F. C, Carlson, K. A, Schroeder, D. R, & Specks, U. Rituximab for refractory Wegener's granulomatosis: report of a prospective, open-label pilot trial. Am. J. Resp. Crit. Care Med. 173, 180-187 ((2006).

[88] Jones, R. B, Ferraro, A. J, Chaudhry, A. N, et al. A multicenter survey of rituximab therapy for refractory antineutrophil cytoplasmic antibody-associated vasculitis. Arthritis Rheum. 60(7), 2156-2168 ((2009).

[89] Stone, J. H, Merkel, P. A, Spiera, R, et al. Rituximab versus cyclophosphamide for ANCA-associated vasculitis. N. Engl. J. Med. 363(3), 221-232 ((2010).

[90] Jones, R. B. Tervaert JWC, Hauser T et al. Rituximab versus cyclophosphamide in ANCA-associated renal vasculitis. N. Engl. J. Med. 363(3), 211-220 ((2010).

[91] Wong, C. F. Rituximab in refractory antineutrophil cytoplasmic antibody-associated vasculitis: what is the current evidence? Nephrol Dial Transplant. (2007). , 22, 32-36.

[92] Cancro, M. P. The BLyS/BAFF family of ligands and receptors: key targets in the therapy and understanding of autoimmunity. Ann Rheum Dis (2006). Suppl. 3):iii , 34-6.

[93] Thien, M, Phan, T. G, Gardam, S, et al. Excess BAFF rescues self reactive B cells from peripheral deletion and allows them to enter forbidden follicular and marginal zone niches. Immunity (2004). , 20, 785-98.

[94] Lesley, R, Xu, Y, Kalled, S. L, et al. Reduced competitiveness of autoantigen-engaged B cells due to increased dependence on BAFF. Immunity (2004). , 20, 441-53.

[95] Baccala, R, Hoebe, K, Kono, D. H, Beutler, B, & Theofilopoulos, A. N. TLR-dependent and TLR-independent pathways of type I interferon induction in systemic autoimmunity. Nat Med (2007). , 13, 543-51.

[96] Krumbholz, M, Theil, D, Derfuss, T, et al. BAFF is produced by astrocytes and up-regulated in multiple sclerosis lesions and primary central nervous system lymphoma. J Exp Med (2005). , 201, 195-200.

[97] Nakajima, K, Itoh, K, Nagatani, K, et al. Expression of BAFF and BAFF-R in the synovial tissue of patients with rheumatoid arthritis. Scand J Rheumatol (2007). , 36, 365-72.

[98] Groom, J, Kalled, S. L, Cutler, A. H, et al. Association of BAFF/BLyS overexpression and altered B cell differentiation with Sjogren's syndrome. J Clin Invest (2002). , 109, 59-68.

[99] Pers, J. O, Daridon, C, Devauchelle, V, et al. BAFF overexpression is associated with autoantibody production in autoimmune diseases. Ann NY Acad Sci (2005). , 1050, 34-9.

[100] Schiffer, L, Bethunaickan, R, Ramanujam, M, et al. Activated renal macrophages are markers of disease onset and disease remission in lupus nephritis. J Immunol (2008). , 180, 1938-47.

[101] Mackay, F, Silveira, P. A, & Brink, R. B cells and the BAFF/APRIL axis: fast-forward on autoimmunity and signaling. Curr Opin Immunol, (2007). , 19, 327-36.

[102] Woodland, R. T, Fox, C. J, Schmidt, M. R, et al. Multiple signaling pathways promote B lymphocyte stimulator (BLyS)-dependent B cell growth and survival. Blood (2007). , 111, 750-60.

[103] Stadanlick, J. E, Kaileh, M, Karnell, F. G, et al. Tonic B cell antigen receptor signals supply an NF-kappaB substrate for prosurvival BLyS signaling. Nat Immunol (2008). , 9, 1379-87.

[104] Von Bulow, G. U, Van Deursen, J. M, & Bram, R. J. Regulation of the T-independent humoral response by TACI. Immunity (2001). , 14, 573-82.

[105] Sakurai, D, Hase, H, Kanno, Y, Kojima, H, Okumura, K, & Kobata, T. TACI regulates IgA production by APRIL in collaboration with HSPG. Blood (2007). , 109, 2961-7.

[106] Furie, R, Stohl, W, Ginzler, E M, et al. and the Belimumab Study Group. Biologic activity and safety of belimumab, a neutralizing anti-B-lymphocyte stimulator (BLyS) monoclonal antibody: a phase I trial in patients with systemic lupus erythematosus. Arthritis Res Ther. (2008). R109.

[107] Hartung, H, & Kieseier, B C. Atacicept: targeting B cells in multiple sclerosis. Ther Adv Neurol Disord. (2010). July; , 3(4), 205-216.

[108] Genovese MC, Schiff M, Luggen M, LE Bars M, Aranda R, Elegbe A, Dougados M. Longterm safety and efficacy of abatacept through 5 years of treatment in patients with rheumatoid arthritis and an inadequate response to tumor necrosis factor inhibitor therapy. J Rheumatol. 2012 Aug;39(8):1546-54

[109] Sibilia, J, & Westhovens, R. Safety of T-cell co-stimulation modulation with abatacept in patients with rheumatoid arthritis. Clin Exp Rheumatol. (2007). Sep-Oct;25(5 Suppl 46):S , 46-56.

[110] Shirota, Y, Yarboro, C, Fischer, R, Pham, T. H, Lipsky, P, & Illei, G. G. Impact of anti-interleukin-6 receptor blockade on circulating T and B cell subsets in patients with systemic lupus erythematosus. Ann Rheum Dis. (2012). Aug 2. [Epub ahead of print]

[111] Ash, Z, & Emery, P. The role of tocilizumab in the management of rheumatoid arthritis. Expert Opin Biol Ther. (2012). Jul 31. [Epub ahead of print]

[112] Rose, J W, Burns, J B, Bjorklund, J, et al. Daclizumab phase II trial in relapsing and remitting multiple sclerosis. MRI and clinical results. Neurology August 21, (2007).

[113] Thomas, A. Waldmann. Immunotherapy: past, present and future. Review.Nature Medicine ((2003).

[114] Lupo, L, Panzera, P, Tandoi, F, et al. October (2008). Basiliximab versus steroids in double therapy immunosuppression in liver transplantation: a prospective randomized clinical trial". Transplantation , 86(7), 925-31.

[115] Unger, L, Kayser, M, & Nüsslein, H G. Successful treatment of severe rheumatoid vasculitis by infliximab. Ann Rheum Dis (2003). , 62, 587-588.

[116] Lepsea, N, Abdulahadb, W A, Kallenbergb, C, & Heeringa, M. P. Immune regulatory mechanisms in ANCA-associated vasculitides. Autoimmunity reviews. December (2011). , 11(2), 77-83.

[117] Clarke, J. B. Mechanisms of adverse drug reactions to biologics. Handb Exp Pharmacol. (2010).

[118] Schneeweiss, S, Setoguchi, S, Weinblatt, M. E, et al. Anti-tumor necrosis factor α therapy and the risk of serious bacterial infections in elderly patients with rheumatoid arthritis. Arthritis Rheum. 56(6), 1754-1764 ((2007).

[119] Kyle BauerBA and Mark Bechtel. A Review of Complications of Biologic Therapy for Psoriasis. Practical Dermatology. December (2009). , 30-36.

[120] Zink, A, Askling, J, Dixon, W. G, Klareskog, L, Silman, A. J, & Symmons, D. P. European biologicals registers: methodology, selected results and perspectives. Ann. Rheum. Dis. 68, 1240-1246 ((2009).

[121] Rubbert-roth, A. Assessing the safety of biologic agents in patients with rheumatoid arthritis. Rheumatology (Oxford). (2012). Jul;51 Suppl 5: , 38-v47

[122] Parakkal, D, Sifuentes, H, Semer, R, & Ehrenpreis, E. D. Hepatosplenic T-cell lymphoma in patients receiving TNF-α inhibitor therapy: expanding the groups at risk.Eur J Gastroenterol (2011). , 23, 1150-6.

[123] Singh, J. A, Furst, D. E, Bharat, A, Curtis, J. R, Kavanaugh, A. F, et al. 2012 update of the 2008 American College of Rheumatology recommendations for the use of disease-modifying antirheumatic drugs and biologic agents in the treatment of rheumatoid arthritis. Arthritis Care Res 2012; , 64, 625-639.

[124] Drug Safety QuarterlyAmerican College of Rheumatology, August, (2012). , 4

[125] Pallavicini, F. B, Caporali, R, Sarzi-puttini, P, et al. Tumour necrosis factor antagonist therapy and cancer development: analysis of the LORHEN registry. Autoimmun. Rev. 9, 175-180 ((2010).

[126] Heldmann, F, Dybowski, F, Saracbasi-zender, E, Fendler, C, & Braun, J. Update on biologic therapy in the management of axial spondyloarthritis. Curr. Rheumatol. Rep. 12, 325-331 ((2010).

[127] Saint Marcoux BDe Bandt M. Vasculitides induced by TNFa antagonists: a study in 39 patients in France. Joint Bone Spine (2006)., 73, 710-3.

[128] Ramos-casals, M, Brito-zeron, P, Soto, M-J, Cuadrado, M-J, & Khamashta, M. Autoimmune diseases induced by TNF-targeted therapies. Best Pract Res Clin Rheumatol (2008)., 22, 847-61.

[129] Ognenovski, V, Clark, T, & Fox, D. Etanercept associated pulmonary granulomatous inflammation in patients with rheumatoid arthritis. J Rheumatol (2008)., 35, 2279-82.

[130] Daien, C, Monmier, A, Claudepierre, P, et al. Sarcoid-like granulomatosis in patients treated with tumour necrosis factor blockers: 10 cases. Rheumatology (2009). , 48, 883-6.

[131] Ashok, D, & Dubey, S. Tomlinson I. c-ANCA positive systemic vasculitis in a patient with rheumatoid arthritis treated with infliximab. Clin Rheumatol (2008)., 27, 261-4.

[132] Simms, R, Kipgen, D, Dahill, S, Marshall, D, & Rodger, R. ANCA-associated renal vasculitis following anti-TNFa therapy. Am J Kidney Dis (2008). e , 11-4.

[133] Douglas, G, Bird, K, Flume, P, Silver, R, & Bolster, M. Wegener's granulomatosis in patients with rheumatoid arthritis. J Rheumatol (2003)., 30, 2064-9.

[134] Hadjinicolaou, A. V, Nisar, M. K, Bhagat, S, Parfrey, H, Chilvers, E. R, & Ostör, A. J. Non-infectious pulmonary complications of newer biological agents for rheumatic diseases-a systematic literature review. Rheumatology (Oxford). (2011). Dec; , 50(12), 2297-305.

[135] Weisman, M. H. What are the risks of biologic therapy in rheumatoid arthritis? An update on safety. J Rheumatol Suppl. (2002). Sep; , 65, 33-8.

[136] Chan, A. T, Flossmann, O, Mukhtyar, C, Jayne, D. R, & Luqmani, R. A. The role of biologic therapies in the management of systemic vasculitis. Aut oimmun Rev. (2006). Apr; , 5(4), 273-8.